MW00453664

The Mediterranean Functional Lifestyle

Food is Life

Creative recipes for healthy diets

Nikos Ligidakis

Foreword by Helene Wechsler, MD

ISBN: 978-0-578-50033-1
Library of Congress Control Number: 2019904666

Published by Inkwell Books LLC
10632 North Scottsdale Road, Unit 695
Scottsdale, AZ 85254
Tel. 480-315-3781
E-mail info@inkwellbooksllc.com
Website www.inkwellbooksllc.com

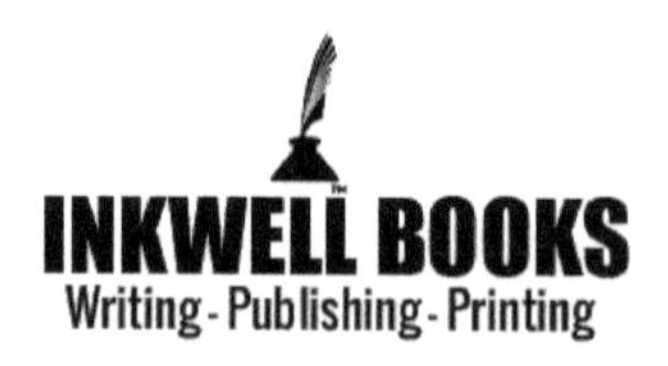

To my amazing wife Helene.
Without her in my life,
this book would not have been possible.

"Let food be thy medicine and medicine be thy food"

Hippocrates 460 - 370 BC

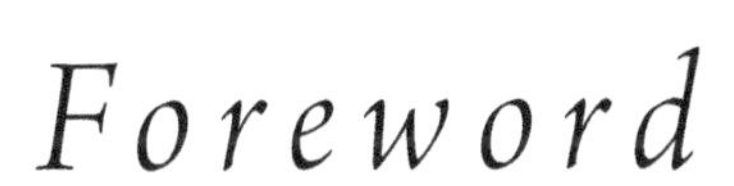

Foreword

By Helene Wechsler, MD

The journey to maximize our health started a couple of years ago. I decided to learn more about Functional Medicine and began attending conferences. It was after one of those conferences that I came home and excitedly explained the nutritional principals to my husband, Nikos (or Nick as I call him). Nick is the cook in our family, he is from Greece and has always followed a Mediterranean style diet. We decided to begin our journey with an Elimination diet. In doing so, we eliminated sugar, alcohol, dairy, eggs, corn and gluten for three weeks. By the end of the third week, Nick and I both lost weight and had much more energy. Nick had so much energy that he decided to let our landscaper go and he started taking care of our large yard himself. He spends hours every morning working outside pulling weeds, trimming bushes and growing a large vegetable garden. Every night we go for long walks. We both felt so much better that at the end of the three-week elimination diet, we decided to add only a few foods back into our diet. In fact, we decided not to call it a diet but a lifestyle and continue indefinitely. Before our elimination diet, we thought that we were eating healthy, but we found out that some of the foods we were eating were not the right foods for us. In order to maintain a diet that worked for us, we had to find ways to make the food more appetizing. I must admit; it is truly wonderful to have a husband who is a creative chef. When I come home every evening after work, I walk through the door and smell the beautiful aroma of a delicious, healthy meal.

Nick has written several cookbooks and is known for his creative, original recipes. After his retirement from the restaurant business, he wrote several other books, but he never intended to write another cookbook. Nick started to create new recipes in order to maintain our new lifestyle. My husband creates recipes in his head and rarely writes anything down. However, when his recipes started to pile up and he noticed more and more health benefits, he decided to write them down and create a cookbook so that he could help others. In addition to recipes he also included all the information that he has acquired over the past couple of years. I have been the fortunate recipient of taste testing his recipes over the past year. Nick's new book is a culmination of over 250 new and unique recipes. I know you will enjoy them as much as I have.

Having been a Family Medicine Physician for over 25 years, I came across Functional Medicine a few years ago. As Dr. Jeffrey Bland, the father of functional medicine, puts it "Functional medicine represents an operational system that focuses on the underlying causes of disease from a systems biology perspective that engages the patient and practitioner in a therapeutic partnership." In Functional Medicine, we try to get at the root of the problem. We evaluate a patient's lifelong history and consider not only their nutritional status but also their stress level and sleep patterns, the quality of their exercise, the health of their relationships, and their unique genetic makeup. We then attempt to bring them all into balance.

The recipes in this book fits well with the philosophy of Function Medicine and the many research studies that has shown us what we need to do to create a healthy lifestyle.

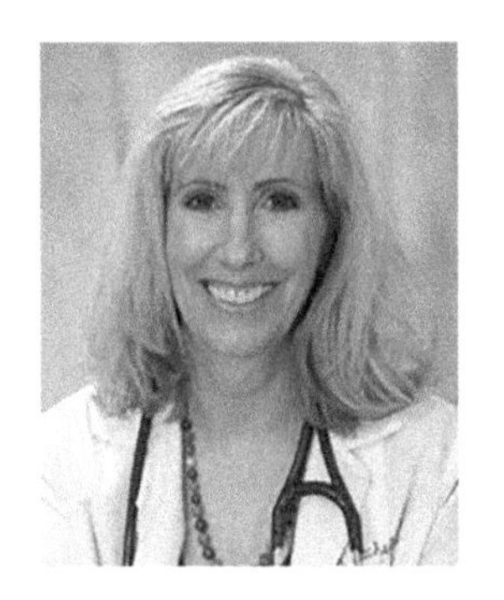

About Dr. Helene Wechsler, MD

Dr. Wechsler is board certified and has had over 25 years of experience in practicing as a Family Physician. In addition, she is also trained in Functional Medicine. For fifteen years, Dr. Wechsler was the co-founder and medical director of Scottsdale Holistic Medical Group, a multidisciplinary group offering conventional and alternative medicine. In 2004 Dr. Wechsler converted her practice to a "concierge" model, thereby limiting her practice to a few hundred patients and giving each her undivided and unhurried attention.

Growing Up Mediterranean

The Mediterranean diet is a diet that evolved over thousands of years. Since ancient times people of the Mediterranean region followed a diet which was mostly shaped by what the earth provided. It was not about one particular food with unique benefits but rather eating mostly plant-based, nutrient-dense foods and limited amounts of meats. Early Hippocratic doctors may have conceived the Mediterranean diet. Following their teacher's theories, rather than attributing illness to a supernatural force, they practiced a healthy diet as a form of medicinal treatment and the maintenance of good health; these are the main characteristics of the Mediterranean diet. The ancient doctors emphasized that their patients use local resources to prepare simple, flavorful foods. Fruits and vegetables that were particularly potent with intense flavors were considered to be a reflection of nutrition value. The ones with a milder taste were important for the body as well but needed flavoring. Therefore, balancing the flavors of foods became a culinary issue. As a result, added flavoring became a vital component of the early Greek diet, with emphasis placed on the use of garlic, olive oil, various herbs, pepper and nuts to improve the taste. Sweet and fatty foods in high quantities were discouraged then as they are today. Meat was not always readily available, which gave rise to a movement towards more plant-based meals.

The method of balancing flavors; using mild spices for the potent foods and strong herbs and spices for the poor tasting ones, is the fundamental principle of creating recipes and the formula used by today's creative chefs to make up new recipes with harmonious flavors. The primary objective is to create a taste so that all flavors "dance" in your mouth rather than just one particular taste overpowering all others. Overpowering a meal is simple, a handful of pepper, half a bottle of hot sauce or a bag of hot peppers would do it. However, to create a taste, spicy or mild, that our palate can identify all the flavors is an art.

Food has always been an essential part of my life and culture.

Throughout the centuries the Mediterranean people used, mainly, foods from the earth, to survive the difficult times during wars and celebrate life's special moments during peaceful times. I was born at a time when Hitler and his gangsters had ravaged our beautiful country. The infrastructure was destroyed, and people's main concern was survival. It was a time that the indomitable human spirit triumphed once again to overcome the torture, the killings and the human suffering. For nursing their family, people searched the fields and hills to find herbs, fruits and vegetables to prepare meals. Looking back at my early childhood, I am amazed by how my parents found the means to feed their five children. During the German occupation, our father walked for miles to find eatables and our mother maintained a small garden to grow a few vegetables. Fortunately, we lived by the sea and from time to time our dad sneaked out to catch some fish. Others, putting their lives in danger, went to the woods to hunt for meat. Trekking up the hills to find eatables from the earth, and relying on the sea to provide foods became the norm for the years to come. Our mother kept growing vegetables and fruits in the back yard, used the milk produced by the goat and eggs from the chickens to feed us. There were tea and herbs from the mountains, olive oil from the mills, food from the sea and occasionally other meats. Our father, running his taverna, went to nearby mountain villages to find the best wines and the purest olive oil, and walked through the farmer's markets to pick fresh vegetables. He visited the local butcher for the prime cuts of meats and waited by the sea to see what the daily catch of the fisherman brought ashore. Those were the ingredients they used to cook for our family and the taverna customers.Since I was a little boy, the people close to me took great pleasure preparing wholesome foods. The expression of pride on my dad's face serving foods he prepared in the taverna is perched at the edge of my consciousness and my mom's smile while preparing meals for special celebrations at home is kept in the safest banks of my memory.

Nearby our taverna in Kiato, there were other restaurants and bakeries with windows full of luscious pastries and ice cream shops to entice children and adults alike. Tempting aromas of various foods draped the neighborhood. There were freshly baked bread and roasted nuts, the exquisite fragrance of chocolate, the distinctive smell of garlic and the exotic scent of cinnamon. The fusion of aromas persuaded my young mind and slowly awakened a mortal fever for food flavorings. Fast forward decades later, I use the earth to grow flowers, vegetables and fruits and I have increasingly become conscious of the quality and origin of foods.

Arriving at the point of getting in the restaurant business wasn't easy. I resisted at every opportunity to get into the restaurant kitchens. Partly because I never thought I could match my parents' cooking and because I saw how hard my parents worked – I did not want that lifestyle. Besides, I had put my engineering degree in a drawer because I was going to be a soccer star. Well, the kid that was supposed to be a soccer star, ended up cooking breakfast in a Chicago grill out of need for survival in an unfamiliar culture. From there, I found myself working in a kitchen of a small restaurant franchise. Soon I became the chef and then I took over the management of the restaurant. Shortly after, I was trusted with the management of all five restaurants of the group. But managing restaurants wasn't in my calling – I wanted to go back to the kitchen. That was where I belonged. I was restless to experience different tastes and techniques. I went from kitchen to kitchen; from Greek diners to English pubs, to steak house, Italian, Jewish, fine dining and everything in between. I wanted to absorb it all, to experience all the new tastes – that was my culinary schooling. And then nothingness. I walked away. I did not want to do cooking like everyone else. I wanted to create my style, one that I had conceived in my head. During that time, I began to study flavors and the chemistry of foods. Four years after leaving the restaurant world, I opened my restaurant in Phoenix.

The five food items written on the blackboard at the opening eventually became hundreds of items in the large menu. The tiny first restaurant grew into an enormous restaurant. The small glass case with the three cakes multiplied into ten large display cases full of desserts. There was so much to explore, so much to learn. My desire to always learn and my passion for creating new tastes was not restrained after leaving the restaurant business. Nearly forty-years after opening my first restaurant I am still learning and creating. Knowledge of how to prepare natural foods and the study of flavor profiles is so vast, it is impossible to learn it all in a lifetime. Learning about the amazing benefits of preparing your own foods is no different; we start with the basics, and we learn from our mistakes.

In no time you will be creating your own recipes in a way you might not have thought possible.

What a great way to develop your culinary skills with healthy foods as your primer.

Some of the foods found in the Greek mountains, during the German occupation.

Armed with a knife and a basket, when people climbed the steep hills they found several items they could use for cooking. Here is some of these items: Horta (leafy greens) dandelions, chestnuts, capers, amaranth, arugula, chervil, mustard greens, mushrooms, oregano, thyme, mint, marjoram, sage. People found wild fruits such as blackberries, pears, and other arbutus fruits, and there was plenty of chamomile and mountain tea.

Nutritional Value of Fruits, Vegetables,Nuts, Spices and Herbs, used in this Book

In general most herbs, vegetables and fruits are loaded with nutrients and are low in calories. The highest calorie count is in dried fruits. The dried fruit is calorie-packed per ounce compared to fresh fruit because of the differences in the water content. The caution in dried fruits is that in many cases chemicals are added to the fruit to maintain freshness and color. Many dried fruits brands add alternative sweeteners, which can also increase calories. The safest dry fruits are the ones you make yourself or ones you find in a reputable health food store. When discussing the health benefits of fruits and vegetables, it's always important to make sure that you have the best quality. Organic is always better but more expensive. EWG.org puts out an annual shopper's guide to pesticides in produce. Every year they test many fruits and vegetables for their pesticide residue and come up with two lists: The Dirty Dozen (contains the highest amounts of pesticides) and The Clean Fifteen (contains the lowest amounts of pesticides). The foods on the Dirty Dozen list should be bought organic. The foods on the Clean Fifteen do not need to be organic. This can save money at the grocery store.

Artichokes

The artichoke originated in the Mediterranean region and has been used for centuries for its potential medicinal properties. Artichokes are packed with powerful nutrients. They are low in fat while rich in fiber, vitamins and minerals. They rank among some of the most antioxidant-rich vegetables. Artichokes are particularly high in vitamins C, K and folate. They supply minerals, such as phosphorus, magnesium, potassium, and iron. Artichokes contain an above average plant-based protein. Artichoke hearts are one of my favorite vegetables to cook with and I use them in many various dishes. The earthy flavor of the artichoke is unique and diverse. Its flavor profile changes according to the way the artichoke is cooked. I use the non-marinated artichoke hearts extensively in my cooking. The fact is that artichokes are unique in flavor; it's difficult to substitute them by any other vegetable. The artichoke is one of the oldest cultivated vegetables. Legend has it that it was made by Zeus himself.

Arugula

Arugula has been cultivated since the times of the ancient Greeks and the Romans. Arugula became more common in the United States during the eighties. The main reasons arugula's popularity around the world increased in the decades to follow has to do with its health benefits and unique taste. This green is a nutrient-dense food that is high in fiber and with several important nutrients. It is loaded with calcium, potassium, vitamins C, K, A and folate, and it is high phytochemicals which contain antioxidants. Arugula maintains its peppery, spicy taste when its leaves are in the early stages, once the leaves mature arugula loses its character and becomes bitter. Using heavy dressings in arugula salads is counterproductive. Arugula's distinctive flavor stands on its own merits. Olive oil and balsamic vinegar pairs best with arugula. Arugula pairs well with nuts, especially pecans and pine nuts, and of course tomatoes and avocado.

Asparagus

Asparagus is also loaded with essential vitamins, minerals and antioxidants. It is an excellent source of vitamins A, C, E, K, folate and riboflavin. Additionally, asparagus has small amounts of protein, potassium, phosphorous, iron and zinc. Asparagus is popular because of its unique taste and it can be used in a variety of dishes. It is low in calories, high in water and rich in fiber, that makes it a weight loss friendly food. Asparagus has a distinctive clean, mild flavor when fresh. It becomes bitter when overcooked. Asparagus can be steamed, roasted, grilled or fried and still maintain its texture and flavor. It can absorb other flavors when cooked with different foods. Asparagus pairs best with chicken, salads, risotto, and pasta.

Beets

Beets contain almost all the vitamins and minerals that we need. It is an excellent source of fiber, folate and vitamin C. Beets are a good source of vitamin B6, magnesium, potassium, phosphorous, manganese and iron. Beets are often recommended to be used by athletes. Several studies suggest that their dietary compounds enhance athletic performance. They are low in calories and high in nutrients, which makes beets a great addition to a healthy and balanced diet. Some people love the earthy taste of beets; others hate it to the point that are not willing to even taste it. The taste of beets has an earthy flavor. Those who love beets embrace its taste like the scent of soil after a rainy day. Those who hate beets compare its taste to eating dirt. Many people also believe that the taste of dirt does not go away even after the beets are thoroughly washed - this is another food myth. Coloring foods with artificial food colors are unnatural and unhealthy. Responsible chefs use natural food coloring for this purpose. Beets and raspberries, for example, can provide deep red colors. Natural food coloring, especially in cakes, is part of the culinary art. Beets are good in salads, and go well with hardy fruits, like apples, citrus and foods with distinctive flavors, like fennel.

Broccoli

A superfood.

Broccoli is another nutritional powerhouse vegetable. It is full of vitamins, minerals, fiber and antioxidants. Broccoli is rich in vitamins C and K and contains proper amounts of potassium, phosphorus, selenium and vitamins A and folate. Broccoli can be eaten cooked or raw; however different cooking methods affect broccoli's nutrient properties. Boiling broccoli, and vegetables in general, reduces some of their beneficial compounds, especially vitamin C. Other than eating it raw, steaming seems to be the best way to prepare vegetables in general. One thing you should never do is to microwave this superfood.

Brussels sprouts

Brussels sprouts are especially rich in antioxidants and fiber. They contain vitamin C, vitamin K, and reasonable amounts of vitamins A, B6, thiamine and folate. Brussels sprouts contain healthy amounts of the minerals; manganese, potassium, iron, magnesium and phosphorus. Brussels sprouts have many health benefits, but their impressive antioxidant content stands out. Also, Brussels sprouts are a good source of omega-3 fatty acids. Eating Brussels sprouts as part of a balanced diet, rich in fruits, vegetables and grains can have a beneficial impact on your health. Brussels sprouts can help supply the antioxidants your body needs to promote good health. They are simple to prepare in a variety of side dishes or main courses. Roasting Brussels sprouts takes away some of their bitterness. Their hardy exterior turns crispy and the insides remain tender. Blending slightly bitter foods with sharper or sweeter flavors and flavorsome herbs creates a balanced taste.

Cabbage

Cabbage's impressive nutrient content does not get the respect it deserves. Cabbage comes with a variety of colors, but the most popular ones are green and red. My personal favorite is red cabbage. I often use it in salads, especially with salads that include fish or lamb. This vegetable has been grown around the world for thousands of years. Kale has, rightly so, become the darling of health-conscious people, broccoli is continually being praised for its powerful nutrient contents and cauliflower is trending with chefs using it in various new recipes. However, cabbage actually belongs in the same cruciferous family of the above-mentioned vegetables and it has similar if not more powerful nutrients. Cruciferous vegetables are a group of vegetables which boost our liver's detoxifying enzymes. Therefore, they are a mainstay in many detox diets. Cabbage is exceptionally high in vitamins K and C and has smaller amounts of vitamins A, B6, folate and riboflavin. Also, cabbage is high in fiber and powerful antioxidants. It contains manganese, calcium, potassium and magnesium. Cabbage is versatile in the kitchen; it can be used in salads, soups and stews. Its outstanding nutritional profile, makes cabbage an exceptionally healthy food to include in your diet.

Capers

If you love to give an unusually lively flavor to your food, capers are one of those ingredients that can accomplish your goal. In my opinion, capers are right up there with lemon and wine when it comes to giving you the necessary acidity for your recipe without an overpowering effect. The Mediterranean region is the caper heaven. Greeks and Italian chefs have used capers since the dawn of time. They are also widely used in Spain and the South of France. Capers grow wild on rocky mountainsides and they are an integral ingredient in Mediterranean cuisines. Various types of capers are available. I believe the best ones are the small ones. They contain less sodium and acidity than the larger capers. Large capers may unbalance the flavors of your food. Carpers are low in calories; two tablespoons of capers contain just two or three calories. Apart from its low-calorie benefit, capers are a powerhouse of vitamins A, K, niacin and riboflavin. They are potent sources of fiber and contain minerals like iron, calcium and copper. Bottom line, capers are a rich source of antioxidants, phytonutrients, and vitamins essential for our health. If, like me, you don't use salt in your cooking, or if you are using limited amounts of salt, capers can give you that salty effect since they contain a good amount of sodium.

Carrots

No one will argue about carrots being one of the healthiest vegetables to eat. Many nutritional experts claim that carrots are the perfect health food. Carrots are a good source of several vitamins and minerals, especially beta-carotene, fiber, vitamin K, vitamin B6, biotin, potassium and antioxidants. They come in many colors, including yellow, white, orange, red and purple. However, the traditional orange carrots get their bright color from beta-carotene. Carrots contain many powerful plant compounds, but the carotenoids are by far best known for their powerful antioxidant activity. There are two kinds of baby carrots; the whole carrots that are naturally small, harvested before they grow large, and the baby-cut carrots, machine cut from larger carrots into the smaller size. Baby carrots are perfect for snacks; they are sweet, crunchy and full of nutrients. There is not much difference in nutrients between large and baby carrots.

Cauliflower

Suddenly the old cauliflower, despised by many for its odd taste, has become trendy among chefs. It is everywhere; side dishes, main courses. There is cauliflower rice packed in the frozen section of supermarkets and then there is the cauliflower pizza crust, cauliflower tortillas, mash, hummus, even mac and cheese! What is up with the cauliflower revolution? I am pleased, however, about the fact that chiefs have found ways to spice up cauliflower because the nutrition profile of cauliflower is impressive. Cauliflower contains a high amount of fiber and provides significant amounts of antioxidants. It is high in choline, an essential nutrient for our body, found only in a few foods. Cauliflower, along with broccoli, is one of the best plant-based sources of choline. Cauliflower contains high amounts of vitamin C, which acts as an antioxidant. It is low in calories but high in fiber and water, perfect for low-fat diets. Besides vitamin C, cauliflower contains vitamins K, B6, folate and pantothenic acid and several minerals, like potassium, magnesium, manganese and phosphorous.

Celery

If you are on a low-calorie diet, add celery to your list. One stalk of celery has just about ten calories. People throughout the decades ate celery because of its low-calorie content. But, celery is an excellent source of antioxidants and contains flavonoids, beta carotene and vitamin C. In fact, there are several kinds of antioxidants found in a single stalk of celery. Celery has a generous amount of dietary fiber as well. It also contains vitamins K and C, folate and minerals like potassium, magnesium and iron. Once celery loses its crunchy, crispy effect, some of these nutrients are lost. This is the case for many vegetables as well. It is a good practice to consume fresh vegetables and a bad practice to overstock your refrigerator with vegetables to be used weeks later. In a perfect world, the best vegetables and fruits are the ones you grow yourself.

Corn

Sweet corn contains a fair amount of fiber and is a decent source of protein. In general, sweet corn is higher in many vitamins than other types of corn and has adequate amounts of minerals. The vitamins in sweet corn are pantothenic acid, folate, vitamin B6 and niacin. Its minerals include potassium, and small amounts manganese, phosphorus, magnesium, zinc and copper.

Cucumber

One of the many reasons nutritional experts recommend consuming fruits and vegetables regularly is due to their antioxidant content. Cucumbers are especially rich in beneficial antioxidants. Antioxidants are molecules that block oxidation, a chemical reaction that forms highly reactive atoms with unpaired electrons known as free radicals. Free radicals have been blamed in many diseases, they cause oxidative stress and damage our cells. Cucumbers are low in calories and have several essential vitamins and minerals. They contain high amounts of vitamin K and moderate amounts of vitamin C, A and minerals like potassium, magnesium and manganese. They also have fiber and high water content. Cucumbers have a mild, refreshing taste. I am not sure if the meaning of the phrase "As cool as a cucumber" is to be calm, or because cucumbers contain hydrating properties that help the body cool off in hot weather. Whatever the reason, I think cucumbers are pretty cool and I use them in many salads and just about on every smoothie. Some of the other fruits and vegetables with high water content are, watermelon, pineapple, lettuce, zucchini, tomatoes, cabbage, eggplant, and the list goes on.

Eggplant

There are many varieties of eggplants that range in size and color. The most common ones are the eggplants with beautiful deep purple skin. Along with their health benefits, eggplants bring into the kitchen a unique texture and multiple flavors. Let me explain. Eggplants taste slightly different depending on how they are cooked and what you cook them with. This wide range of potential flavors is one of the reasons that I love to cook with eggplants. The main reason that eggplants change their character is their ability to absorb high amounts of liquids; hence eggplant adopts high quantities of other flavors. But whatever different flavor penetrates the eggplants, they never lose their luxurious taste. Some people complain that eggplants are bitter or spongy, but when eggplants are adequately cooked, they achieve tastes that no other fruit or vegetable can. In addition to bringing a unique texture and flavors to recipes, eggplant brings a host of potential health benefits. They are a nutrient-dense food. Eggplants provide a good amount of fiber, vitamins and minerals in a few calories. They contain Vitamins K, C, B6, thiamin, folate and minerals like manganese, potassium, magnesium, copper and niacin. Also, eggplants boast a high number of antioxidants. Eggplants are incredibly versatile and can be easily incorporated into your diet. I use them for grilling, baking, salads, or soups. I've heard of many tricks to prepare eggplant for cooking; peel the skin, salt the eggplant for several hours, wash and place it between paper towels, and so on. Losing the peel, drenching them with salt or washing them will cause you to lose the essential character of the eggplant – its bitterness, which is its most exciting feature. I do none of that – I handle eggplants straight forward. I am careful with the oil used and when I grill them outdoors, I will often dip them in a mustard vinaigrette. There are several eggplant recipes in this book, I encourage you to try some of them.

Endives

There are different types of endives, for instance Belgian endives are curly. Escarole is known as a broad-leafed endive. Endives belong to the chicory family, known for their bitterness - radicchio is a part of this group. In other words, when using the chicory family vegetables, you must embrace their bitterness, and be able to "doctor them up" with the right techniques and spices. With the right combination of herbs and spices they can be delicious and healthy. Belgian endives are high in fiber, iron, calcium, potassium, folic acid, niacin, copper and thiamin. Also, they contain large amounts of beta carotene, riboflavin, vitamin E, C and moderate amounts of vitamins K and A.

Fennel

Fennel has been trendy lately among skilled chefs who understand how to take advantage of its exciting citrus, licorice flavor which can easily overpower the taste of your recipe. Fennel is a Mediterranean native. Italian and Greek cooks have used fennel for hundreds of years. Fennel is unique in a sense that has two different characteristics; the bulb is crunchy and citrusy, while the seed is aromatic and extremely licorice. Both bulb and seeds of the fennel plant are highly nutritious. All parts of the fennel plant are rich in powerful antioxidants and are packed with nutrients: fiber, vitamin C, calcium, iron, magnesium, potassium and manganese and are low in calories. However, the most impressive benefits of all parts of fennel come from the antioxidants and potent plant compounds that they contain.

Kale

Love it or hate it, Kale is a superfood.

And, suddenly, there was the invasion of kale. It came along with an impressive nutrition profile. Kale was introduced to the United States during the nineties and, shortly thereafter, became a staple in the farmer markets. For the last decade it has gone from farmer markets to the top of the super healthy greens. Kale is nothing new to the rest of the world. The Greeks cultivated kale over two thousand years ago and the Romans made it a staple on their dinner table. Kale has always been an essential part of people's diets during difficult times, mainly because it is so easy to grow and is resistant to cold temperatures. Kale lives up to the hype surrounding it: it delivers more nutritional benefits for fewer calories than nearly any other item at the market. Eating more kale is a great way to increase the total nutrient content of your diet dramatically. Kale is extremely high in vitamin C, in fact, one cup of kale contains more vitamin C than an orange. Kale is one of the world's best sources of vitamin K, a cup of kale containing almost seven times the recommended daily amount. Kale is also loaded with vitamins A, and many powerful antioxidants are found in kale. It also provides moderate amounts of vitamin B6, thiamin, riboflavin, niacin. Kale is high in minerals; it is an excellent plant-based source of calcium and magnesium. Other minerals like manganese, copper, potassium, iron and phosphorous are found in kale. To avoid the bitterness of kale, use it with slightly sweet foods and flavorful herbs and spices. Most of kale's bitterness is concentrated in its stem; therefore, you want to avoid using its stem. The same, using leaves only, goes for parsley as well. Adding kale to your diet is simple; add it to your salad or a smoothie. There is no doubt that kale is one of the healthiest foods on the planet.

Lettuce

Generally, all types of lettuce are good for you. They provide fiber, vitamins, minerals and phytochemicals and are very low in calories. Lettuce is a source of folate and vitamin K. It also has potassium and a little calcium. It is a good source of phytochemicals, like beta-carotene, a powerful antioxidant and lutein. But all lettuces are not created equal. Leafy green lettuce, as is the case with darker green vegetables, are a better choice when it comes to vitamins. The one exception is romaine lettuce which is on the top of the list of being one of the healthiest types of lettuce. In my opinion, it is one of the top three best tasting lettuce. The combination of the slightly bitter crunchy leaves and the sweeter softer center rib provides a robust flavor to your salad. Romaine lettuce can be used in recipes as well. Growing up in Greece, I remember the wonderful nights when there was Lamb Fricassee on the dinner table. The lamb, romaine lettuce, artichokes and egg lemon dill sauce created a celebration of tastes – I can still taste it. Red leaf and butter lettuce are not far behind the romaine lettuce. The texture of fresh red leaf lettuce is crispy and succulent. Its taste is mild and slightly bitter and earthy flavor. Butter lettuce comes with a sweet buttery flavor and delicate leaves. The lettuce section of the grocery stores has grown as there are many more lettuce varieties today. Among the many types, there is oak leaf lettuce, frisee, summer crisp, mache lettuce, and the always present iceberg lettuce which is on the bottom of my list when it comes to nutrients. The theory of why iceberg has the least nutrients overall is because it grows in a tighter head, so the inner leaves get less sunlight. However, the bottom line is that all lettuces are good for you – they are low in calories and are good sources of essential nutrients. But no one will be able to convince me a wedge of iceberg lettuce laden with blue cheese dressing and bacon is healthy for you.

Mushrooms

Most mushrooms provide around the same amount of nutrients. They are rich in B vitamins such as riboflavin, folate, thiamine, pantothenic acid and niacin. The minerals in mushrooms are copper, iron, phosphorous, selenium and potassium. Mushrooms are naturally low in sodium, fat, calories, and are high in fiber and protein content. Even though mushrooms have similar nutrients contents, they vary in tastes. The Portobello mushroom, a fully mature cremini mushroom, is higher in potassium and it is often used in place of meat in many dishes. Mushroom are versatile in the kitchen and go well with just about every other food. There are thousands of species of edible mushrooms grown all around the world. Picking wild mushrooms can be a dangerous hobby if you do not know what you're doing. Many wild mushrooms are highly poisonous and, alternatively, there are many medicinal mushrooms that have healing properties.

Okra

Okra is low in calories and has a high fiber content and antioxidant qualities. For a long time, okra has been a favorite food for health-conscious people. It is a good source of protein, riboflavin, niacin, phosphorus, potassium, zinc and copper, and an excellent source of dietary fiber, vitamins A, C, K, thiamin, vitamin B6, folate, calcium, magnesium and manganese. Okra is an old stable food and was used by many cultures. Its origination is not certain. It was cultivated in South Asia, Ethiopia, West Africa and the ancient Egyptians used it. Okra arrived in the Caribbean and the United States in the seventeen hundreds. Today okra is used in many dishes in the Middle East, Mediterranean, the Caribbean and South America. Okra is commonly associated with Southern, Creole, and Cajun cooking.

Onions

Onions come with impressive health benefits. The importance of health benefits in onions is significant because onions, along with tomatoes and garlic are consumed by the general public more than any other vegetable or fruit. Onions are packed with vitamins, minerals and potent plant compounds. Their medicinal properties have been known since ancient times when onions were used to treat various ailments. Onions are unusually high in vitamin C and rich in B vitamins, including vitamins B6 and folate, and they are an excellent source of potassium. Onions, especially the red onion, are loaded with antioxidants. The health benefits of onions seem endless. Onions are a staple in kitchens around the world. They are versatile and can be used to increase the flavor in many foods. Making the onions part of your diet is an easy way to benefit your health.

Green Peas

Green peas have an impressive nutrition profile. They are relatively low in calories and contain just about every vitamin and mineral you need, in addition to significant amounts of antioxidants and fiber. What makes green peas unique from other vegetables is their high protein content. Green peas are high in vitamins A and K; they contain moderate amounts of Vitamin C, folate, thiamin, manganese, iron and phosphorous.

Bell peppers

Bell peppers are low in calories and exceptionally rich in vitamin C and other antioxidants. Bell peppers come in various colors; green, red, yellow, and orange. The green bell pepper has a slightly bitter flavor than the other three. All bell peppers have similar nutrients. Bell peppers are mainly made up of water and carbs and are an excellent fiber source. Bell peppers are loaded with vitamins and minerals and are extremely rich in vitamin C. They also contain vitamins B6, K1, E, A and folate and moderate amounts of potassium. Bell peppers are rich in various antioxidants, especially carotenoids. My favorite bell pepper to cook, roast and used in salads is the red ones. They provide the mild sweetness to give the rest of the food a bit of an exotic flavor. Red bell peppers are ripened green peppers, and it is the reason for their sweetness. They also contain more amounts of vitamin C than the green peppers.

Potatoes

Potatoes are native to South America. They were brought to Europe in the sixteenth century and are now grown in countless varieties worldwide. Potatoes are incredibly versatile in the kitchen: They can be eaten fried, boiled, baked, or mashed. Potatoes are a good source of many vitamins and minerals, such as potassium and vitamin C and contain moderate amounts of protein and fiber. The main dietary component of potatoes is carbohydrates. Potatoes lose some of their nutrients during the cooking process, but the reduction of nutrients can be minimized when baked or boiled with the skin on. Here are the vitamins and mineral in potatoes; vitamin C, B6, folate and potassium. Potatoes are rich in antioxidants; however, the potato antioxidants are mostly concentrated in the skin. Eating potatoes is generally healthy depending on how the potatoes are prepared. Obviously, baked and boiled is healthier than fried.

Shallots

Shallots are a member of the onion family although their flavor is closer to garlic. They look like a yellow onion but when peeled are separated into cloves, like garlic. Interesting vegetable. Sautéing shallots in olive oil brings out their best character; a soft texture with a mild, less potent flavor than either onion or garlic. But make no mistake about this, shallots are neither onions nor garlic. I believe that the only other vegetable that comes remotely close to shallots in texture and flavor, are the red onions. Shallots are great for baking with other vegetables or with chicken. I like the texture and the complex character that shallots add to various dishes; sweeter and milder than yellow onions with a slightly garlicky hint. And, as is the case for most foods, slow cooking brings out a more intense flavor. The amazing fact about cooking shallots with various foods is that it takes on slightly different tastes determined by the items they are cooked with. In a baked chicken recipe with other vegetables and various herbs, I thought I tasted a slight apple flavor in the shallots! Shallots are rich in dietary fiber, protein, vitamins C, A, B6, folate, potassium, iron, copper and manganese, and they have a high content of antioxidant compounds. Shallots are native to Asia and are believed to have been introduced to Europe from crusaders during the eleventh century. Today shallots are used worldwide and are no longer a specialty item; they are available on every food market.

Spinach

A superfood.

Spinach originated in central Asia and was enjoyed by the ancient Persians. Later, they became popular in the Mediterranean and from there they spread to the rest of Europe. Spinach is loaded with nutrients and antioxidants, and is one of the healthiest foods to eat. Spinach is an extremely nutrient-rich vegetable. It is low in carbohydrates and high in insoluble fiber. It is an excellent source of vitamins A, C, K1, folate, as well as iron. Spinach also contains several other vitamins and minerals, such as vitamins B6, B9 and E and minerals such as potassium, magnesium. Spinach contains several important plant compounds as well. The antioxidants found in spinach are linked to numerous health benefits. Spinach is best when it's color is between medium and dark green. The nutrients in spinach are most dominant when the vegetable is fresh. Raw spinach used in salads or blended into a smoothie is the best way to consume all the vitamins and minerals contained in the vegetable. Although spinach is versatile in the kitchen, the mild bitterness in spinach shines when blended with pungent foods, like feta cheese. Hence the extremely popular spanakopita. Some health experts suggest boiling the spinach before eating, to reduce the presence of oxalic acid found in many greens, while other health experts have no concern about the small amounts of the acid in spinach. Boiling spinach by itself to serve as a side dish, is committing a culinary crime. Bottom line; spinach is one of the healthiest foods to eat. And, no, spinach does not build massive forearms – contributes to health for the entire body. And, another no, do not eat spinach from a can. And yes, spinach is a superfood.

Sweet potatoes

Sweet potatoes are excellent source of vitamin A and C, manganese, copper, pantothenic acid and vitamin B6. They are also a good source of potassium, fiber, niacin, vitamin B1, B2 and phosphorus. Sweet potatoes come in a variety of sizes and colors. The most popular ones are the orange sweet potatoes. They are rich in antioxidants, and soluble and insoluble fiber . The unique sweetness in this potato gives power to creative chefs to imagine endless tastes in every meal of the day. This makes the sweet potato one of the most versatile vegetable in the kitchen; it can be prepared in both sweet and savory dishes, and pairs well with extreme flavors, such as cinnamon and garlic. Healthy, versatile and gluten-free is a powerful tool to have in your kitchen. In this book I use sweet potatoes in many recipes; in pancakes, with stews, salads, mashed, baked, and I use the skin for various stuffings. The skin of the potato is where the nutrients are more concentrated . The sweet potato was cultivated in North America when Columbus arrived. Because of the unique taste, the nutritional value and easy agricultural production, sweet potatoes are now a favorite vegetable around the world. It wasn't that long ago when sweet potatoes were used as a staple in Thanksgiving to make the classic, delicious dish covered with marshmallows. Today sweet potatoes can be prepared in many different ways – but, when you are ready to cook sweet potatoes, please, save the marshmallows for Thanksgiving.

Pumpkin

Pumpkin is a good source of vitamin E, magnesium, phosphorus, potassium and copper, and an excellent source of dietary fiber, vitamin A, vitamin C, vitamin K, iron and manganese. Roasting a pumpkin brings out its sweetness. Pumpkin is useful as a puree to be used as the main ingredient to make pancakes, muffins or quick bread. Pumpkin shines when it is spiced with exotic spices, especially cinnamon, cloves, nutmeg, ginger or cardamom – pumpkin pairs exceptionally well with white chocolate. Its puree makes a creamy, delicious pie. There are, however, creative ways to use pumpkin. A few decades ago I made a pumpkin white chocolate cheesecake that became an instant favorite. Just before Thanksgiving, our kitchen was busy producing that cheesecake to fill up the many requests. At Thanksgiving, it is the first item on our family's request list.

Zucchini

Zucchini is a good source of protein, vitamins A, C, K, B6, folate, magnesium, potassium, manganese, thiamin, niacin, copper and phosphorus. Zucchini also boasts several antioxidants that provide various health benefits. The highest antioxidant levels are found in its skin. Zucchini is rich in water and fiber. Even though raw zucchini does not have much taste, it is versatile in the kitchen. The main reason is its mild flavor, it can be blended and spiced with just about everything. You can make zucchini bread, fritters, stuffed zucchini, bake it with other vegetables, or use it in soups. Some of the herbs and spices that are best with zucchini are basil, oregano, black pepper, thyme, garlic. It pairs well with lemon, tomatoes, onions, feta and ricotta cheese, as well as with white meats, seafood, olive oil and nuts.

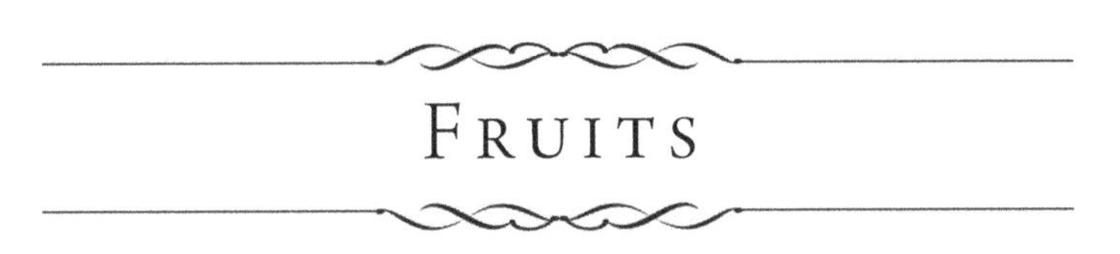

FRUITS

APPLES

A super-fruit.

You might want to re-think before removing the skin from the apple. The skin of the apple contains large amounts of vitamin C, potassium, calcium and fiber. The skin of many other fruits and vegetables also contain various nutrients. The problem with the skin of fresh produce is the pesticide. It is one of the many reasons that many fruits and vegetables we eat should be organic. Apples are a good source of fiber and several antioxidants. Apples used in salads, smoothies, cooking and baking. Apple pairs well with almond, walnuts, caramel, cinnamon, raisins, ginger. The tree originated in Central Asia and have been grown for thousands of years around the world.

APRICOTS

Apricots are an excellent source of vitamins A and C, copper, fiber and potassium. When ripe and fresh, apricots are both sweet and tart. Apricots go well with chicken and can be grilled. They can be used in many baking recipes. The origin of the apricot is unsettled. Most likely it originated around the Russian-Chinese borders. They were cultivated in Armenia in ancient times, but China is credited for its domestication. Other sources claim that were cultivate in India first, from where Alexander introduced it to Greece. One thing is sure, apricots have been grown since antiquity. Today they are popular in the Mediterranean and the Middle East.

AVOCADOS

Avocados are loaded with nutrients, many of which are lacking in modern diets. They are rich with fiber, powerful antioxidants and monounsaturated fatty acids. Avocado consumption in Mexico goes back almost ten thousand years. Back then, humans were merely eating wild avocados. The avocado cultivation began over five thousand years ago. The Incas and the Mayas grew domesticated avocado trees and since then it has been a part of the Mexican diet. The Spanish explorers were the first Europeans to taste the avocado in the sixteenth century. By that time the avocados had spread through the rest of the Americas. Avocados are low in sodium, cholesterol free and rich in healthy fats. They can be used in place of butter and are a good substitution for mayonnaise or sour cream. Because of its taste and texture the avocado is extremely versatile in the kitchen. It is excellent in salads, spreads, sandwiches, sauces, smoothies, or it can be grilled. Bottom line, the multitude of ways you can use avocados are endless. It provides texture, taste and nutrients. My favorite hummus is made with avocados and feta. The smooth buttery taste of avocados and the tangy, salty and creamy flavor of real feta cheese is the perfect union of tastes.

BANANAS

Bananas contain vitamins B6, C, A, as well folate, riboflavin, niacin, manganese, potassium, magnesium, iron, protein and fiber. Bananas have been part of our diet for about two-thousand five hundred years. Bananas are the most popular fruit in the world. The origin of bananas is placed in Southeast Asia. From there it spread to the Philippines and Africa. Bananas are the perfect snack; they are nutritious, inexpensive and safe, protected by its thick skin. It is excellent in smoothies, bread, cakes, with pancakes and oatmeal, and of course with peanut butter.

BLUEBERRIES

Another super-fruit.

This super-fruit has an impressive nutrition profile. Blueberries have the highest antioxidant content of the most commonly consumed fruits. Flavonoids appear to be the blueberries' antioxidant with the most significant impact. They contain high amounts of fiber, vitamin C, vitamin K and manganese, and decent amounts of folate, choline, vitamins A and E, and manganese. Blueberries are versatile in the kitchen. They can be used in salads, smoothies, with yogurt, in baking, or just eat them by the handful. Native Americans used blueberries for centuries. They ate blueberries fresh and dried them to preserve them for the winter. Blueberry juice was used by Native Americans for medical reasons and to dye their clothes and baskets. Its leaves were used to make a medicinal tea. English settlers tried unsuccessfully to cultivate blueberries since the early sixteen-hundreds, but it wasn't until 1910 that farmers were successful in growing blueberries. Finally, in 1916, blueberries made their way to the American dinner table.

CANTALOUPES

Cantaloupes are extremely high in beta-carotene, vitamins C and A, and a good source of potassium, copper, folate and vitamins B1, B3 and B6. When ripe, cantaloupe's flesh is sweet and juicy. It is extremely aromatic. The cantaloupe that is grown in the United States is a type of muskmelon rather than the European cantaloupe. The true cantaloupe is a European melon with a rough surface, soft flesh and, even before opening it, you can smell its distinctive aroma. Cantaloupes need plenty of sunshine. They are grown mainly in the Mediterranean area, where the summers are hot and the winters are mild. The original cultivators of cantaloupes are thought to be ancient Italians and Greeks. The commercial farming in the United States began toward the end of eighteen-hundreds.

CHERRIES

Cherries are a good source of vitamin C, vitamin A, calcium, protein and iron and very high in potassium. It seems like cherries have been present around the globe since ancient times. The Chinese, Greeks and Romans used cherries for centuries. Cherries pits were brought to America by French colonists in the sixteen-hundreds. The French grew cherries along the Saint Lawrence River and the Great Lakes. Today, cherries grow into different colors and tastes. The tart cherries are bright red, and the most common sweet cherries are the bing cherries. Bing cherries come in various colors as well. They are mostly dark, and sometimes are black or purple. Because of its different flavors, today's chefs find creative ways to use them. Cherries can be used in sweets, smoothies, breakfasts, in sauces, desserts, and with some grains. In this book, I have a pancake recipe made with buckwheat flour, cherries and pears.

FIGS

Figs are rich in minerals including potassium, calcium, magnesium, iron and copper and a good source of the antioxidant vitamins A, E and K that contribute to health and wellness. Firmenich, the world largest privately-owned fragrance and flavor company, named the fig as the 2018 flavor of the year. Because of this, it expected that more people, outside the Mediterranean, are about to discover the tremendous nutritional value, remarkable versatility of the complex sweet, smooth and silky tasting fig. The history of figs is as fascinating as is its taste. The word sycophant, from the Greek sykophantes; from *sykon* "fig" and *phainein* "to show, make known." Many stories have been created over the years to give sense to the composition of this word. Whatever reason, this word was created for those who illegally exported figs did not pay taxes for the fig sales or harmed the fig trees. As stories evolved, figs and the word sykophantes described shady people. Figs were loved in ancient Greece so much that sycophant offenders were arrested and prosecuted. The love of the fig has not changed much over the years in the Mediterranean. Firmenich used over ten flavors trying to describe the taste of fig. These descriptors will not make sense unless you've eaten fresh figs at peak ripeness. I get it. Growing up in Greece, I had the privilege to consume tons of figs during the hot summer months. Figs can be used as appetizers, salads, and in both cooking and baking. In the late eighties, I created a fig pie with raspberries and dark chocolate. In the 1993 "Best of Phoenix" awards by the New Times the author noted; "In Nick's restaurant, there is a monstrous dessert selection, including a wicket Fig Berry Pie with raspberries and dark chocolate." In Greece, the ultimate compliment to a chef when asked about the taste of the food is to say, "It was just like a cold fig."

GRAPES

Grapes contain a fair amount of vitamins C and K and they are high in antioxidants. Some foods, throughout the centuries, shaped the course of history by taking a life of their own in a popular culture. Among them are grapes and cocoa beans. Grapes were a part of the earlier human civilization in literature, arts and religion. Wine and religion are ageless companions. From the Egyptian patron god of wines, Hathor, to the bad boy Greek god of wine Dionysus, or Bacchus by the Romans. Christ turned water to wine and the Christians symbolize the blood of Christ with wine. In history, Homer in the Odyssey mentioned how wine forces even a wise man to laugh and sing and dance and bring forth unspoken words. In the symposiums, Socrates suggested that wine should be drunk in small cups and diluted with water to reach a state of amusement, instead of being forced into drunkenness. Shakespeare's plays are full of wine quotes; "Good wine is a good familiar creature if it be well used." The grape's most significant contribution is wine, but there's so much more. Grapes are the most produced fruit in the world. Grape culture is as old as civilization. Humans began growing grapes over eight thousand years ago. Grapes appeared during the Neolithic and Paleolithic periods, in Asia Minor and through the Nile Delta of Egypt and the Babylonians. The Hittites of the ancient Anatolia migrated to Bosporus, Crete and Thrace, and brought their grapes along. From there the Greeks and the Phoenicians brought the grapes to Sicily. And, the grape culture spread fast to the rest of Italy, France and Spain. Over twenty-four million people have visited the breathtaking wine country of California. Even after devastating fires, the number of visitors is expected go be back to normal. California is the fourth most wine producer in the world. Over 80% of the wine in the United States is being produced in California. It will take many pages to talk about all the types of grapes out there. Today, besides the wine, grapes have become a significant contribution to the culinary world. They are used in many dishes and salads; grapes pair well with chicken, seafood and fine grains like quinoa and millet. They are a great partner to feta, arugula and yogurt. Raisins, black or blond, are extremely useful in recipes that you need to sweeten and balanced bitter tastes, they are also great with breakfast grains and with nuts. Yes, grapes are one of those foods that helped to shape the world in which we live today.

Mango

Mangos are high in vitamins C and A. They contains goodly amounts of vitamins B6, K, folate, potassium, calcium, copper and iron, as well as antioxidants and beta-carotene, and small amounts of protein. Mangoes are native to India. They were cultivated for the first time around five thousand years ago. Fortunately, the cultivation of mangoes spread to all tropical regions of the world. Because of their exquisite and unusual flavor mangoes are regarded as the king of the tropical fruit. Mango can be used to make a sweet and sour salsa and chutney; it is great with yogurt and in smoothies. In this book, I have a fruit relish recipe with mango and pineapple. Also, I use it in a salad with quinoa, yogurt and other fruits. While in the restaurant, I created a white cake with mango mousse and kiwi white chocolate. Today it is the most requested cake for family birthdays.

Pears

Pears are high in vitamins C, K, and potassium. They have small amounts of calcium, iron, magnesium, riboflavin, vitamin B-6, and folate. Pears are popular as appetizers and desserts. They can be served with hard or soft cheese and salads. Their subtle, distinct flavor works well with dark chocolate, sweet sauces and baked goods. There are thousands of pear varieties grown in countries with temperate climates. Like bananas, pears are not tree-ripened, they are sold when firm, but to get their full flavor they must be ripened before serving. Pears are one of the world's oldest cultivated fruits. In The Odyssey, Homer praises pears as a "gift of the gods." The Roman farmers documented extensive pear growing and pears have been a muse in the works of Renaissance masters. Pears are versatile and have a long storage life.

Pineapple

The pineapples is loaded with vitamin C, Vitamins A, B6, folate, thiamin, pantothenic acid and riboflavin. It contains calcium, magnesium, manganese, potassium, as well antioxidants. Fresh pineapple is the only known source of an enzyme called bromelain, which is an anti-inflammatory. The pineapple is known to the Europeans as ananas, from its botanical name *ananas comoros*, and to most Spanish speaking countries as *pina*. The pineapple was first cultivated in Hawaii, the Caribbean, Central America, and Mexico where the Aztecs and Mayans cultivated it. From there it made its way to India, Asia and West Indies. When the pineapple is ripened is exceptionally juicy with an intensely sweet and tangy tropical flavor. Pineapples pairs well with red meats, chicken and shrimp. They are best with baking recipes, breakfast, salads and smoothies.

Pomegranates

Nothing like it on earth.

Pomegranates contain large amounts of Vitamins C and K, folate, fiber, potassium and even some protein. The pomegranate is a fruit unlike anything else on earth. Although all the different colors of its seeds have a similar taste, I believe that the common deep red ones are the ones with the most complex taste. They are sweet with a sour and tart undertone. To get the most of its complex flavor, pomegranate seeds are best eaten alone or with mild foods. Pomegranate seeds are a real treat. Pomegranate trees are known for their ability to withstand lengthy droughts. Pomegranates come with a long and colorful history. Their origin is not well known. They appeared at the same time in the Middle East, Afghanistan and the Mediterranean and from there they migrated to China. Today, they are commonly grown in California. Pomegranates have been both enjoyed in cooking and in medicine throughout the centuries. They appear in many historical events and mythological tales. Based on excavations of the early Bronze Age, it is believed that the pomegranate was one of the first cultivated fruits. Ancient Egyptians thought that the pomegranate juice had healing abilities, they used the blossoms as a red dye and the peel was used for dyeing leather. In Ancient Rome, pomegranates were depicted in Roman mosaics. In ancient Persia, pomegranates were associated with fertility and pomegranate trees were planted in the courtyards of Zoroastrian temples as a symbol of eternal life. In Buddhism, the pomegranate is one of the three blessed fruits and represents the essence of favorable influences in Buddhist art. The completion and printing of the first bible included the references to pomegranates and pomegranate trees decorated the temple of the founder of Zen. In paintings by Sandro Botticelli, the Virgin Mary appears with the infant Christ and a pomegranate. Pomegranates were part of various modern artistic movements; Cezanne, Matisse, Picasso and Salvador Dalí all portrayed pomegranates in their work. In Greek myths, the pomegranate appears in several tales – the most famous involved Persephone, daughter of Zeus and Demeter, who was abducted by Hades. Once in the underworld, Hades tempted her with a juicy pomegranate. When she tasted the fruit, Persephone stayed in the underworld. Demeter, the goddess of the harvest, mourning the loss of her daughter, prevented the earth from bearing fruit unless she saw her daughter again. Zeus arranged a compromise with Hades for Persephone to live with Hades for one-third of the year and the other two thirds with Demeter. The arrival of spring is marked each year by the return of Persephone from the underworld. After several decades of California's cultivation of pomegranates, American consumers rediscovered this ancient fruit. I have a special affinity for pomegranates. In our back yard, my mother grew vegetables, flowers and there were several fruit trees, among them was a pomegranate. As a young boy, I remember, after the bright red blossoms appeared on the tree, waiting with great anticipation for the fruit to grow. Our hands and faces were permanently red when the fruit finally ripened. We could not get enough of that magical taste. I remember the flavor all too well; it is one of those fascinated tastes that has haunted my culinary brains. It is most likely the only one that I know I do not want to spoil it with other flavors. So I only use it in salads and side dishes where the taste of pomegranate seeds is the dominant one. Pomegranate is one of my weaknesses. Maybe it is because it is nothing like I had tasted before. Perhaps because it reminds me of the wonder of the earth in which my mother grew endless foods for us to eat. When opened, the pomegranate reveals a dense collection of seeds nestled among a white membrane. The seeds are easily separated. Cut the pomegranate in half, break them with your hands and drop the seeds and parts of the membrane into a bowl of water and discard the shell. The seeds will sink in the bottom and the lighter membrane on the top. Pick the membrane pieces out and drain the water.

Raspberry

Raspberries are rich in vitamin C and K and contains good amounts vitamin E, iron, potassium, manganese and lesser amounts of thiamin, riboflavin, niacin, pantothenic acid, vitamin B-6, calcium. Natives of Asia Minor and North America collected raspberries as a food source for centuries. By the Middle Ages, wild raspberries had many uses. Artists used raspberry juice in paintings and physicians recommended the fruit, leaves, and roots for various medical reasons. When the first European settlers migrated to America, Native Americans were drying raspberries to preserve them. Since the early eighteen-hundreds raspberries are made into preserves and syrups. Raspberries seem to have originated in Asia. Since then, raspberries have been widely bred, with a multitude of varieties. Raspberries were long considered a luxury, as only the rich were able to enjoy this delicate fruit. Today, raspberries rank high on the list of the world's most popular berries. Raspberries are extremely versatile fruits and can be used in sauces, jams, smoothies, ice cream, salads, pies, cakes, or pancakes. I use raspberries for my baking – they partner well with dark chocolate. Some decades ago I created a recipe for breakfast called Raspberry Stuffed Toast. It is a staple in every one of our family gatherings for brunch.

STRAWBERRIES

Strawberries contain iron, copper, magnesium, phosphorus, vitamin B6, vitamin K and vitamin E. Strawberries are a good source of vitamin C, manganese, folate and potassium. Strawberries are the most cultivated berry in the United States. Most commercial strawberries in the United States are grown in California or Florida, where the climate helps to extend the strawberry growing season. The best strawberries are brightly colored, plump and have fresh green caps attached. Strawberries do not ripen after being picked, so if you buy the partly white ones, it means that they were not ripe when picked. Here is a good time to talk about pesticides. For the past three years strawberries have topped the Environmental Working Group's dirty dozen list of fruits and vegetables with the most pesticide residues. While others, including the alliance for food and farming, view the report with skepticism. Following the dirty dozen list is spinach in which most of the samples contained pesticide residues. Among the fruits and vegetable making a list are some other favorite items, including apples, grapes, tomatoes and cherries. There are several fruits and vegetables free of pesticides and safe to eat. My question is this, even if the report is not entirely accurate, why take the chance? The simple solution is to buy organic, at least the items on the list. There is a theory that you can wash out pesticides with various methods, like a long wash or with vinegar. I am not convinced that any of that works. Some people have noted that it is difficult to find organic products and they are more expensive. It is true that not all organic fruits and vegetables are always available in your supermarket. However, they are almost always available in special farmers markets. It is also true that organic products are more expensive. I am known to be a smart shopper; I watch prices and quality. What I have noticed lately is that when a particular fruit and vegetable is in season, there is not much difference in costs between organic and non-organic. Even though I am trying to get the best for my money, I maintain the belief that there is no price for my health.

WATERMELON

A super-fruit.

Watermelon contains thiamine, riboflavin, niacin, vitamin B-6, folate, pantothenic acid, magnesium, phosphorus, potassium, zinc, copper, manganese, selenium, choline, lycopene, and betaine. The origins of watermelon have been traced back to over four thousand years to the continent of Africa. Watermelon is unique in terms of anti-inflammatory and antioxidant benefits. The depth of its nutrition profile is impressive. More in-depth research for additional information about the number of nutrients and health benefits of the watermelon will convince anyone about the great importance of this fruit. From a nutrient perspective, watermelon seeds are every bit as nutrient rich as the flesh. Watermelon is best tasting and fuller in nutrients when ripe. To select a ripened watermelon check for its heaviness, the water content of a watermelon will typically increase along with ripening. Also look for a slightly flattened spot. More ripened watermelons will have sat on the ground more extended periods. If all this fails, use the sound technique; a ripe watermelons will have a deep hollow sound, rather than a solid and shallow one. Watermelon is excellent by itself, but it can give a fruit salad an extra crispness and freshness. In this book, there is a watermelon salad with feta. It is unique and refreshing.

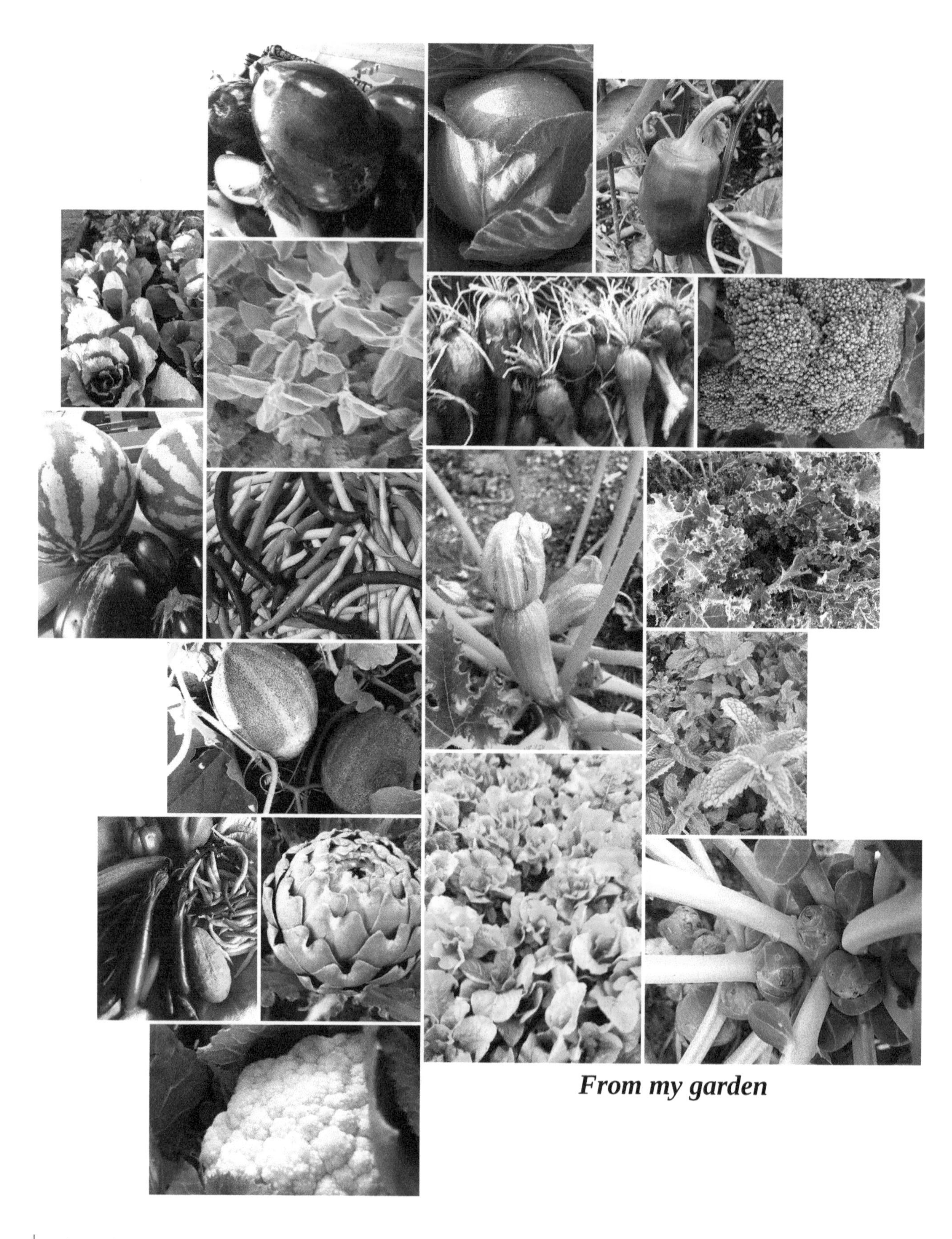

From my garden

Nuts

Most nuts are high in omega 3 fatty acids. Also, nuts contain high amounts of fiber, protein, Vitamin E, and a variety of essential minerals. Raw nuts contain the highest numbers of these healthy nutrients. Roasting nuts reduce the antioxidant content and can reduce the amount of healthy fats. Nuts are a common snack food and can be used as a vegetarian protein source. Because nuts are quite high in calories, they are a naturally compact source of energy, which is perfect for traveling. Since ancient times, grounded nuts were used, in some cultures, to thicken various sauces. I use this method in some of my creamy sauces.

Almonds

Almonds deliver a massive amount of nutrients: Fiber, manganese, magnesium, vitamin E, copper, riboflavin and phosphorus.

Chestnuts

Chestnuts are high in manganese, vitamin C, vitamin B6 and copper and vitamin C.

Hazelnuts

Hazelnuts are high in magnesium, calcium and vitamins B and E.

Pecans

Pecans are high in healthy unsaturated fat. They also contain vitamins A, B, and E, folic acid, calcium, magnesium, phosphorus, potassium, and zinc.

Pine Nuts

Pine nuts contain nutrients that help boost energy, including monounsaturated fat, protein and iron. They are also a good source of magnesium and potassium.

Pistachios

Pistachios are extremely rich in potassium. They are high in protein, fiber and antioxidants.

Walnuts

Walnuts contain good fats. They also contain iron, selenium, calcium, zinc, vitamin E.

Seeds

Seeds are good sources of healthy fats, rich in protein, fiber and antioxidants. They are naturally low in sodium. Seeds are extremely easy to add to salads, yogurt, oatmeal and smoothies, an easy way to add healthy nutrients to your diet.

Flaxseed

Flaxseed is a rich source of healthy fats, antioxidants, and fiber. The seeds contain protein, lignans, and the essential fatty acid omega-3.

Poppy seeds

Poppy seeds are a rich source of thiamin, folate, and several essential minerals, including calcium, iron, magnesium, manganese, phosphorus and zinc.

Sesame seeds

Sesame seeds have beneficial nutrients and is rich in many minerals and vitamins which includes selenium, calcium, phosphorus, zinc, copper, dietary fiber, protein, molybdenum, folate, magnesium, iron, manganese, vitamin B1 and B6.

Sunflower seeds

Sunflower seeds are an excellent source of vitamin E, copper, manganese, selenium, phosphorus, magnesium, vitamin B6, B1, folate and niacin.

Oats

Oats are high in manganese magnesium, copper and vitamin B1. They contain good amounts of iron, zinc, folate and vitamin B5.

Herbs and Spices

In book II, *On the Soul,* Aristotle discusses the perception of taste. He establishes four basic tastes that the tongue is sensitive to; sweet, sour, bitter and salty. In my opinion, those are the four tastes that allow you to balance food flavors. Since the time of Aristotle, tastes have been studied and contemplated. New tastes were discovered; one of them is umami. Umami, a Japanese word meaning savory, applies to the sensation of savoriness. Savory is considered a popular taste in Japan and China but is not discussed as much in western cuisine. The action of umami receptors explains why foods treated with monosodium glutamate often taste better. MSG is a flavor enhancer. The FDA has classified MSG as a food ingredient that's "generally recognized as safe." However, its use remains controversial. The FDA has received many reports of harmful reactions to foods containing MSG. From a personal perspective, when I eat foods that contain MSG, my mouth dries up and I get severe headaches. The question is why use it if there is a chance that is harmful to your health? There are so many natural ingredients that you can enhance the flavor of your foods. It is essential that the exploration of new tastes continues, but I am content to base my creativity around the four original tastes – it fits my style of cooking. In every one of my recipes, I try to combine as many as the four flavors without one overpowering the others. The day that I can combine the four tastes in harmony, I will have invented the perfect taste.

Basil

Everyone's favorite.

Besides being calorie-free, Basil is a rich source of antioxidants and phenolics, vitamin K, zinc, calcium, magnesium, potassium and dietary fiber. Basil is sweet, highly aromatic with peppery and licorice undertones. Basil shines when fresh or dried. When dried it takes a minty flavor.

Cardamom

Cardamom contains calcium, potassium and vitamins B and C. It also contains small amounts of protein, fiber, and fatty acids. Cardamom has a sweet and light lemony flavor, with a fruity robust aroma.

Cinnamon

The healing superspice.

Cinnamon is another good healing superspice that contains large amounts of highly potent polyphenol antioxidants. It is so powerful that cinnamon can be used as a natural food preservative. Cinnamon also includes a small amount of vitamin E, niacin, vitamin B6, magnesium, potassium, zinc and copper. Sweet, aromatic and spicy flavors. Cinnamon is both sweet and spicy which is the reason it does well in both baking and cooking. It is extremely aromatic as well. Cinnamon is a personal favor.

Cumin

Cumin contains an excellent amount of iron and a good source of calcium, manganese, magnesium, phosphorus and vitamin B1. Cumin has a very distinct smoky and earthy flavor with hints of lemon and nutty and spicy undertones. Cumin seeds are greatly underrated, they are packed with flavor and, when roasted, have a warm aroma.

Cloves

Cloves contain fiber, vitamins and minerals. Among them vitamin K and C, calcium, magnesium and potassium. Cloves have a bitter, intense aroma and fruity, woody undertones. Cloves contain high consternation of oil which during cooking or baking time releases a sweet warm flavor.

Dill

Contains excellent amounts of fiber, niacin, phosphorus, copper, riboflavin, vitamin B6, magnesium, and potassium. Dill is a light herb with sweet, grassy and anise undertones.

Fennel

It is an excellent source of vitamin C, fiber, potassium, manganese, copper, phosphorus and folate. It is a good source of calcium, pantothenic acid, magnesium, iron and niacin. Fennel has a warm, licorice type aroma with a flavor that is slightly sweet with camphor undertones.

Ginger

Another superspice.

Ginger is an excellent natural source of vitamin C, magnesium, potassium, copper, and manganese. Ginger is fierce and peppery with lemon/citrus aroma undertones. When cooked has a mild sweetness with warm flavor. Its complex flavor makes ginger versatile for both baking and cooking.

Mustard, Ground

Mustard seeds are an excellent source of selenium and a very good source of omega-3 fatty acids and manganese. They are also a good source of phosphorus, magnesium, copper and vitamin B1. Yellow ground mustard is ideal for tempering mustard flavor. It has a mellow spiciness and strong mustard flavor.

Mint

Mint contains potassium, magnesium, calcium, phosphorus, vitamin C, iron and vitamin A. Mint is sweet with an intense refreshing flavor and grassy, bitter undertones. It is surprisingly versatile for such an intensely flavored herb.

Oregano

A superherb.

I've heard people saying that oregano should be in the medicine cabinet, right along with garlic. Oregano contains calcium, iron, magnesium, manganese, potassium, vitamin K. It is high in antioxidants. Oregano has a dominant earthy and peppery flavor with some lemony and bitter flavors.

Paprika

Paprika is a good source of thiamin, magnesium, phosphorus, copper and manganese. It also contains Fiber, vitamins A, C, E, K, B6, riboflavin, as well niacin, iron and potassium. Paprika has slightly sweet, earthy flavors with mild spicy and smoky undertones.

Parsley

Another superfood.

Parsley is a concentrated source of nutrition and antioxidants, and more. It is incredibly high in vitamin K and vitamin C. Parsley is also a good source of vitamin A, folate and iron. Parsley is grassy, slightly bitter flavor with woody and citrus undertones.

Rosemary

Rosemary provides a bit more of everything: fiber, iron, calcium, vitamin C, and vitamin A. Rosemary is most likely the most complex flavor of all herbs. It has strong lemon-pine flavor and a distinct minty one. There is a noticeable peppery taste with hints of eucalyptus. Rosemary isn't a shy herb when it comes to aroma – it is strong. It is extraordinary that this incredibly unique flavor profile is something that works extremely well with a vast array of various dishes.

Pepper

Part of my superspice team.

Pepper is incredibly popular among spices since ancient times. Black pepper is an excellent source of manganese and vitamin K, an excellent source of copper and dietary fiber, and a good source of iron, chromium and calcium. There is a distinct and undeniable earthiness to the flavor of black pepper. It is packed with a mild heat and depth of flavor. Its aroma is pungent and sharp. It goes well with nearly any dish.

Turmeric

Superspice.

Turmeric is a member of my superspice team. Every label of turmeric should have a giant red S to identify this superspice. Turmeric contains curcumin, a powerful antioxidant. It is also a good source of vitamin C and magnesium, and an excellent source of dietary fiber, vitamin B6, iron, potassium and manganese. Turmeric adds a rich, woody with somewhat bitter and earthy flavor. When cooked it has a warm, peppery flavor. It comes with an intense color.

Thyme

A member of my superherb team.

Along with basil and oregano, thyme is one of my favorite herbs. It contains thymol, a potent antioxidant. It is an excellent source of vitamin C, vitamin A, fiber, riboflavin, iron, copper, and manganese. It also contains calcium and manganese, vitamin B6, folate, phosphorus, potassium, and zinc. Thyme is another one with a complex flavor. It is somewhat spicy and minty and has a strong fresh, lemony flavor. It has a subtly dry aroma with bitter and piney undertones.

Tarragon

Tarragon is high in potassium and a good source of calcium and magnesium. Tarragon has a pungent licorice flavor with hints of mint. When cooked it adopts a sweet, spicy taste.

Tomatoes

Tomatoes are the primary dietary source of the antioxidant lycopene, one of the most powerful antioxidants. Other vegetables and fruits with lycopene are guavas, watermelon, papaya, grapefruit, sweet red peppers, asparagus, red cabbage, mango and carrots. Tomatoes are also a great source of vitamin C, potassium, folate and vitamin K.

If there is a low-acid red tomato I have not found it yet. The only ones that might have a bit less acidic are the bright red, ripe organic tomatoes. The firmer tomatoes contain more acid. There is also green, yellow, purple, orange, white and so on, but we are talking about real tomatoes here - unless you are making a multicolor tomato sauce. The conventional wisdom about how to avoid acidity in your tomato sauce is to use sugar and/or baking soda. But I have sworn to the cooking gods to never use sugar or baking soda in my tomato sauce or any other sauce in that matter; somehow sugar and baking soda belong to my baking pantry. Here is what works for me; I select ripe Roma tomatoes and use as much fresh herbs as possible, and plenty of fresh basil – you can never have too much basil. The use of onions and garlic helps as well. In some dishes, like lasagna, I add a bit of cinnamon to my tomato sauce, it pairs well with ricotta. I remember my father use to peel the tomatoes to be used for his sauce. My mother would ask; Why are you peeling the tomatoes? His answer was; They taste sweeter this way! Peeling the tomatoes might work as well. I do not peel my tomatoes. I chop the tomatoes in small pieces to break the skin. Tomato skins contain important amino acids and, especially the seeds, have a high amount of minerals. They also have monounsaturated fatty acids and antioxidant compounds. Most mushrooms have a mild sweet taste and using mushrooms for the quick tomato sauce, takes away some of the acidity. The best mushrooms to use are the cremini mushrooms. They are similar to the white mushroom in shape and size but firmer to the touch. The portobello mushrooms work as well. Portobello is a fully mature cremini mushrooms, but they have a meaty texture and flavor that might overpower all other ingredients in your sauce. The good thing about portobello mushrooms is that they are much higher in protein than the white or cremini mushrooms. Switching Parmesan grated cheese to Romano helps as well. Romano, especially the pecorino Romano, has a sharper and saltier taste than Parmesan. I use both or a combination of both in various recipes. There is an intense debate out there, usually between the tomato canning companies and the purists of fresh foods. The discussion between canned or fresh tomatoes has strong arguments on both sides. The one side claims that canned tomatoes are safe to eat. On the other side there are concerns about BPA and additives. Canned tomatoes often contain salt, sugar and preservatives like citric acid and calcium chloride, all safe to eat. There are benefits for using canned tomatoes; they are quick, convenient and full of nutrients, but you cannot substitute freshness. The safest way is choosing the healthiest ingredients that go into your body.

Tomatoes from my garden

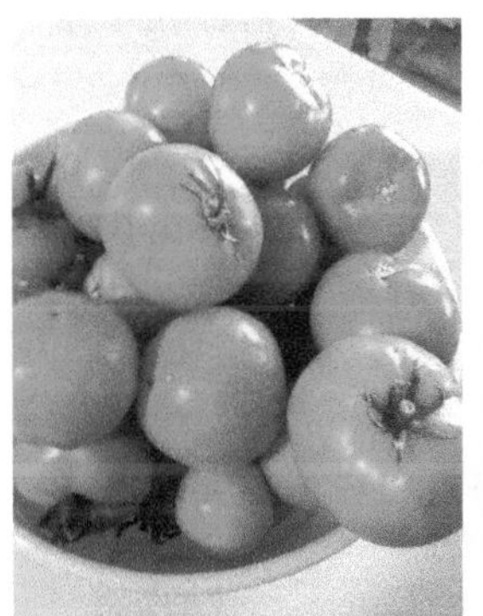

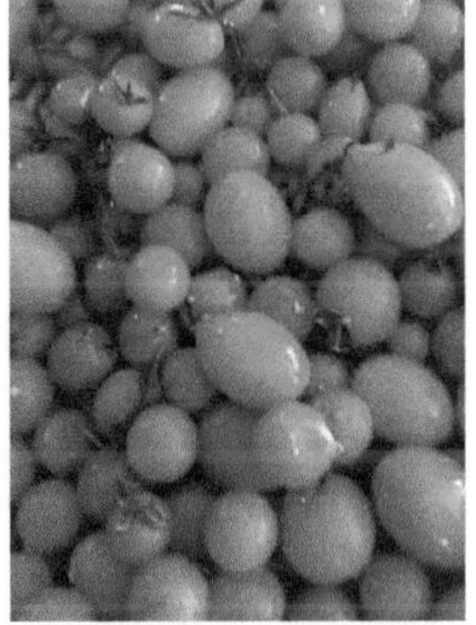

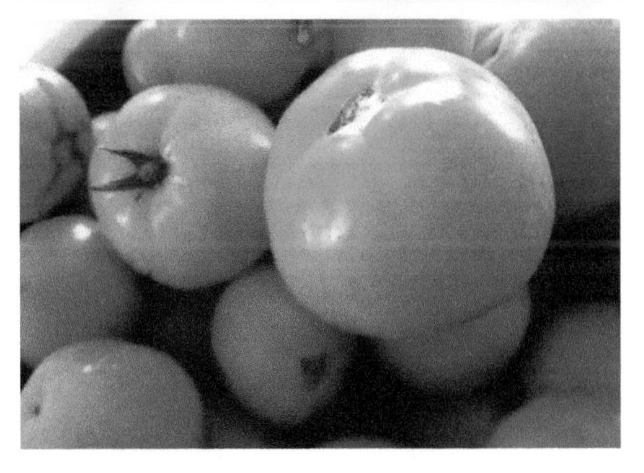

Sun-dried tomatoes

Sun-dried tomatoes are loaded with antioxidants, vitamins and minerals. Most importantly, sun-dried tomatoes unique flavor brings another dimension to the art of cooking. I've been using sun-dried tomatoes since the early eighties, many years before they became a sensation in creative recipes. The best sun-dried tomatoes are when the tomatoes are ripe and dried slowly by the sun and packed in olive oil. In places without much sun, there is a recipe for sun-dried tomatoes in this book.

Garlic

The ultimate superfood.

In my humble opinion, garlic is the superfood of all the superfoods. When Hypocrites said, “Let food be thy medicine, and medicine be thy food,” most likely he was holding a head of garlic in his hand. Historians note that Hippocrates used to prescribe garlic to treat a variety of medical conditions. Modern science has now confirmed the beneficial health effects of garlic. Even though I have done much research about garlic, covering all the incredible health benefits of garlic, it is beyond the scope of my expertise to discuss the beneficial effects of different nutrients in various illness. Garlic contains multiple nutrients, just about of almost everything we need. Among these nutrients are, plentiful amounts of vitamin C, vitamin B6 and manganese. It also contains fiber, selenium and small amounts of calcium, copper, potassium, phosphorus, iron and vitamin B1. Additionally, there is a long list of other compounds in garlic. The conversion of 1/2 tsp should equal one medium garlic clove. However, since garlic gloves vary in size, it is difficult to determine the exact conversion. What do I do? I like to add a bit more garlic I use fresh garlic or garlic in oil according to the recipe. In recipes that are not cooked, like hummus, pesto, etc. I often use roasted or garlic in oil for a smoother more delicate taste. Roasted garlic takes away the garlicky aftertaste. When using garlic, even if you love it as much as I do, you must be careful not to overpower your recipe. One thing I never do though, I never use garlic powder in my recipes – it is disrespectful to this superfood.

Extra virgin olive oil

Nothing like it in the entire planet.

Most research experts agree that extra virgin olive oil it may be the healthiest fat on earth. Olive oil is most definitely a superfood. It is a significant part of the Mediterranean diet and has been a dietary staple since ancient times. There is quite a bit of research behind the health benefits of olive oil. It is rich in healthy monounsaturated fats and contains a moderate amount of vitamins E and K and has antibacterial properties. Extra virgin olive oil is loaded with antioxidants. Studies have shown that extra virgin olive oil has potent anti-inflammatory properties, it may help prevent strokes and is protective against heart disease. It may fight Alzheimer, reduce type 2 diabetes risk and help treat rheumatoid arthritis. When using olive oil, it is essential to use extra virgin olive oil. All other olive oils have been diluted and processed with cheaper oils.

Kalamata olives

The earliest cultivation of olive trees were recorded in the western Mediterranean at about five thousand years ago. Kalamata olives are only found on the Peloponnese peninsula in southern Greece. Kalamata olive trees have much larger leaves than other types of olive trees and absorb more sunshine. It is from where this dark purple fruit takes its dense texture and unique flavor. There is a reason why this olive is considered to be one of the healthiest foods on earth: It contains an impressive range of health-protective compounds and health-promoting vitamins and minerals. Kalamata olives are particularly high in iron and vitamin A and a good source of fiber, calcium, vitamin C, and K. They also provide some magnesium, phosphorous, potassium and B vitamins. Kalamata olives, like pure Greek olive oil, contain phenolic compounds, which are natural antioxidants. Olive oil and olives are the cornerstones of the Mediterranean diet. Health benefits aside, it is impossible to overlook this olive’s irresistible taste.

Feta cheese

Feta is a big part of the Mediterranean cuisine. In the Greek regions, feta is usually made with pasteurized milk from sheep and goats raised on local grass. The grass-fed environment is what gives the cheese the unique characteristics of sharpness and creamy texture. Feta cheese is a low-calorie, low-fat cheese. It is also a good source of B vitamins, high amounts of calcium and phosphorus, and decent amounts of vitamins A and K. Additionally, feta contains beneficial bacteria and fatty acids, but it has a higher sodium and lactose content than some other cheeses.

Seafood

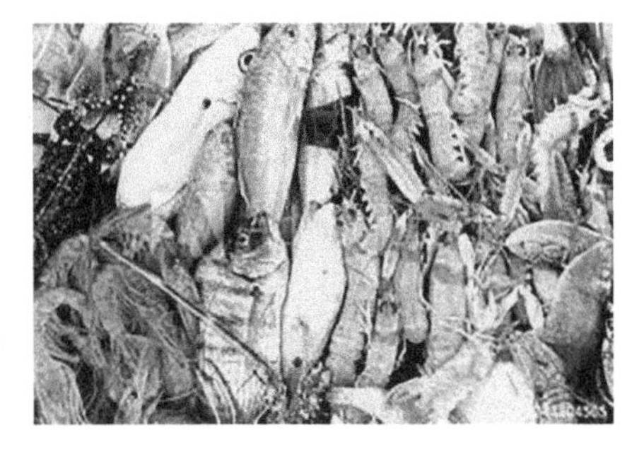

Seafood has been an essential part of a healthy diet since the human existence. It is the primary source of healthful long-chain omega-3 fatty acids and is also rich in other nutrients such as vitamin D and selenium, high in protein, and low in saturated fat. However, our environment has changed over the centuries. Modern conveniences of our lifestyle have led to the polluting of our earth. The environmental contamination in marine life is severe. Since most of the seafood we consume comes from the body of oceans, seas, lakes and rivers, various pollutants make their way from these waters into our dining table. The downside of the amount of fish you eat is the exposure to mercury, a toxin that can affect our health. Consumer Reports recommends getting our omega-3s from low-mercury fish. In general, research is vital for seafood consumption, as we should do with all other foods.

Here is a list so that you can choose the right seafood to eat and to determine how many portions to eat per month:

Least mercury: Anchovies, Catfish, Clam, Crab, Flounder, Haddock, Herring, Mullet, Oyster, Perch, Pollock, Salmon, Sardines, Scallops, Shrimp, Sole, Calamari, Tilapia, Trout, Whitefish, Whiting, North Atlantic Mackerel.
Moderate mercury: Striped Bass, Carp, Cod, Atlantic and Pacific Halibut, Lobster, Mahi Mahi, Perch, Snapper, Tuna.
High mercury: Bluefish, Grouper, Spanish and Gulf Mackerel, Chilean Sea Bass, Albacore and Yellowfin Tuna.
Avoid: King Mackerel, Shark, Orange Roughy, Marlin, Swordfish, Ahi and Bigeye Tuna, Tilefish.

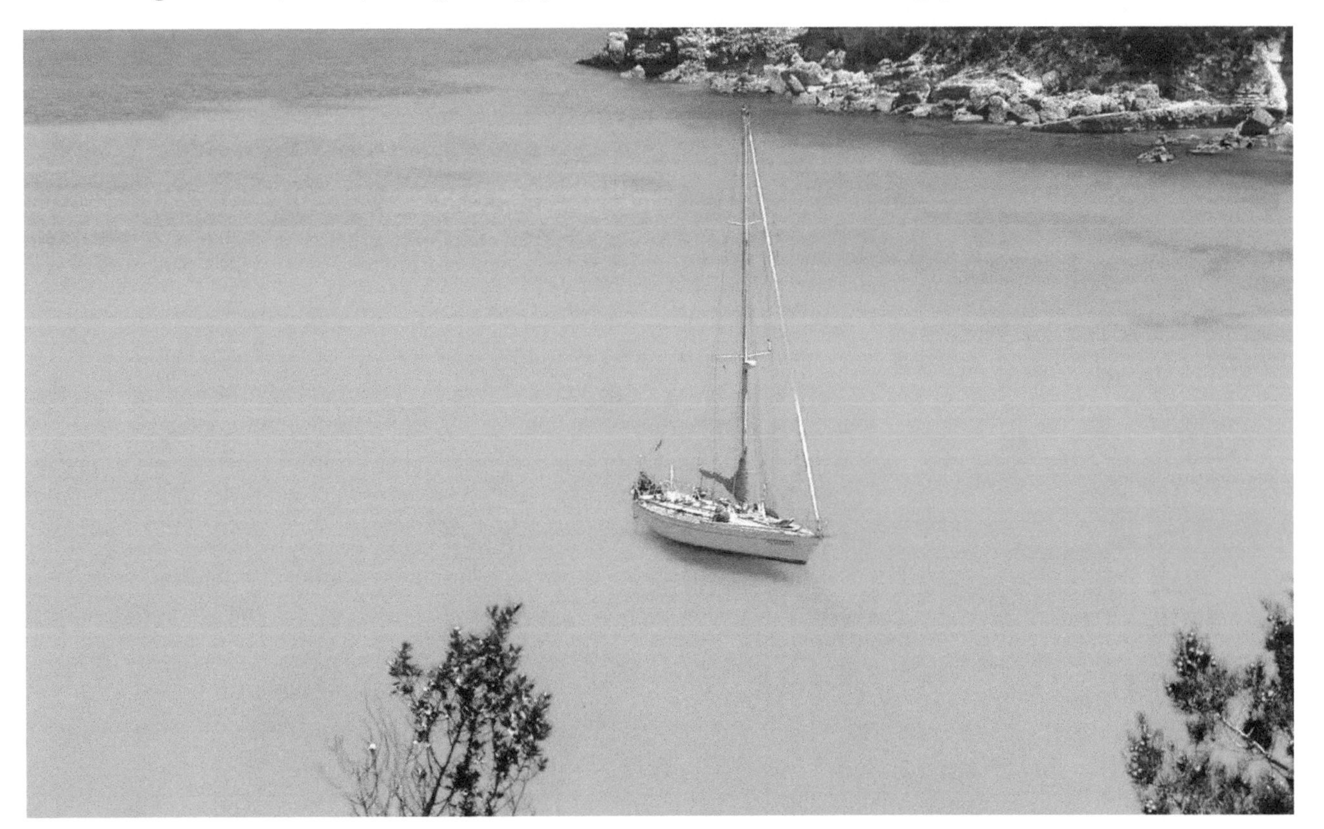

The Myth of Cooking Beans

Somehow the simple process of cooking beans became a complicated science. Soaking beans overnight is an unnecessary step; it is a waste of time and water. There is also the thought that beans lose some of their nutrients while being soaked overnight. Another myth is always keeping the bean soup covered while cooking. The only reason for covering is to shorten the cooking time, a process that takes away much of the food flavor. The idea of soaking beans is to shorten your cooking time as well. However, unsoaked beans take 10 to 15 minutes longer to cook. It is true that soaking beans helps the digestive process because all legumes contain phytic acid. The hard beans like kidney beans or navy beans include oligo-saccharides, (as do some other foods in lower levels) a complex sugar challenging to digest. This is an entirely different subject and mainly concerns those who have digestive issues. It is best to consult with your physician about this issue. It is hard to ignore the nutritious benefits of eating beans. Beans are rich in cleansing and detoxifying fiber, plant-based protein, vitamins and minerals. Additionally, organic beans are very affordable compared to other foods that contain the same or fewer nutrients. You could either cook the beans directly or do a quick soaking. A quick soaking does the same job as the overnight soaking, and in my humble opinion, a quick soaking is the best way to cook beans. You should cook the beans, as you should do with most foods, longer on medium heat. In some recipes I add a bit of apple cider or red wine vinegar in the beans. It gives some extra flavor, and some research is showing that vinegar breaks down the complex sugar. It is true that the idea of cooking beans with the lid on shortens the cooking time by 10 to 15 minutes and produces a creamier bean but cooking with the lid off and cooking a bit longer intensifies the flavor. I will take a flavorful bean with a bit of bite at any time.

Cooking with Grains

It is difficult to determine the exact amount of time it takes to cook grains and legumes. The cooking times listed in any recipe (in this or any other cookbook) is an approximate time. Cooking time for grains and legumes depends on several factors; the initial temperature of the water, size, quality and origin, preferable texture, or if the grain or legume is cooked by itself or with several other ingredients:

- I like to slow cook foods, this method extends the cooking time a bit longer. I believe "al dente" is the ideal consistency. When grains or pasta is overcooked it loses its identity.
- Using familiar ingredients and techniques helps to determine the cooking time of grains and legumes.
- For a more intense flavor, in some recipes, I like to cook grains with other ingredients. This slows down the cooking time versus when grain or legumes are cooked by themselves.
- Watch and cook your grain a bit less or longer to bring it to your desired texture.

Another issue is the amount of liquid used for each recipe:

- During the cooking process with vegetables, some vegetables absorb more liquid than others.
- Origin and size of grain/legume can make a difference in the amount of liquid used.
- Boiling versus simmering will determine the final amount of liquid. By boiling more liquid evaporates.
- After a particular stage of cooking, you must watch the liquid content of your food and if need add more hot water or broth to bring it to your desired consistency.

Why simmering? Simmering is a cooking method gentler than boiling and requires you to be more attentive with your cooking. The simmering technique cooks food gently and slowly. It is an approach for more flavorful outcome than boiling, especially when the food is simmered in flavored liquid, such as broth or wine. Generally, in cooking, there is no scientific formula for exact cooking times or liquid contents. Only your experience can determine the outcome of these two issues. Baking is another story. In baking, you must be accurate with both measurements and techniques. This is the main reasons that only a handful of chefs can master both cooking and baking; they are two different mindsets. When potential chefs ask my advice for success, my initial reaction is; to use quality ingredients and to be consistent – two elements which we can only control individually.

TASTES, TEXTURE AND HISTORY OF VARIOUS GRAINS AND LEGUMES

AMARANTH

A flower for the ages.

Amaranth cultivation is dated at about 7,000 years ago. During its long history, amaranth was cultivated by the Mayans and later by the Aztecs. Before amaranth was included in our pantheon of the ancient superfoods, it was a superfood for the Aztecs, during the height of the Aztec civilization. The Aztecs worshiped amaranth as much as they worshiped the cocoa beans. The myth goes that the Aztec god Quetzalcoatl disappeared in the great ocean-while walking east, towards the morning sun. When a strange bearded creature, clad in iron and carrying fire appeared across the vast sea from the east, people thought he was their lost god returning home. But it was none other than conquistador Herman Cortes. The year was 1519. Even though the Aztecs kindly received Cortez, his mission was to conquer the land, find treasure and convert the Aztecs to Christianity. The Spaniards had to destroy all that the Aztecs worshiped. They burnt the amaranth fields and sent shipments of the cocoa beans to Europe. Then they forbade the use of amaranth and cocoa beans. A few years earlier, Columbus, in his fourth voyage to Americas, sent cocoa beans to Spain. However, nobody knew how to rid of their bitterness. Cortez, after tasting chocolate as a liquid, brought back the knowledge of how the Aztecs treated the bean. Fortunately for the world, a few amounts of amaranth grains survived. Now there are over fifty varieties of amaranth cultivated around the world. This historic grain was introduced to the United States in the 1970s. Amaranth prefers high elevation, but it is adaptive to almost any altitude and any temperate climate. Amaranth can thrive in places where the water supplies are low and there are no frequent rainfalls. This makes amaranth a good environmental plant. I was first attracted to amaranth because of the familiarity of the name. Amaranth (from the Greek amaranthos, meaning "unfading"). It is a green that grows wild in gardens all over Greece. In a popular Greek dish called Vlita, the amaranth greens are boiled and served with olive oil and lemon. In various parts of the country, some of the amaranth recipes include zucchini, onions, garlic, tomatoes, beans or potatoes. When different amaranth varieties are in full bloom, the gold, deep red, light green and purple colors are spectacular. Amaranth's small grains have a subtle nutty, earthy flavor. The closest resemblance I can think is to brown rice. Many, mostly mild, foods and spices compliment amaranth. Looking at the tiny, pale seeds of amaranth it is difficult to believe that they packed such power: they are rich in fiber and protein. Excellent source of manganese, magnesium, phosphorus, iron, selenium, copper, zinc, vitamins C, thiamin, riboflavin, niacin, vitamins B12, B6, A, and folate. Amaranth is also an excellent source of health-promoting antioxidants. On top of these rich nutrients, amaranth is earth friendly and a gluten-free grain.

BARLEY

Greatly misunderstood.

I don't get it why more chefs do not use barley in their menu. Barley, when cooked has a nice nutty, subtle flavor, a chewy texture and it is not overbearing in taste. The closest texture I can think is similar to farro. Granted, barley is one of the three primary gluten-based grains, but for those, like myself, who are not in an all gluten-free diet, barley is an excellent addition to your diet. The gluten-based grains are Wheat, which is the primary gluten grain. Barley is the second most common gluten grain and Rye which is commonly found in some breads. Even though remains of barley were discovered and dated at about 10,000 years ago, it became widely farmed starting at 6,000 years ago, in West Asia, North Africa, Southern Europe and from there on to the rest of the world. Barley deserves some respect, at least from those who love their beer and whiskey (drinks made partially from barley) and for those of us who love their history. It is good to know that during the rebirth of civilization, following the middle ages, barley flour was the main flour used to make bread. Barley is an ancient grain and like most ancient grains, barley grows in various varieties. Barley is used as a grain, flour, flaked, for malting or brewing. Most of the barley used for food is pearled barley. Just about everything can go with barley: walnuts, pecans, almonds, beef, chicken, lamb, mushrooms, onions, green peas, sage, celery, carrots, kale, thyme, lemon, pepper, cumin, turmeric, various fruits like apricots and apples and grated cheese like Parmesan and Romano. In some recipes, I pair barley with mung beans, amaranth or lentils. Barley, as a grain, has some powerful beneficial nutrients. It contains lignans that act as antioxidants. It is a rich source of fiber, manganese, selenium, thiamine, niacin and copper. It has high levels of plant-based protein and some riboflavin, iron, potassium and zinc. When I try to get my friends to eat barley, I can picture them saying, "But I get it in my beer and whiskey." Guys, it does not count.

Farro

In a class of its own.

Farro is an ancient grain that's been around longer than most other grains. It has only recently surged in popularity. This ancient grain originated in the fertile crescent and was brought from travelers to the region that is now Italy. In this new land, farro produced three varieties of heirloom grains; einkorn, spell and emmer wheat. But, all we really need to know is that farro comes in three sizes; piccolo, medio and grande – small, medium and large. To avoid confusion on what type you use in various recipes, I have simplified my choice. I choose the large size for its intense flavor, and it is suited better for the style of my cooking. Although farro is a form of wheat, it is not the same as the conventional wheat but a plant and grain all its own. Farro is not gluten-free. It is, however, low in gluten and easier to digest compared to modern wheat. When cooked right farro has a taste of its own, it's difficult to compare with other grains. Most experts say that it tastes a bit like lighter brown rice. I can't disagree with that point since farro has the same complex, nutty taste of brown rice. But farro has undertones of oats and barley. To me, farro looks like large barley and the flavor and texture is closer to barley than any other grain. However, farro has a bit of sweetness to it, something that barley has not. It is that sweetness that gives farro its elegant taste. Farro, like barley, is a bit chewy when cooked. Faro is excellent in stews, salads, pilafs, soups, and combines with other grains exceptionally well. Farro is loaded with fiber and protein. It is rich in magnesium, zinc and vitamins A, B, C and E. The larger farro is the whole grain variety and packs more nutrients than the other two. The myth of farro being challenging to cook has some food experts recommending substituting farro for wheat berries or spelt. Because your head is probably spinning by now, I want to make this clear: Farro is not spelt. The only grain that comes even close to a substitute for farro with is barley. Farro is cultivated in Italy and spelt, the one found in the grocery stores, is usually farmed in the United States. Spelt does not taste nor cooks like farro. And speaking of farro being challenging to prepare, keep this in mind: Farro is a grain, and like all grains, farro is uncompromising when it comes to cooking; is done when it's done.

Millet

Easy to fall in love with.

Millet, like quinoa and amaranth, belongs to a small group of small-seeded plants. Those "tres amigos" are widely grown around the world as either cereal crop or seeds. Millet has a mild flavor and a delicate texture. Because of it has the mild and nutty-flavor of traditional grains, it can combines well with a wide variety of dishes. The cultivation of various types of millet is mentioned in several countries, starting 7,000 years ago. The Chinese people were the first ones to claim the domestication of millet. Later on, during the Indian bronze age, around 6,500 years ago, millet consumption was widespread in India and Africa. Soon after, its cultivation spread to Europe. How to use millet? For me, it is an easy choice. I use millet in place of couscous or orzo, not only because it is tasty but mainly because millet is gluten-free. Millet is an environmentally friendly plant. It is resistant to drought. I believe millet will be a perfect crop in California and other places with frequent droughts. It is, after all, the main reason that it was popular in ancient times. Millet is high in antioxidants, iron, magnesium, zinc and calcium. It is a good source of protein, fiber and vitamins B. I hope that after you've read about the health benefits of millet, you no longer think that millet is just for the birds.

Quinoa

Star power. A Superfood.

Quinoa, the darling of health-conscious people has now carried its star power into the general population. Sometimes it is difficult to determine if a trend will continue. But, make no mistake about this one. Quinoa is here to stay. It is loaded with nutrients, versatile in the kitchen, easy to cook, tastes great, and it blends well with just about any other food. Quinoa is easy to grow and harvest and its natural defense system against plant pests reduces the need for pesticides. Just as the amaranth was the sacred grain to the Aztecs, quinoa was a sacred grain to the Incas. Quinoa originated in Peru, Chile and Bolivia, about 7,000 years ago. It reached the height of its cultivation in pre-Colombian civilizations. By the time explorer Francisco Pizarro sailed dawn to Peru in 1531 with his Spanish army, quinoa was the mother grain for the Inca empire. During their conquest, the Spaniards suppressed quinoa cultivation because of its use in religious ceremonies. All quinoa fields were destroyed, but a few seeds survived on the mountains. It wasn't until the 1970s that quinoa was introduced to the modern world and about 40 years later has risen into a superfood giant. Quinoa, like amaranth, can thrive in places where the water supplies are low and there are no frequent rainfalls. This makes quinoa an excellent environmental plant. Quinoa is high in protein, has a nutty flavor and a slight bitterness. I've heard some complaints about its bitterness, but so many other foods like kale, artichokes, broccoli, asparagus, eggplant and even chocolate are somewhat bitter before being ready to be consumed. The slight bitterness of quinoa is not something that a little lime juice while cooking it or a nice rinse before cooking, cannot fix. It is this challenging mild bitterness that is exciting for me. Quinoa is gluten-free and one of a few plant foods that is considered a complete protein, and it is high in fiber content compared with other grains. Among the gluten-free diet plants, quinoa provides the highest amounts of antioxidants. Quinoa also offers large quantities of manganese, calcium, fiber, iron and magnesium, as well as antioxidants, vitamins B and E. Bottom line; It is difficult to ignore the powerful nutrients in this tiny grain. It is higher in nutrients and quality protein than most other grains. On top of these rich nutrients, quinoa is earth friendly and gluten-free grain.

Sorghum

A hidden gem.

This grain is a superfood on the rise. It is an environmentally friendly ancient grain, among the most efficient crops in the conversion to solar energy and decreasing water use. It is known as a high-energy, drought tolerant crop. Sorghum is a powerhouse regarding nutrients. It provides large amounts of protein, vitamins B6, niacin riboflavin, and thiamin, high levels of iron, calcium, magnesium, copper, phosphorus and potassium and a significant amount of fiber. Sorghum contains a wide variety of beneficial phytochemicals that act as antioxidants in the body. It actually contains significantly higher amounts of antioxidants than plums, blueberries and strawberries. This gluten-free grain also contains the phytochemicals lignans, phenolic acids and phytic acid. The earliest known record of the domestication of sorghum, dated 9,000 years ago, is from Northeastern Africa. Sorghum then spread to various tribal groups throughout Africa, and along the way, adapted to a wide range of environments. From Africa was spread to India and China and eventually worked its way into Australia. The first known record of sorghum in the United States was in the late 1700s.

Chia

The lost treasure.

This tiny seed comes in black or white. The only difference is the color since there is no difference nutritionally. Chia was another superfood for the Aztecs. The cultivation of chia declined with the arrival of Spanish colonists in the 1500s. For the next 500 years, chia seeds fell into obscurity. During that period chia was cultivated in some regions of Mexico, which is is how this miracle seed kept alive. Aztecs and Mayans used chia seeds to make flour and oil as well. These ancient cultures considered chia seeds to be magical because of their ability to increase stamina and energy. Due to the efforts of a South and North American science team, Chia surfaced into the modern world during the 1990s. The reason chia has climbed to superfood status is that it is among one of the healthiest foods on the planet. The nutritional benefits of chia include fiber, omega fatty acids, antioxidants and so much more. It is also loaded with protein, calcium, manganese, magnesium and phosphorous. It is amazing that this tiny seed packs such nutritious power. And you thought that this super-grain only purpose was to make chia pets, the popular potted pets during the eighties and nineties.

Rice

Part of a healthy diet.

Consumer Reports published an article stating that while arsenic is naturally present in a variety of foods, it is more likely to contaminate brown rice because brown rice absorbs a great deal of water containing arsenic while growing. However, the Food and Drug Administration analyzed over 1,000 rice samples, and in 2014 stated, "the arsenic levels that FDA found in the samples it evaluated were too low to cause any immediate or short-term adverse health effects." The FDA advised maintaining a diet that includes a variety of whole grains. Additionally, those concern about arsenic levels can cook their rice in six times the normal amount of water and reduce the arsenic level by about half, according to the FDA. Considered a whole grain, brown rice is less processed than white rice, which has had its hull, bran and germ removed. Brown rice only has the hull removed, leaving the nutrient-packed bran and germ. As a result, brown rice retains the nutrients that white rice lacks such as vitamins, minerals, and antioxidants.

Bottom line: Arsenic content of rice varies greatly depending on the type of rice and where it was grown. White basmati rice from California, (along with India, and Pakistan) has half of the inorganic-arsenic amounts of most other types of rice. According to consumers reports, different types of rice from other parts of the United States contain the highest levels of inorganic arsenic. Brown rice is the entire whole rice grain and contains the fiber-rich bran, the nutrient-packed germ and the carbohydrate-rich endosperm. White rice is stripped of its bran and germ, leaving just the endosperm. In general, brown rice has higher amounts of vitamins and minerals and fewer calories and carbs per cup than white rice and twice as much fiber. Brown rice contains more antioxidants and essential amino acids. White rice is more processed but is still not necessarily bad. It is enriched with vitamins to improve its nutritional value. Even though brown rice is the best choice regarding nutritional quality and health benefits, either rice can be part of a healthy diet.

To reduce arsenic intake from rice: Wash before using. Boil in plenty of water. Do not use as often. Substitutions for rice; quinoa, millet, buckwheat.

Black Rice

The Forbidden Rice.

In ancient China, black rice was reserved solely for the royal family and it was forbidden for anyone else to eat it. Black rice originated in China somewhere around 10,000 years ago. Recently black rice has gain popularity worldwide because of its high levels of antioxidants, fiber, and valuable anti-inflammatory properties. It is well documented that colored rice is more nutritious than white rice. Like brown rice, black rice has similar nutrient levels, but it contains higher amounts of antioxidants, protein and fiber. Black rice has substantial mineral content including potassium, iron and copper, and high levels of vitamin E and zinc. Its deep, beautiful dark color is due to an excess of anthocyanin, a powerful antioxidant, found in other darkly colored foods, like eggplants, blueberries, purple cauliflower or dark grapes. Like different rice varieties, black rice naturally contains no gluten. Bottom line: This powerhouse grain is loaded with enormous health benefits, which makes it a perfectly healthy option for your diet. A few years ago, I started cooking with black rice and loved its texture and remarkable nutty flavor.

Arborio Rice

The Italian pearl.

I love to cook with Arborio rice and basmati rice. Arborio is a short, fat oval shaped grain and has a pearly white exterior. When Arborio is cooked right, it is firm, creamy and chewy. Arborio undergoes less milling than ordinary long-grained rice; therefore, it retains more of its natural starch content. Cooking it releases this starch, giving risotto its creamy consistency. Because of its starch and shape, Arborio rice can absorb much more liquid than any other rice without becoming mushy. This process of releasing starch and slow-cooking is key to risotto's creaminess. Because Arborio absorbs so much liquid, it must be watched during the cooking process and you need to add more hot water as needed. This unique grain, when cooked slightly al dente, oozes creaminess out of each grain. Arborio is the classic choice for risotto. However, my goal with this book is to introduce more whole grains into your diet; therefore, I tried other options for risotto in my recipes. I found that, with the right combination, other grains are rich and creamy. Other than Arborio rice, the best grain to make creamy risotto might surprise you – Barley. Yes, barley that "I get no respect grain" cooks creamy and flavorful which makes it perfect for another risotto option. Its taste is a mixture of grain and pasta. Other options for risotto are farro, buckwheat and brown rice. Arborio rice was grown in Italy since the fourteenth century. It contains a good amount of protein and most of its calories comes from its carbohydrate content. Arborio rice is a better source of fiber from the long-grain rice and it is sodium-free. It contains a small amount of iron and it is packed with vitamins A and C and easy to digest.

Buckwheat

The beautiful flower and practical seed.

Buckwheat originated in Southeast Asia around 6,000 years ago. From there it found its way to Central Asia, Europe and the Middle East. Buckwheat flowers produce hundreds of small brown seeds, protected by an outer shell much like a sunflower seed. The buckwheat plant endures harsh weather to create a white flower. With time the color changes to purple and finally into a striking dark red color. Buckwheat flowers are admired everywhere they grow. Several buckwheat festivals are held around the world, with the most famous one in the Provence of Ha Giang in northern Vietnam. Thousands of beauty enthusiasts travel to this mountainous region to attend the annual celebration of their iconic buckwheat flower. The visual aspect of nature excels in this northern Vietnam region during October through December when buckwheat flowers are in full bloom. The purple-pink buckwheat wildflowers disperse over the mountainside, across villages and fields, and into the green forest to create a multi-cored plateau. Buckwheat grows best in a cool, moist climate and is easy and economical to produce. It requires little to no fertilizer or pesticides and it grows quickly. Russia, China and Kazakhstan are currently the world's largest producers of buckwheat. Buckwheat was brought to North America in the 1600s from northern European immigrants. It is a rich source of protein and dietary fiber. It has high amounts of potassium, manganese, phosphorus, magnesium and reasonable amounts of zinc, copper, selenium and iron. It contains decent amounts of folate, riboflavin, niacin and pantothenic acid vitamins. Don't let the name fool you. This flower brings beauty to our earth and its grain and flour are versatile in the kitchen and suitable for every meal of the day, easy to cook and it is gluten-free.

Lentils

The ageless wonder. The superfood.

There is so much to say about lentils; it could take an entire chapter to write about their long history and nutritious benefits. There is even an identity controversy with lentils. Some call it a grain and others argue that it is a legume. I'm not sure that I care what you call it so, to keep the peace, I will call it a grain legume. One thing I am certain though is that I am impressed with this "old timer" grain legume. Lentils are in a category of their own – literally. Although its earlier popularity is recorded in the Mediterranean area, lentils have been a source of food since prehistoric times. Archaeologist dated lentils to the Paleolithic layers of Franchthi Cave in Greece, around 13,000 years ago. The first crops were grown in the Mediterranean area about 9,000 years ago. That makes lentils the oldest pulse crop and one of the earliest domesticated grains or legumes. Lentils contain important nutrients: protein, fiber, vitamins and minerals – you name it, lentils are loaded. Protein accounts for one-quarter of lentils calories. They are packed with both soluble and insoluble fiber. They are extremely high in manganese, magnesium, thiamin, folate and vitamin B6 and have good amounts of phosphorus, iron and potassium. Lentils have been an essential nutritious food through the ages for a good reason. Besides their highly nutritious value, lentils are the most versatile grain legume out there. With their rich, earthy flavor, soft texture, and beautiful appearance, lentils make a great base for just about any dish. Throughout history, lentils have developed into different types and shapes. The most common variety today are the brown, green and red lentils. My personal preference is the brown lentils. Today lentils are a major part of a healthy diet. They were introduced to America by European explorers in the sixteenth century, but it wasn't until the nineteen-forties that lentils were widely used. Their use back then wasn't mainly for nutrient reasons but rather for an alternative for meat during the economic crisis of World War II. Today the general population is becoming more conscious about the foods we eat, so I understand the reason why foods like quinoa, farro and kale, to name a few, have become trendy. However, while most of us acknowledge lentils for their incredible nutritious value, others are concern about being fashionable; lentils are not trendy. They come with baggage, carrying their reputation as "hippie food" since the sixties. Lentils get a bad rap from some "foodies"; therefore, they are skeptical when it comes to tagging them as superfoods. Lentils are my personal choice for the best super-grain-legume. The word superfood is thrown around loosely nowadays to describe an item that is healthy for you. But let's sit back and think about what deserves the label "superfood." Lentils have stood the test of time. They contain an extremely dense concentration of vital nutrients. They have a positive effect on your body, improving physical health. Those are some of the elements that make a superfood. I'd also like to add lentils to the list plants that are good for the earth. They can be grown with limited irrigation and are essential in areas with frequent droughts. Lentils can draw their nitrogen from the air and don't require loads of synthetic fertilizer, which are a potent contributor to global warming. Lentils mentioned in ancient Greek as lathyrus, meaning a type of pea, on to Latin lathyrus genus name to lenticula, diminutive to today's lens; shaped like the double rounded lentils. From the classical era of Greece to the Romans into the Renaissance, numerous writers and poets referred to lentils as a healthy food. Including the great poet Aristophanes who said, "You, who dare insult lentil soup, sweetest of delicacies." There is no question about lentils being a superfood. The question shouldn't be why eat lentils? But why you are not eating them.

Garbanzo

Much more than hummus.

The Spanish word garbanzo and chickpea is the same thing. The only reason I use the word garbanzo in my recipes is that I like it better. Garbanzos have been grown around the world for more than 7,000 years. The ancient Greeks and the Romans ate roasted garbanzos as snacks. They've been popular in the Mediterranean, India, Asia and Latin American kitchens for a long time. In recent years they became popular in the USA mainly because of the immense popularity of hummus brought to you by the waves of health consciousness. I grew up eating garbanzo soup (revithia) and eating roasted garbanzo beans (stragalia.) There was not a movie intermission without stragalia, the equivalent of popcorn in America. Movie intermissions back then, occurred in the middle of the movie so the viewers could get a snack. A vendor will go around selling stragalia and drinks. Garbanzo beans are naturally gluten-free and come with an impressive collection of nutrients. They are rich in plant-based protein, fiber, folate, phosphorus, potassium and with decent amounts of magnesium and calcium. They provide smaller amounts of manganese, zinc, selenium, iron and vitamin K. Garbanzo nutrition also provides some copper, vitamins A, C, E, B6, riboflavin, pantothenic acid and niacin.

Black Beans

The black beauty.

I believe beans are some of the most underrated foods. Black beans are a good source of protein, very high in dietary fiber, magnesium, potassium, phosphorus and folate. Black beans also have high levels of flavonoids, which have antioxidant abilities. They also contain omega-3 fatty acids. They are a great source of folic acid and have incredibly high levels of the rare compound molybdenum, which is very difficult to find in any other food. Black beans have long been a protein-rich staple food of many Latin American cultures. Because of their incredibly high protein content, black beans are great for vegans and vegetarians. Black beans date back at least 7,000 years when they were a staple food in the diets of Central and South Americans. They remain a popular food in many households in the Americas. Black beans are mostly associated with Mexican cooking in the United States. However, black beans are common in Cuban, South American, Spanish, and Caribbean dishes. They are popular in stews, soups, and salads and frequently served with rice. Black beans have an intense earthy flavor. Latin American and Caribbean cooks rarely soak their dried beans. Soaking may speed up cooking time and improve texture, but it can cause beans to lose their flavor and color. Traditional they simmer beans slowly and long in a clay pot.

Mung Beans

The great discovery.

There are impressive health benefits in mung beans. Since mung beans are healthy and versatile, I am surprised that mung beans are not very popular with the general population. They are packed with antioxidants and rich in potassium, magnesium,folate and fiber. They also contain manganese, phosphorus, iron, copper, potassium, zinc, selenium and vitamins B1, B2, B3, B5, B6. The mung bean originated in India and can be found in many different cultural recipes throughout Southeast Asia. They were domesticated in India as early as 3,500 years ago before spreading throughout Asia, the Middle East and finally to the United States.

Cranberry Beans

More than good looks.

Cranberry beans, a light-colored beans with red speckles and are more delicate and sweeter than your common beans. Their nutty, rich flavor and creamy texture make this bean a perfect legume for Mediterranean style cooking. Cranberry beans have been cultivated for many centuries, originally from Colombia and are now grown around the world. Also known as Borlotti, Roman or Madeira bean. They are extremely popular in Italian, Greek and Portuguese cuisines. The cranberry bean is not just a pretty face. Besides its unique taste, it has an impressive array of nutrients. Cranberry beans have one of the highest contents of essential nutrients of any plant-based food. They are a rich source of dietary fiber, extremely high in protein, packed with B-complex vitamins, essential minerals and various components of antioxidant properties. Besides being a plant-protein powerhouse, cranberry beans are versatile in the kitchen. It can be used in salads, soups, stews, with pasta, grains, and with an array of vegetables and herbs. Cranberry bean's combination of taste and nutritious value makes it an essential part of any diet.

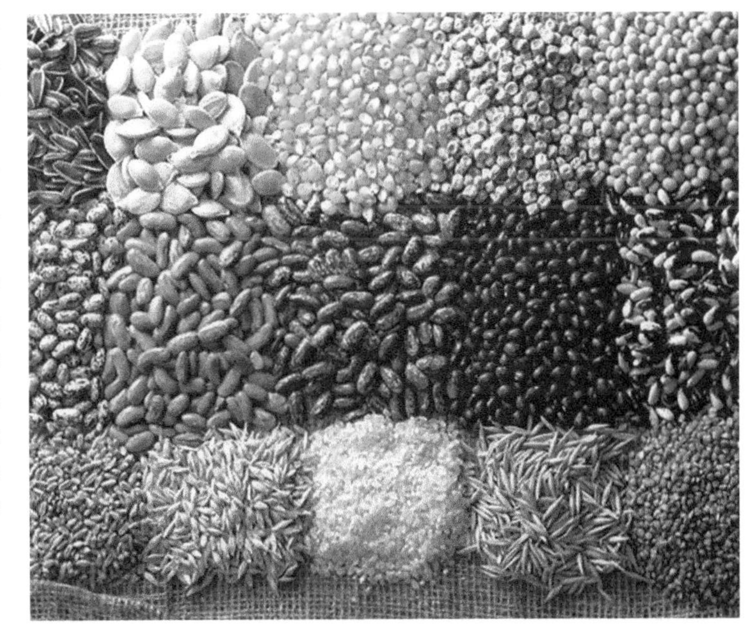

Stock and Broth

The difference between stock and broth is a subject that some people find perplexing. Vegetable broth is made by clean, trimmed vegetables and it has a lot fewer calories and significantly higher doses of vitamins and minerals. Vegetable stock is made with all parts of vegetables, including roots, skins and leaves and is more concentrated with flavor. I used broth because I like a more soothing taste in my food and by using organic, clean, trimmed vegetables, I protect my food from pesticides. Stock is primarily used for sauces or heavy soups and is too overpowering for my taste. The same goes for chicken and red meat broths. The broth is made by simmering meat with vegetables and herbs in water. The stock is made by boiling mainly bones with vegetables in water for many hours. This gives the stock a thicker consistency than broth. Whether you choose to use broth or stock depends on how you will use it in your cooking.

Making bone broth is nothing new; my parents made it by the gallons to be used in their cooking. I remember a boiling pot filled with water, vegetables and bones simmering for endless hours on top of the stove of my father's taverna. When I asked my dad about it, he would say, "It makes the soups taste better and it is good for you, it is like nectar." That was over 60 years ago, and I am thinking - how did they know? They knew what is good for you and what not to eat. There was no scientific research back then, just folk wisdom. Today things are different; you can find information about any food and make educated decisions as to what food you put in your body. You cannot turn a blind eye on the things that are harmful to your health. And so, today, around town, there is a buzz about the miracle of bone broth. Being the curious person that I am, I decided to do some research about this new phenomenon, partly because I like to learn and partly to understand what my parents and their parents knew about this "nectar." Bone broth is the new terminology for chicken or beef broth. However, it is cooked a bit different. The difference is, with bone broth you must roast the bones before making bone broth and it takes much longer to cook, sometimes up to 24 hours. After doing some careful reading about bone broth, I will have to say that the hype about this broth is entirely overblown. I am sorry about my skepticism, but I have a difficult time believing that any single food is a cure-all miracle. The health benefits from nutrients and minerals that are claimed to be miraculous in bone broth could be found in abundance in many other foods: Bone broth contains less protein, potassium and calcium from many plant-based foods, such as beans and kale or any leafy vegetables. Many plants are rich sources of the phytonutrients, including vitamin C, a powerful antioxidant, found in all citrus fruits, berries and vegetables, such as broccoli and bell peppers. Vitamin E found in almonds, sunflower seeds, broccoli and spinach, and vitamin A found in carrots, squash, sweet potatoes, fruits such as apricots and cantaloupes, and many leafy greens. Bone broth contains the amino acid glycine. However, amino acids such as glycine, proline and lysine are found in vegetables, soy, legumes, nuts and seeds. Also, garlic, onions, cabbage are among some of the foods that contain sulfur. There are plenty of plant foods that have the same benefits of bone broth to keep your bones strong and your joints and gut healthy. So, what am I missing here?

Bottom line: is the bone stock or broth good for you? *Of course, it is.*

Is it a miracle cure? *I don't think so.*

Should we use stock or broth in our cooking? *Absolutely.*

Will I sit around sipping bone broth? *I don't think so.*

My preference has always been the vegetable broth.

My dad's "nectar" remains a beneficial food for our health, but like it was back then, there are plenty of other foods that have the nutrients included in the bone broth. There is a recipe for vegetable and chicken broth in this book, but, really, you could mix and match any vegetables you want and make your recipe.

What's Next

Plant-based protein foods. Foods to benefit both our body and the planet. I believe that more restaurants will start serving foods with plant-based protein. Some of these foods are lentils, quinoa, garbanzo, sorghum, amaranth, oats, brown rice, chia, broccoli, spinach, asparagus, artichokes, sweet potatoes, Brussels sprouts, blackberries, seeds and nuts. I also believe that restaurants that continue to serve foods that are tenderized for texture or use unhealthy products to enhance the taste will lose popularity. There is a reason that restaurants began to have a healthy section in their menu and are listing nutrients under each dish. Grocery items with unhealthy preservatives will have to replace them with items that use natural preservatives. The main reason that major food chain stores, that have monopolized the grocery markets, now have large sections of healthy and gluten-free items, is because health food markets have threaten their business. The health food markets are no longer little stores in the neighborhood shopping center but have become giant chains, as more consumers demand to know the quality and origin of the foods they're about to consume.

Cooking is a Responsibility

"Never serve food you wouldn't *eat yourself"*

This is what I used to say to my cooks and to potential chefs. When I was doing cooking classes or training interns out of culinary schools, my goal has always been to educate potential chefs about the chemistry of foods, encourage them to create their own style of cooking and to respect the quality and wholesomeness of the food they serve. Furthermore, to simplify the cooking process and not to be intimidated about various unnecessary fancy terminologies some chiefs use. In this book my goal remains the same; learn how to create new tastes, and above all to recognize that the paramount step to every chef's success is the use of quality ingredients.

The Importance of Slow Cooking

I have followed the method of slow cooking religiously since the eighties. Culinary "experts" secretly rolled their eyes and some openly scorned me when I was invited to speak to their students about cooking. "This is not what we teach our students." I've heard it too many times. But with all the respect I have for teachers, you cannot argue with the results. I remember one instructor in particular who visited me in my restaurant, to make a point about his way of teaching. I remember smiling and telling him, "To be a good teacher, first you have to be a good student, and adapt to new ideas." He argued his point and of course, I was never invited again to speak to his students. I believe in facts and logic. And the point is that slow cooking rarely failed me. Let's talk now about risotto that needs to be continuously stirred to absorb the liquid, to be creamier and flavorful. The fact is that using more liquid and cooking slowly accomplishes the same goals as the constantly stirring to make risotto. The idea of slow cooking is to allow the grain or legume to absorb the liquid slowly. You will notice throughout this book that I use much more liquid that the "traditional" measurements. There is a reason for this. It is because boiling on lower heat the grain or legume absorbs more liquid; therefore, it is creamier, more tender and flavorful. Scientifically, it only takes a few minutes longer to cook on lower heat. High heat boiling cooks mostly the outer part of the food. Your grain will become spongy or sticky. In the slow cooking method the grain will rarely be mushy or lumpy if overcooked for a few extra minutes. The same belief goes for cooking with the cover on. It suffocates the food, unlike with the lid off it gives the grain a chance to "breath" and "swim" in the liquid. My belief is to sauté foods on lower heat, with rare exceptions, like deep frying. This gives the ingredients time to absorbed one-another's flavor. The reason I use much less oil and more vegetable broth in most of my recipes is to accomplish several goals – the use of less oil, cut down the calories and diminish the oily aftertaste while using flavorful broth which boosts the flavor. As much as I love olive oil, too much of the good thing it can be counterproductive.

The Convenient Truth About Convenience

Unhealthy cookware and cluttered kitchen.

For several decades I've been using stainless steel sauté pans. The main reasons I used them is that stainless steel heats up very fast and hold the heat well. Also, it is durable and lasts for a long time. I still have, and use for home cooking, some of the stainless steel pans used in my restaurants. My children have a few of them and most likely they will hand them down to their children. Several years after using stainless steel cookware, I was pleased to discover that stainless steel is one of the healthiest cookware to use. Today I use cast iron stock pots as well. Cast iron cookware is probably the safest and most effective cookware in the kitchen. While cast iron is relatively heavy and takes a while to heat up, it holds heat very well and is oven-safe.

Glass cookware tends to be mostly for baking and is entirely non-toxic. Glass isn't the most dynamic cooking material and it's somewhat limited in its use in the kitchen. However, to be used as baking dishes, there aren't many materials more safe and affordable than heatproof glass.

Ceramic cookware is non-toxic as well, as long as they are correctly glazed with a glass-like surface. Glass and ceramic are durable and versatile. They could be moved from stove top to the oven and to refrigerator or freezer.

Using non-stick cookware, such as Teflon, for convenience is most likely the most dangerous cookware to use. The non-stick properties of Teflon cookware are coated with polytetrafluoroethylene (PTFE), a plastic polymer that leaches toxins when heated on high heat. Aluminum and copper cookware can be very toxic when used in high temperatures also. These heavy metals are released into foods during cooking and end up in your body. Please do your research about the cookware you are using.

During my years in the restaurant business, everyone in the kitchen knew my fixation about having an organized, clean and declutter kitchen. Organization in your kitchen, knowing where everything is, allows you to speed up your cooking process and keep an inventory of foods.

I don't like my kitchen to be crowded with gadgets that I will use once in a long while. Why do I need things like a garlic peeler, strawberry huller, citrus zesters, food chopper, melon ballers, or a banana slicer? There is nothing these things can do that I cannot accomplish with my knives. Not sure why I would need an egg separator, or a rice cooker or an electric steamer.

Besides the obvious items, like knives, mixing bowls, serving spoons, etc., the essentials needed while using my cookbook are various sizes of stock pots, baking and sauté pans. Use a small or medium stock pot, unless specified to use a large one. Same with the sauté and baking pans. The equipment which are used continuously in my kitchen are my food processor, mixer, and blender.

Some of the rules that make my life easier in the kitchen are:

- After using an item, I don't put it down. I put it away where it belongs.
- I clean as I go, especially the countertops.
- I try to leave my kitchen as I found it – organized.

My Superfood Team

Herbs and spices

Cinnamon, Turmeric, Ginger, Oregano, Garlic, Thyme, Parsley, Black Pepper.

Grains

Quinoa, Lentils.

Fruits and Vegetables

Blueberries, Apples, Watermelon, Pineapple, Kale, Broccoli, Spinach.

Ancient Grains used in this book

Amaranth, Barley, Farro, Millet, Quinoa, Sorghum, Chia, Black Rice, Buckwheat.

Symbols used throughout this book

tbsp - tablespoon
tsp - teaspoon
oz – ounce
lb - pound
GF - Gluten free
EL - Safe for elimination diet
VT - Vegetarian diet
VG - Vegan diet
CL - Celebrate Life's special moments

VEGETABLE CUTS USED IN MY RECIPES:

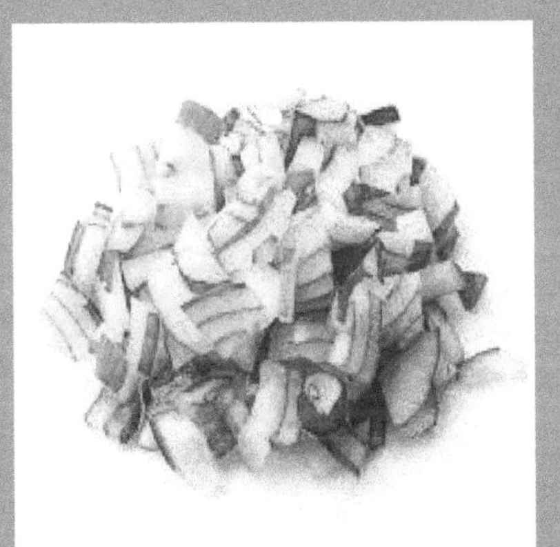

Chopped

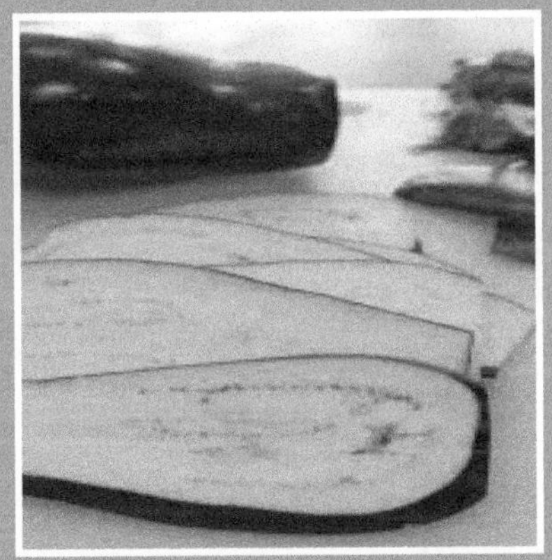

Sliced lengthwise

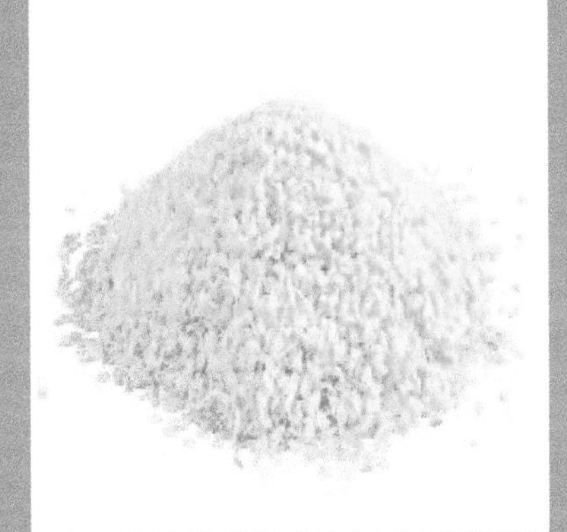

Minced

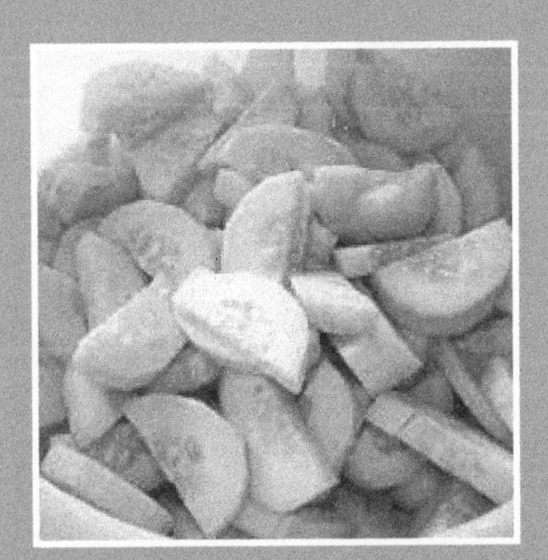

Half sliced

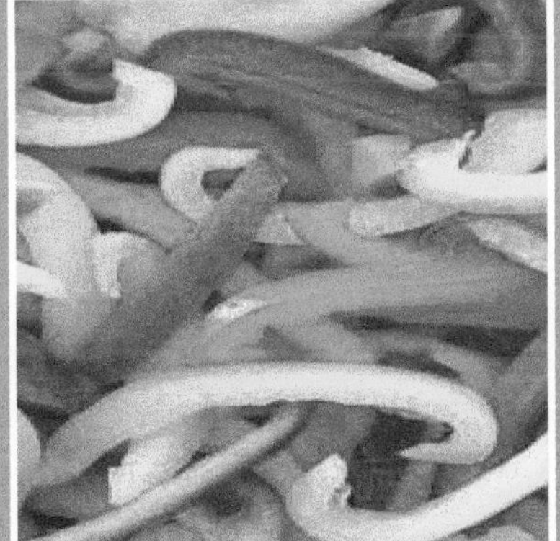

Sliced

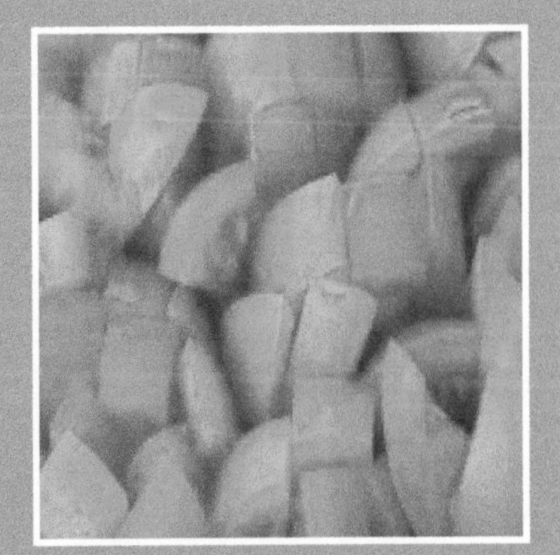

Large cut

Recipe Format

More than a few times people asked me to explain recipes written in various cookbooks or magazines. Even someone like me who spent most of my life in the kitchen gets confused with the multiple formats and additional long explanations. In my previous cookbooks, I created a recipe format easy to follow and avoids repeating annoying details in every recipe. It is common sense to peel the onion before chopping it, how to boil water or wash your vegetables before using them. In my format, I list the ingredients and directly below, to the right, the step necessary on how to use these ingredients.

Please read the recipe before using it so you can understand the steps and so you can have all the items necessary for the completion of your recipe.

To simplify my recipe format, here are some common steps that are not going to be repeated on every recipe.

- Wash vegetables, grains and legumes before using.
- Use the quick soak method when the legume calls for soaking: Cover the legumes with water and bring them to a quick boil. Remove from the heat and let them soak for about 1 hour. Do not discard the water. Place the pot back on the stove and continue your cooking.
- Always use the slow cooking method; medium heat and gently boil, unless specified otherwise.
- Pulsing allows you to regulate the texture of your food. The pulsing function on a food processor works by turning the blade a few turns at the time. Pulsing in a food processor for one second is about the right time. Any longer the food is either mashed or liquefied.
- Use organic foods, especially in foods that are more exposed to chemicals and are listed in the dirty dozen report.
- Use fresh ingredients.
- Use plenty of liquid when you cook grains or legumes.
- Artichoke hearts are not marinated unless specified.
- Sun-dried tomatoes are packed in oil.
- Olive oil is always extra virgin.
- For recipes that call for sweet potatoes, use the orange sweet potatoes. Use the white sweet potato for stuffed potato skins; it is more stable.
- When a recipe calls for cooked black beans, use BPA- free canned and rinse and drain well.
- When recipe calls for cooked garbanzo beans, use BPA- free canned and rinse and drain well.
- Green Onions, use the white and light green parts, unless specified otherwise.
- For roasted garlic choose a garlic head that is short and "fat" it most likely will have evenly matched cloves. Best way to mince crushed garlic or crush nuts is to use a wooden mortar and pestle.
- The conversion of 1 clove garlic equals ½ tsp of chopped garlic.

Other Tips:

The use of extra broth is to limit the use of oils, limit calories and enhance flavors.

If you choose to eat out choose a busy restaurant – the busier, the better which means their foods are fresher.

Don't be afraid to ask questions; when a restaurant in a desert town like Phoenix tells me that they get their seafood flown in daily, I have questions about that. Or a restaurant that has a few salads in their menu tells me that they just got their produce. I am not sure I believe it. Ask if the dressings and sauces are homemade, if the kitchen uses added salt, sugar or processed oils. Remember knowledge gives you the power to demand what goes into your body.

Make your vegetable broth. Cook plenty of it, refrigerate it and use as you go along. It is far superior, healthier, and more economical than the store-bought one.

There is plenty of information in this book to help you with your cooking and a healthy diet. My advice is to do what I do when I cook: Play my favorite music, relax, enjoy, and put a lot of love into my cooking.

Appetizers and Side Dishes

"Nick creates dishes like Mozart made music, all in his head able to picture the final result without writing it down or tasting it first."

Arizona Republic

"This culinary heaven is a tribute to the chef/owner's skills, innovating spirit and dedication to freshness with the use of quality ingredients."

Destinations of the Southwest

The Salty Truth

And the three principles

The salt controversy is nothing new. Throughout the years there have been several debates about the harmful health effects of consuming too much salt. The reports published in recent years about salt intake should be enough to convince the skeptics about the harm that salt does to your health. The recent Lancet Report, *Health effects of dietary risks in 195 countries, 1990-2017: a systematic analysis for the Global Burden of Disease Study 2017*, published in April 3, 2019, points out that; "High levels of unhealthy red and processed meats, sugar-sweetened beverages, trans fatty acids and salt – all known to be health risks – were compared with the effects of a diet low in many healthy foods. In fact, more than half of all global diet-related deaths in 2017 were due to just three risk factors: eating too much salt, not enough whole grains and not enough fruit. Those risks held true regardless of socioeconomic level of most nations." Ashkan Afshin, the lead author of the 27-year global diet analysis published in the Lancet journal points out, "In many countries, poor diet now causes more deaths than tobacco smoking and high blood pressure."

When I decided to become a chef, I understood that cooking for the public comes with great responsibility. I contemplated my options before opening the doors of my first little restaurant. I decided that my new journey's priority should be about a culinary exploration of new tastes. My initial thoughts were to focus on three principles: I wanted my food to be Fresh, to be Wholesome, and to have Character. I wasn't naive to think that amidst the grueling, high-pace restaurant activity I would have the time to perfect all my goals at first. The dilemma was how much you compromise while trying to maintain your principals. I was confident that I could manage the freshness, that was the most natural part. I defined wholesomeness to be about healthy, nutritious foods. I understood that this was an ongoing process since the research about foods was constantly updated. I also realized that to develop the character of my foods would be a never-ending process. My definition of "food character" included the essence of flavors and then the perception of tastes. Research in those days was difficult. After the long daily shifts in the kitchen, there was not much time to spend on research. I had to rely on experience and memories; what I had learned working in restaurants and what I remembered growing up. It is true that creativity unfolds by adding to familiar tastes. And it is true that the behavior of each food changes according to what it is blended with. I mentioned in another note that my parents knew things because of common sense and folk wisdom, but eventually, we had scientific research; there was functionalism and undeniable truths about how some foods are harmful to your health. Slowly I began to limit or to eliminate food items that seemed to be unhealthy. The most recent report mentioned some of the foods that cause more deaths, than smoking or drinking! Are we supposed to ignore this, because we know better? From my perspective, I was never a big fan of processed meats, I had not had a sugary soda since the early nineties, and salt was not even an issue. Growing up I don't remember the use of salt in cooking. In my father's taverna, I can still smell the oregano, the thyme, and the rosemary, and there was basil, olive oil and garlic. I do not remember salt. At home, there was a box of salt in the corner of my mother's cabinet. When I left my hometown to go to school in Athens, it was still there. When I started my first restaurant, not using salt in my cooking was not by design; I merely didn't like the taste of salt. To improve the character of my foods I use lemon or wine rather than using salt. However, the more I start learning about salt in the years to come; it was apparent that I was doing the right thing. I understand that salt is needed sometimes, especially in baking, where salt helps to activate the yeast. But, eventually, I found a way around it. I discover that the egg whites could activate the yeast the same as salt does. It is common when you approach your business from the unconventional, innovative perspective, to cause some controversy. Refusing to follow the formulate restaurant model some critics characterized me as idiosyncratic and resolute. The vast popularity of my restaurant and the loyalty of our frequent patrons suggest otherwise. To always embrace the new, like this new healthy lifestyle, has helped me to improve my already good health. The lesson here is that never be afraid to try the new and the different and that positive changes are necessary for our growth. This book is the brainchild of this attitude.

Eggplant Spread

2 tbsps olive oil
Heat in a large saute pan.
1 red onion, chopped
4 cloves garlic, chopped
1 large eggplant, large cut
5 Roma tomatoes, chopped
1 red bell pepper, chopped
Add to the pan and cook for 8 to 10 minutes.
½ cup vegetable broth
1 tbsp red wine vinegar
1 tbsp Italian parsley, chopped
1 tbsp cumin
1 tsp black pepper
1 tsp dry thyme
Add to the pan and continue cooking for another 5 to 6 minutes, until liquid is absorbed.
Place mixture into a food processor and pulse 3 or 4 times.
Serve eggplant dip cold or warm.

6 servings

EL – GF – VT - VG

Calories of the main ingredients per serving: Olive oil 30. Eggplant 14. Total 44.

In addition to bringing a unique texture and flavors to recipes, eggplant brings a host of potential health benefits. They are a nutrient-dense food. Eggplants provide a good amount of fiber, vitamins and minerals in a few calories. They contain Vitamins K, C, B6, thiamin, folate and minerals like manganese, potassium, magnesium, copper and niacin. Also, eggplants boast a high number of antioxidants.

• *Tomatoes are the primary dietary source of the antioxidant lycopene, one of the most powerful antioxidants. Other vegetables and fruits with lycopene are guavas, watermelon, papaya, grapefruit, sweet red peppers, asparagus, red cabbage, mango and carrots. Tomatoes are also a great source of vitamin C, potassium, folate and vitamin K.*

Kalamata Olive Paste

1 cup pitted Kalamata olives
½ cup pitted green olives
1 tbs capers
2 tbsp olive oil
3 cloves garlic, roasted
1 tbsp walnuts
½ tsp fresh rosemary
1 tsp dried thyme
Place in a food processor and pulse 2 or 3 times.
Serve with gluten-free crackers or chips.

8 servings

GF - EL – VG – VG

Calories of the main ingredients per serving: Kalamata olives 35. Green olives 8. Olive oil 30. Walnuts 18. Total of 91.

The earliest cultivation of olive trees was recorded in the western Mediterranean at about five thousand years ago. Kalamata olives are only found on the Peloponnese peninsula in southern Greece. Kalamata olive trees have much larger leaves than other types of olive trees and absorb more shine. It is from where this dark purple fruit takes its dense texture and unique flavor. There is a reason why this olive is considered to be one of the healthiest foods on earth: It contains an impressive range of health-protective compounds and health-promoting vitamins and minerals. Kalamata olives are unusually high in iron and vitamin A and a good source of fiber, calcium, vitamin C, and K. They also provide some magnesium, phosphorous, potassium and B vitamins. Kalamata olives, like pure Greek olive oil, contain phenolic compounds, which are natural antioxidants. Olive oil and olives are the cornerstones of the Mediterranean diet. Health benefits aside, it is impossible to overlook this olive's irresistible taste.

Sun-Dried Tomatoes Spread With Hearts of Palm

5 hearts of palm
½ cup sun-dried tomatoes
1 tbsp olive oil
4 cloves garlic, roasted
1 tsp sesame seeds
½ tsp black pepper
⅓ cup feta cheese
⅓ cup fresh mint leaves
1 tbsp capers
2 tbsp grated Romano cheese
Combine all ingredients in a food possessor and mix until smooth.
Serve with gluten-free crackers or chips.

8 servings

EL – GF – VT

Calories of the main ingredients per serving: Hearts of palm 5. Sun Dried tomatoes 9. Olive oil 15. Feta 17. Romano 5. Total of 51.

• *Sun-dried tomatoes are loaded with antioxidants, vitamins and minerals. Most importantly, sun-dried tomatoes unique flavor brings another dimension to the art of cooking.*

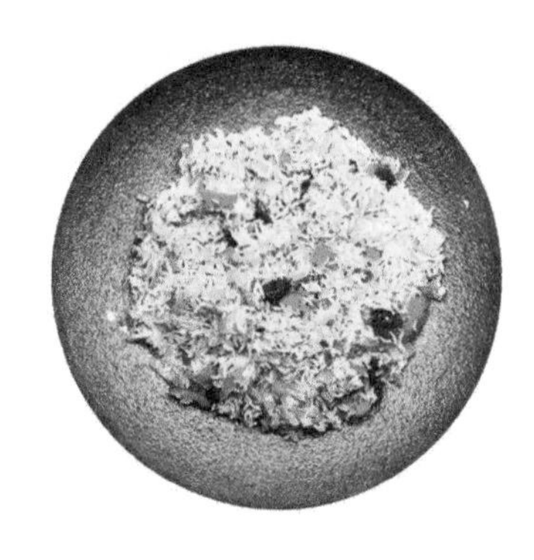

Basmati White Rice Pilaf

2 tbsp olive oil
Heat in a stock pot on medium heat.
¼ red onions, sliced
6 mushrooms, chopped
1 roasted red peppers, sliced
4 artichoke hearts, chopped
2 roasted garlic cloves, minced
1 tsp dry thyme
1 tsp black pepper
½ tsp ginger root, minced
½ tsp turmeric
1 tsp of lemon juice
¼ cup sliced almonds
Add to the pot and simmer for 5 minutes.
2 and ½ cups of vegetable broth
Add to the pot and heat for 2 minutes.
1 cup of basmati white rice
Add to the pot and cook for about 20 to 22 minutes, until rice is tender.
Different brands of rice varied in cooking time. Check the rice after 18 minutes. You might have to adjust the time of cooking or add a little hot water.

4 servings

GF – EL – VT – VG

Calories of the main ingredients per serving: Basmati rice 160. Olive oil 119. Artichokes 76. Almonds 20. Total of 375.

• *Ginger is an excellent natural source of vitamin C, magnesium, potassium, copper, and manganese. Ginger is fierce and peppery with lemon/citrus aroma undertones. When cooked has a mild sweetness with warm flavor. Its complex flavor makes ginger versatile for both baking and cooking.*

Mediterranean Avocado Dip

6 ripe avocados, peeled
In a large bowl mash the avocados with a potato masher.
Juice of half lemon
½ red onion, chopped
2 cloves garlic, minced
⅓ cup sun-dried tomatoes, chopped
1 small tomato, chopped
1 tsp oregano
6 kalamata olives, chopped
1 tsp black pepper,
1 tbsp fresh basil, minced
⅓ cup grated Parmesan cheese
1 cup black beans.
Add the rest of the ingredients to sweet potatoes and mix well.
Refrigerate before serving.
Serve with gluten-free crackers or chips.

8 servings

GF – EL – VT

Calories of the main ingredients per serving: Avocados 242. Black beans 79. Parmesan cheese 19. Total of 340.

• *Avocados are loaded with nutrients, many of which are lacking in modern diets. They are rich with fiber, powerful antioxidants and monounsaturated fatty acids. They contain vitamins A, C, E, K, B6, thiamin, riboflavin, niacin, folate, pantothenic acid. Avocados are rich in potassium, magnesium, copper and manganese.*

Brown Rice Pilaf

STEP 1

2 cups vegetable broth
4 cups water
In a stockpot bring the liquid into a boil.
1 cup of brown rice
Add to the pot, reduce heat to medium and simmer for about 35 to 40 minutes.
Although brown rice usually requires 35 to 40 minutes of cooking, I suggest starting checking it after 30 minutes.
Remove from heat and drain the liquid.

STEP 2

1 medium-size sweet potato.
Place in a pot with boiling water and cook for about 16 to 18 minutes. Sweet potatoes come in many different sizes. The potato is ready when tender with a pierce of a fork.
Remove, cool, peel and cut the potato into small pieces.
While the rice and sweet potato are being cooked, prepare the vegetables.

STEP 3

2 tbsp olive oil
Heat in a saute pan under medium heat.
1 cup broccoli florets, chopped
½ red onions, sliced
1 red bell pepper, sliced
3 cloves garlic, minced

¼ cup raisins
1 tsp dry thyme
1 tsp black pepper
Add to the pan and cook for about 6 to 7 minutes.
2 tbsp white wine
½ cup vegetable broth
1 cup baby spinach, chopped
Cooked brown rice
The cooked sweet potato
Add to the pan and simmer for 4 to 5 minutes longer.

4 servings

GF – EL – VT – VG

Calories of the main ingredients per serving: Brown rice 162. Vegetable broth 7. Olive oil 60. Sweet potato 31. Raisins 28. Total of 288.

• *Broccoli is a nutritional powerhouse vegetable. It is full of vitamins, minerals, fiber and antioxidants. Broccoli is rich in vitamins C and K and contains proper amounts of potassium, phosphorus, selenium and vitamins A and folate.*

Millet Pecan Risotto

1 cup millet
Place millet in a small saute pan and toss for about 5 minutes under medium heat, frequently stirring, until the millet is lightly golden. This process brings out the millet's nutty flavor.
2 cups vegetable broth
1 cup of water
Heat in a stock pot, bring to a gentle boil. Turn heat to medium and add the millet. Cook for about 18 to 20 minutes, until millet is tender. Remove from heat and drain excess liquid, if any.
While millet is being cooked prepare the risotto.
2 tbsp olive oil
Heat in a large saute pan.
½ onion, chopped
Add and saute on medium heat for about 2 to 3 minutes.
2 tbsp white cooking wine
1 large portobello mushroom, sliced
2 cloves roasted garlic, minced
½ cup pecan pieces
½ tsp fresh rosemary, chopped
1 tsp fresh basil leaves, chopped
1 tsp dry thyme
1 tsp black pepper
¼ cup vegetable broth
Add to the pan and cook for about 5 to 6 minutes.
Cooked millet.
¼ cup unsweetened almond milk
Add to the pan and cook for 3 to 4 minutes longer, until the liquid is absorbed.

2 servings

EL – GF – VT – VG

Calories of the main ingredients per serving: Millet 189. Olive oil 119. Pecans 180. Total of 488.

Millet is high in antioxidants, iron, magnesium, zinc, and calcium. A good source of protein, fiber and vitamins B.

• *Portobello mushroom are an excellent source of protein, dietary fiber, magnesium, zinc, manganese, thiamin, vitamin B6, folate. It is also an excellent source of riboflavin, niacin, pantothenic acid, phosphorus, potassium, copper, and selenium.*

• *Pecans are high in healthy unsaturated fat. They also contain vitamins A, B, and E, folic acid, calcium, magnesium, phosphorus, potassium, and zinc.*

Arborio Rice Risotto

2 tbs olive oil
Heat in a stock pot.
½ onion, chopped
2 cloves garlic, chopped
Add to the pot and saute on medium heat for 5 to 6 minutes.
¼ cup white cooking wine
8 cremini mushrooms, sliced
1 tsp black pepper
1 tsp fresh parsley, chopped
1 tsp fresh basil, chopped
1 tsp fresh rosemary, chopped
1 tsp dry oregano
1 tsp dry thyme
Add to the pot and cook for 2 to 3 minutes.
2 cups vegetable broth
1 ½ cup of water
Add to the pot and cook for 2 minutes until water is hot.
1 cup Arborio rice
Add and cook for about 20 to 22 minutes longer.

2 servings

GF – VT – VG

Calories of the main ingredients per serving: Olive oil 119. Arborio Rice 358. Total of 477.

Grecian Grilled Vegetables

12 asparagus, discard tough ends,
2 red bell peppers, sliced
1 eggplant, slice lengthwise
2 yellow squash, slice lengthwise
Set aside
¼ cup olive oil
⅛ cup balsamic vinegar
2 cloves garlic, chopped
1 tsp fresh mint, chopped
1 tbsp dry oregano
1 tsp dry thyme
1 tsp dry basil
1 tsp black pepper
1 tbsp dry mustard
Mix ingredients in a large ball. Heat your outdoor grill, dip vegetables in the dressing and grill well on both sides. Serve whole or cut into large pieces.
2 tbsp fresh mint, minced
Sprinkle on top of the vegetables.
4 servings

GF – EL – VT – VG

Calories for main ingredients in this recipe: Olive oil 119. Asparagus 9. Eggplant 29. Total of 157.

• *Bell peppers are low in calories and exceptionally rich in vitamin C and other antioxidants. Bell peppers come in various colors; green, red, yellow, and orange. The green bell pepper has a slightly bitter flavor than the other three. All bell peppers have similar nutrients. Bell peppers are mainly made up of water and carbs and are an excellent fiber source. Bell peppers are loaded with vitamins and minerals and are extremely rich in vitamin C. They also contain vitamins B6, K1, E, A and folate and moderate amounts of potassium. Bell peppers are rich in various antioxidants, especially carotenoids.*

Lemony Artichoke Hearts

2 tbsp olive oil
Heat in a saucepan.
2 cups artichoke hearts, quartered
Add to the pan and saute for 4 to 5 minutes.
Juice of ½ lemon
½ red onion, sliced
1 clove garlic, chopped
Add and saute for 4 to 5 minutes longer.
1 tbsp fresh rosemary, chopped
1 tbsp fresh Italian parsley, chopped
1 tsp dry thyme
1 tsp dry oregano
½ tsp black pepper
Add and cook for 2 to 3 minutes.
¼ cup grated Parmesan cheese
Turn off the heat, add Parmesan into the pan, steer well.
4 servings

GF – VT

Calories in the main ingredients: Artichoke hearts 45. Parmesan cheese 27. Total of 72.

• *Artichokes are packed with powerful nutrients. They are low in fat while rich in fiber, vitamins and minerals. They rank among some of the most antioxidant-rich vegetables. Artichokes are particularly high in vitamins C, K and folate. They supply minerals, such as phosphorus, magnesium, potassium, and iron. Artichokes contain an above average plant-based protein.*

• *Onions are packed with vitamins, minerals and potent plant compounds. Their medicinal properties have been known since ancient times when onions were used to treat various ailments. Onions are unusually high in vitamin C and rich in B vitamins, including vitamins B6 and folate, and they are an excellent source of potassium. Onions, especially the red onion, are loaded with antioxidants. The health benefits of onions seem endless.*

Black Rice Pilaf

¼ cup of olive oil
Heat in a stock pot on medium heat.
½ red onion, sliced
2 cloves of garlic, minced
Add to the pot and cook for 3 to 4 minutes.
2 tbsp red cooking wine
4 cremini mushrooms, sliced
2 small tomatoes, chopped
¼ tsp fresh ginger, minced
1 tsp black pepper
1 tsp dry thyme
½ tsp cumin
Add to the pot and cook for 3 minutes longer.
2 cups of water
1 cup vegetable broth
Add to the pot and cook for 2 minutes.
1 cup of black rice. Rinse well before cooking.
Add to the pot and cook for 20 to 22 minutes on medium heat, until rice is tender.
2 servings

GF – EL – VT – VG

Calories of the main ingredients per serving: Black rice 108. Olive oil 119. Total of 227.

• *Black rice is known as the "Forbidden Rice." In ancient China, the black rice was reserved solely for the royal family and was forbidden for anyone else to eat it. A few years ago, I started cooking with black rice and loved its texture and the nutty flavor. Black rice is a rich source of antioxidants, fiber, and anti-inflammatory properties. It contains substantial mineral content including iron and copper, and a good source of plant-based protein.*

• *Cumin has an excellent amount of iron and a good source of calcium, manganese, magnesium, phosphorus and vitamin B1. Cumin has a bitter taste with earth and nutty undertones. Cumin has a very distinct smoky and earthy flavor with hints of lemon and nutty and spicy undertones. Cumin seeds are greatly underrated, they are packed with the same flavors and when roasted they have a warm aroma.*

• *Pepper is incredibly popular among spices since ancient times. Black pepper is an excellent source of manganese and vitamin K, an excellent source of copper and dietary fiber, and a good source of iron, chromium, and calcium. There is a distinct and undeniable earthiness to the flavor of black pepper. It is packed with a mild heat and depth of flavor. Its aroma is pungent and sharp. It goes well with nearly any dish.*

Spinach and Butternut Squash Quinoa

2 tbsp olive oil
Heat in a large saute pan.
1 shallot, chopped
4 green onions, chopped. Use only the white and the light green part of the onion.
2 cloves garlic, minced
Add to the pan and saute on medium heat for about 3 to 4 minutes.
2 ½ cups vegetable broth
Add to the pan and heat on medium heat for 2 minutes.
1 cup three color quinoa
2 tbsp golden raisins
2 tbsp pecan pieces
2 cups butternut squash, peeled and chopped.
Add to the pan and cook for about 15 to 18 minutes.
1 ½ cups baby spinach, chopped
Add in, stir well, cook for another minute. Remove from heat.

4 servings

GF – EL – VT – VG

Calories of main ingredients per serving: Olive oil 60. Quinoa 159. Raisins 15. Pecans 12. Butternut squash 32. Total of 278.

• *Butternut squash is a good source of vitamin E and B6, thiamin, niacin, folate, pantothenic acid, and manganese and high in potassium.*

• *Spinach is loaded with nutrients and antioxidants, and considered to be one of the healthiness foods to eat. Spinach is an extremely nutrient-rich vegetable. It is low in carbs and high in insoluble fiber. They are an excellent source of vitamins A, C, K1, folate, as well as iron. Spinach also contains several other vitamins and minerals, such as vitamins B6, B9 and E and minerals such as potassium, magnesium. Spinach contains several important plant compounds as well. The antioxidants found in spinach are linked to numerous health benefits.*

Raisin and Cashew Buckwheat

2 tbsp olive oil
Heat in a large saute pan.
1 small onion, chopped
½ red bell pepper, chopped
2 cloves garlic, chopped
Add to the pan and saute on medium heat 4 to 5 minutes.
2½ cups vegetable broth
Add to the pan and heat for 2 to 3 minutes
1 cup buckwheat groats
½ tsp cumin
½ tsp ground cardamom
1 tsp ground mustard
½ tsp turmeric
½ tsp black pepper
1 tsp Italian parsley, chopped
¼ cup golden raisins
¼ cup cashews, chopped
Add to the pan and cook for 13 to 15 minutes.

2 servings

GF – EL – VT – VG

Calories of the main ingredients per serving: Olive oil 119. Buckwheat 284. Raisins 55. Cashews 80. Total of 538.

Nutrients in Buckwheat. It is a rich source of protein and dietary fiber. It has high amounts of potassium, manganese, phosphorus, magnesium and reasonable amounts of zinc, copper, selenium and iron. It contains decent amounts of folate, riboflavin, niacin and pantothenic acid vitamins. Don't let the name fool you. This flower brings beauty to our earth and its grain and flour are versatile in the kitchen and suitable for every meal of the day, easy to cook and it is gluten-free.

Turmeric contains curcumin, a powerful antioxidant. It is also a good source of Vitamin C and Magnesium, and an excellent source of dietary fiber, vitamin B6, iron, potassium and manganese. Turmeric adds a rich, woody with a somewhat bitter and earthy flavor. When cooked has a warm, peppery flavor. It comes with intense color.

Contains calcium, potassium and vitamins B and C. It also contains small amounts of protein, fiber, and fatty acids. Cardamom has a sweet and light lemony flavor, with a fruity, robust aroma.

Ginger Dill Carrots

2 tbsp olive oil
Heat in a saute pan.
2 large carrots, sliced.
Add to the pan and cook on medium heat for 6 to 7 minutes.
Juice of ½ lime
1 tsp dry thyme
1 tbsp fresh dill, chopped
1 tsp dry mustard
½ tsp fresh ginger, minced
Add to the pan, lower the heat and cook for another 3 to 4 minutes

2 servings

GF – EL – VT – VG

Calories for main ingredients in this recipe: Olive oil 119.

• *Dill contains excellent amounts of fiber, niacin, phosphorus, copper, riboflavin, vitamin B6, magnesium, and potassium. Dill is a light herb with sweet, grassy and anise undertones.*

• *Ginger is an excellent natural source of vitamin C, magnesium, potassium, copper, and manganese. Ginger is fierce and peppery with lemon/citrus aroma undertones. When cooked has a mild sweetness with warm flavor. Its complex flavor makes ginger versatile for both baking and cooking.*

Grilled Endives, Fennel and Radicchio

STEP 1

3 heads Belgian endives, cut in halves lengthwise
2 heads radicchio, quartered through the core
2 fennel bulbs, thinly sliced lengthwise
2 tbsp olive oil
On a flat grill use the olive oil to grill the vegetables. Pour the olive oil on your cooking surface and add the endives, radicchio and fennel, and grill for about 6 to 7 minutes, until lightly brown. Remove and arrange on a large serving plater.

STEP 2

1 tbsp olive oil
1 tsp balsamic vinegar
1 roasted garlic clove, chopped
1 tsp grated orange peel
2 tbsp pomegranate seeds
2 tbsp pistachios, chopped
1 tbsp fresh basil, chopped
Place in a mixing bowl, mix well with a spoon and pour over grilled vegetables. Serve as an appetizer/side dish.

4 servings

GF – EL – VT – VG

Calories of main ingredients per serving: Olive oil 89. Pomegranate 18. Endives 65. Radicchio 12. Fennel 14.

Pistachios 22. Total calories per serving: 220.

• *Belgian endives are high in fiber, iron, calcium, potassium, folic acid, niacin, copper and thiamin. Also, they contain large amounts of beta carotene, riboflavin, vitamin E, C and reasonable amounts of vitamins K and A.*

Nutrients in pistachios: Pistachios are rich in potassium, much higher than bananas, and contain high amounts of protein, fiber, antioxidants, and vitamin B6.

All parts of the fennel plant are rich in powerful antioxidants and are packed with nutrients and are low in calories; fiber, vitamin C, calcium, iron, magnesium, potassium, and manganese. However, the most impressive benefits of all parts of fennel come from the antioxidants and potent plant compounds that they contain.

Steamed Ginger Vegetables

1 cup broccoli florets
1 cup cauliflower florets
6 baby carrots

Heat the water in a steamer basket. Add vegetables into the basket and steam for 2 minutes.

1 red bell pepper, sliced lengthwise
1 cup pea pods, remove strings and cut sliced
1 yellow squash, sliced
1 tsp fresh ginger, chopped

Add to the basket and steam for another 2-3 minute

Remove and place in a mixing bowl.

Juice of ½ lemon
1 tbsp olive oil
1 tbsp fresh Italian parsley, chopped
1 tbsp fresh dill, chopped
1 tbsp sesame seeds

Add to the mixing bowl, toss and serve as a side dish.

2 servings

EL – GF – VT – VG

Calories for main ingredients in this recipe: Olive oil 60.

• *Ginger is an excellent natural source of vitamin C, magnesium, potassium, copper, and manganese. Ginger is fierce and peppery with lemon/citrus aroma undertones. When cooked has a mild sweetness with warm flavor. Its complex flavor makes ginger versatile for both baking and cooking.*

• *Parsley is a concentrated source of nutrition and antioxidants, and more. It is incredibly high in vitamin K and vitamin C. Parsley is also a good source of vitamin A, folate and iron. Parsley is grassy, slightly bitter flavor with woody and citrus undertones.*

Zucchini and Sweet Potato Fritters

2 large zucchinis, large cut
1 large sweet potato, large cut
1 clove garlic, chopped

Place in the food processor and pulse 2 or 3 times. Transfer into a mixing bowl.

1 tsp fresh dill, chopped
1 tsp black pepper
1 tsp fresh Italian parsley, chopped
1 tsp dry oregano
½ cup feta cheese, crumbled
1 egg, beaten
¼ cup grated Parmesan cheese
¼ cup buckwheat flour

Add ingredients to the mixing bowl and mix well with a spoon. It is best to refrigerate for at least one hour. With a large ice cream scoop, scoop out the mixture and form tennis size balls. Press together into firm balls. You should have 8 to 10 fritters.

1 cup almond meal. Place in a mixing bowl.

Roll each ball into almond meal to lightly coated and press it to form a thick patty.

¼ cup olive oil

Heat on a flat grill. Grill the zucchini patties until lightly brown on both sides, about 5 to 6 minutes on each side. Serve with sun-dried tomato sauce.

While the zucchini mixture is refrigerated, make the sauce.

4 servings

GF – VT

Sautéed Shallots with Carrots

2 tbsp olive oil
5 medium carrots, sliced
5 purple carrots, sliced
5 shallots, large cut

Heat the olive oil in a medium sauté pan. Add the vegetables, turn the heat to medium.

Sauté for about 5 to 6 minutes.

Juice of ½ lime
1 tbsp fresh dill, chopped
½ tsp white pepper

Add to the pan and sauté for another 2 minutes.

4 servings

GF – EL – VT – VG

Calories for main ingredients in this recipe: Olive oil 60.

• *Shallots contain a good amount of protein, fiber, protein, vitamin C, potassium, folate, vitamin A and B6, and manganese.*

• *Dill contains excellent amounts of fiber, niacin, phosphorus, copper, riboflavin, vitamin B6, magnesium, and potassium. Dill is a light herb with sweet, grassy and anise undertones.*

Sun-Dried Tomato Sauce

1 tbsp olive oil

Heat in a sauté pan.

¼ onion, chopped
1 clove garlic, chopped

Sauté on medium heat for 3 to 4 minutes.

2 large Roma tomatoes, chopped
¼ cup sun-dried tomatoes, chopped

Add to the pan and cook for 6 to 7 minutes

¼ cup white cooking wine
¼ cup chicken broth
1 tsp dry thyme
1 tsp dry oregano
½ tsp black pepper

Add to the pan and continue cooking for another 4 to 5 minutes.

EL – GF – VT – VG

Calories of the main ingredients in the sauce per serving: Olive oil 30. Sun-dried tomatoes 15. Roma tomatoes 11. Total 56.

Calories of main ingredients in zucchini fritters per serving: Sweet potato 29. Feta 50. Egg 20. Parmesan cheese 27. Buckwheat flour 25. Almond meal 138. Olive oil 119. Total at 408.

• *Sub-dried tomatoes are loaded with antioxidants, vitamins, and minerals. Most important, sun-dried tomatoes savory flavor bring another dimension to the art of cooking.*

Steamed Broccoli

3 cups of broccoli florets

Heat the water in a steamer basket. Add broccoli and steam for 3 to 4 minutes.

Juice of ½ lemon
2 tbsp olive oil
2 roasted cloves garlic, chopped
¼ cup toasted slivered almonds. To toast almonds, place in a baking pan and roast in a 375-degree oven for about 5 to 6 minutes.

Place in a mixing bowl, toss together with broccoli and serve.

4 servings

GF – EL – VT – VG

Calories for main ingredients in this recipe: Olive oil 60. Almonds 52. Broccoli 22. Total of 134.

• *Broccoli is a nutritional powerhouse vegetable. It is full of vitamins, minerals, fiber, and antioxidants. Broccoli is rich in vitamins C and K and contains proper amounts of potassium, phosphorus, selenium, and vitamins A and folate. Broccoli can be eaten cooked or raw; however different cooking methods affect broccoli's nutrient properties. Boiling broccoli, and vegetables in general, is reducing some of its compounds, especially vitamin C. Other than eating it raw, steaming seems to be the best way to prepare vegetables in general. One thing you should never do is to microwave this superfood.*

• *Almonds deliver a massive amount of nutrients: Fiber, manganese, magnesium, vitamin E, copper, riboflavin and phosphorus.*

Roasted Garlic

Discard the outer layers of the whole garlic bulb. Slice off the top each head of garlic to expose some of the cloves inside. Drizzle with olive oil and wrap it with aluminum foil – Bake in a preheated 400-degree oven for about 30 minutes. Cool and remove garlic cloves from their skins. Keep refrigerated.

GF – EL – VT – VG

• *Modern science has now confirmed the beneficial health effects of garlic. Even though I have done much research about garlic, covering all the incredible health benefits of garlic, it is beyond the scope of my expertise about the effects of nutrients in various illness. Garlic contains amounts of multiple nutrients, just about almost everything we need. Among these nutrients are, plentiful amounts of vitamin C, vitamin B6 and manganese. It also contains fiber, selenium and amounts of calcium, copper, potassium, phosphorus, iron and vitamin B1. Additionally, there is a long list of other compounds in garlic.*

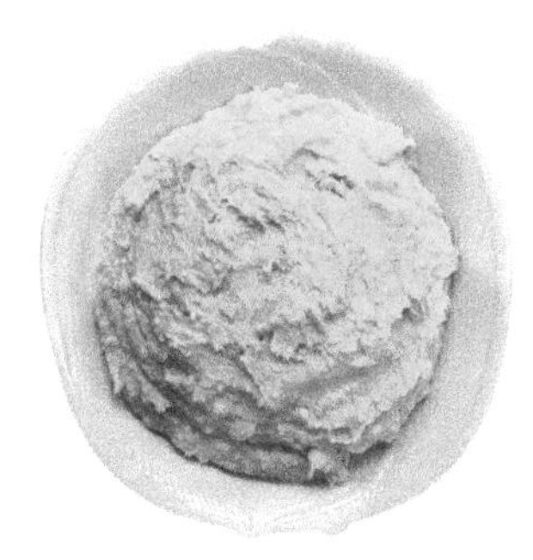

Hummus with Sun-Dried Tomatoes

Add to the hummus recipe:
¼ cup sun-dried tomatoes, packed in olive oil.

GF – EL – VT – VG

Calories per serving: dried tomatoes 4. Humus 220. Total of 224.

Sun-dried tomatoes savory flavor bring another dimension to the art of cooking.

1 tsp lemon juice

Add to the pan and sauté for about 5 to 6 minutes on medium heat.

2 servings

GF – EL – VG – VG

Sautéed Asparagus

2 tbsp olive oil
12 asparagus, discard tough ends

Heat on a sauté pan.

2 large portobello mushrooms, sliced
2 roasted cloves of garlic, chopped
4 Kalamata olives, sliced
½ tsp black pepper
6 fresh basil leaves, chopped
½ tsp ground mustard
¼ cup slivered almonds
1 tsp lemon juice

Add to the pan and sauté for about 5 to 6 minutes on medium heat.

2 servings

GF – EL – VG – VG

Calories per serving 114.

• *Asparagus is an excellent source of fiber, folate, vitamins A, C, E, and K, as well as chromium.*

• *Mustard seeds are an excellent source of selenium and an excellent source of omega-3 fatty acids and manganese. They are also a good source of phosphorus, magnesium, copper and vitamin B1. Yellow ground mustard is ideal for tempering mustard flavor. It has a mellow spiciness and strong mustard flavor.*

• *Almonds deliver a massive amount of nutrients: Fiber, manganese, magnesium, vitamin E, copper, riboflavin and phosphorus.*

• *Besides being calorie-free, basil is a rich source of antioxidants and phenolics, vitamin K, zinc, calcium, magnesium, potassium and dietary fiber. Basil is sweet, highly aromatic with peppery and licorice undertones. Basil shines when fresh or dried. When dried it takes a minty flavor.*

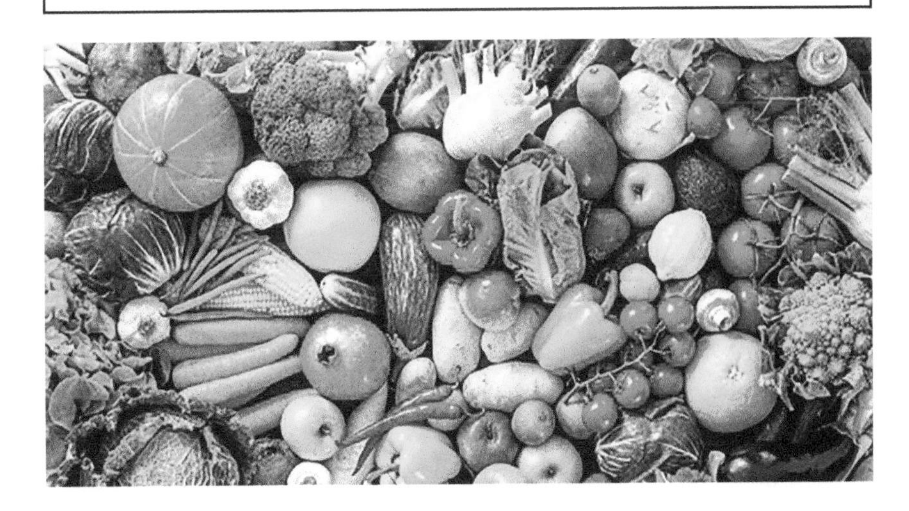

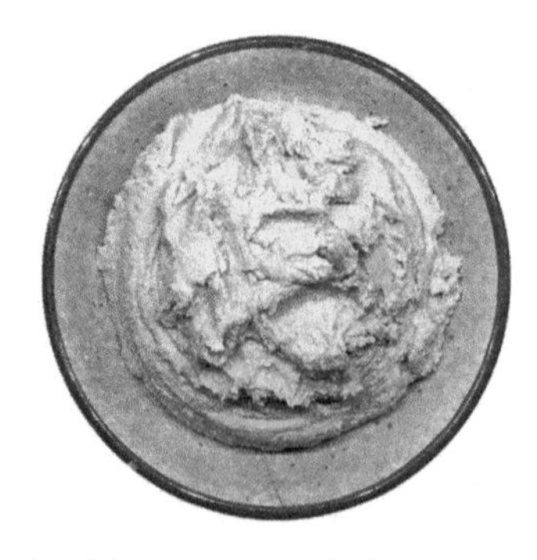

My Favorite Hummus

Add to hummus recipe:
1 Avocado, peeled and chopped
4 oz Feta cheese

GF – EL – VT

Calories per serving: Avocado 27. Feta cheese 26. Hummus 187. Total of 240.

In this recipe, the smooth buttery taste of avocado and the tangy, salty and creamy flavor of real feta cheese is the perfect union of tastes.

Feta Pesto Mushrooms

Preheat oven to 350-degrees,
8 large cremini mushrooms

Take off the stem of the mushrooms, place mushrooms caps in a baking dish, open cavity up, and bake on the oven for about 10 minutes

Since mushrooms contain water, you might have water in the caps – discard the water.

Hummus Recipe

6 cups of cooked garbanzo beans
Juice from 1 large lemon
4 roasted cloves garlic or 3 raw cloves
1 cup of olive oil
1 tsp sesame seeds
¼ tsp white pepper

Run ingredients in a food processor until mixture is smooth. Refrigerate.

12 servings

Cook your garbanzo beans, (I do not recommend it) or use canned or frozen garbanzo beans.

To boil garbanzo beans takes more two hours. 3 cups of dry beans equals about 8 cups of cooked beans.

If you are using canned beans for this recipe, you must drain them well and might have to adjust the amount of the olive oil. For a smoother taste, I use roasted garlic or 1 and ½ tbsp garlic in oil – see index for the recipe of Garlic in Oil.

GF – EL – VT – VG

Calories of main ingredients per serving: Garbanzo beans 68. Olive oil 119. Total of 187.

Garbanzo beans vitamins: C,E,K,B6 thiamin, folate, Riboflavin, Pantothenic Acid.

Minerals – calcium, iron, magnesium, potassium, phosphorus, zinc, copper, manganese, selenium.

• *Garbanzo beans contain antioxidant and significant amounts of fiber. They are packed with nutrients and rich in plant-based protein. A recent study on garbanzos and fiber suggests that the fiber benefits of garbanzo beans go beyond the fiber benefits of other foods. Garbanzo beans are low in saturated fat and very low in cholesterol and sodium, and contain high amounts of folate and manganese.*

Hummus with Kalamata Olives

Add to the hummus recipe:
12 pitted Kalamata olives

GF – EL – VT – VG

Calories per serving: Kalamata olives 5. Humus 220. Total of 225.

Feta Pesto Sauce

1½ cups of fresh basil
3 cloves of roasted garlic
¼ cup of olive oil
1 tbsp Parmesan cheese
¼ cup walnuts
4 oz feta cheese

Mix in a food processor until smooth. Store remaining pesto in a glass jar in your refrigerator.

4 servings

GF – VT

Calories of main ingredients per serving: Olive oil 119. Walnuts 33. Feta 25. Total at 177.

• *Besides being calorie-free, in addition to antioxidant vitamins and phenolics, basil is a rich source of vitamin K, zinc, calcium, magnesium, potassium and dietary fiber. Basil is sweet, highly aromatic with a peppery and licorice undertones. Basil shines when fresh or dried. When dried it takes a minty flavor.*

Pumpkin Walnut Pesto

1 cup green pumpkin seeds, unsalted
½ cup walnut pieces
⅓ cup sun-dried tomatoes
½ cup kale leaves, large cut
1 and ½ cups fresh basil
3 tbsp olive oil
Juice of ½ lemon
3 cloves garlic, chopped
½ tsp black pepper
1 cup low-fat real Greek yogurt

Place all ingredients in a food processor and mix until smooth.

6 servings

EL – GF – VT

Calories of the main ingredients of this recipe: Pumpkin seeds 48. Walnuts 44. Sun-dried tomatoes 13. Greek yogurt 30. Total of 120.

• *Pumpkin seeds are a source of essential nutrients like zinc, magnesium, manganese, copper. Pumpkin seeds are a rich source of various antioxidants, healthy fats and fibers.*

• *Kale is one of the healthiest foods on the planet. It delivers more nutritional benefits for fewer calories than nearly any other item at the market. Eating more kale is a great way to increase the total nutrient content of your diet dramatically. Kale is exceptionally high in vitamin C, in fact, one cup of kale contains more vitamin C than an orange. Kale is one of the world's best sources of vitamin K, a cup of kale containing almost seven times the recommended daily amount. Kale is also loaded with vitamins A, and many powerful antioxidants are found in kale. It provides proper amounts of vitamin B6, thiamin, riboflavin, niacin. Kale is also high in minerals; it is an excellent plant-based source of calcium and magnesium. Other minerals like manganese, copper, potassium, iron and phosphorous are found in kale.*

Sun-Dried Tomatoes Recipe

40 ripe plum tomatoes.

Slice the tomatoes lengthwise. Line a baking sheet with parchment paper place then on a baking sheet. Slice tomatoes in half and place them on the sheet, cut side.

6 tbsps olive oil
½ tsp black pepper 2 cloves garlic, chopped
1 tsp dried oregano
1 tsp drained basil.

Mix ingredients in a bowl and brush the top of the tomatoes with it.

Place sheet in a 200-degree oven and bake for about 3 hours.

Turn oven off and let them dry in the oven for a couple of hours

Pack the tomatoes in a one-pint class, add a few basil leaves between the tomatoes, fill it with olive oil.

Refrigerate for at least a week before using.

Making sun-dried tomatoes is time-consuming. If you are using as many sun-dried tomatoes as I use, It is easier to buy them already cured in jars. There are many brands of sun-dried tomatoes in jars carried by all groceries stores.

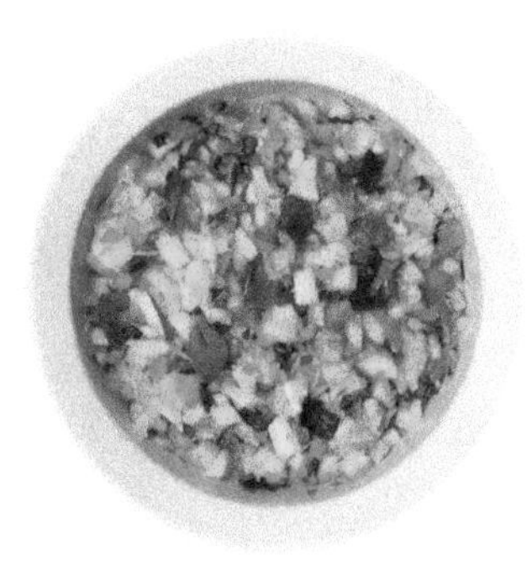

Mango Relish

2 mangoes, chopped
1 roasted red pepper, chopped
½ cup red onion, chopped
1 cup pineapple, chopped
1 tbsp fresh basil, chopped
Juice of ¼ lemon
1 tsp olive oil

Place ingredients in a mixing bowl and mix well by hand.

6 servings

GF – EL – VT – VG

Calories of main ingredients per serving: Mango 36. Pineapple 14. Olive oil 7. Total 57.

• *Mango is high on vitamins C and A. It contains reasonable amounts of vitamins B6, K and folate. Suitable amounts of potassium, calcium, copper and iron, as well as antioxidants and beta-carotene, and small amounts of protein.*

Avocado Relish

3 avocado, diced
1 small red bell pepper, chopped
1 small red onion, chopped
1 Roma tomato, chopped
½ cup frozen corn kernels, defrosted
Juice from ½ lime
1 tbsp red wine vinegar
1 tbsp olive oil
1 tsp black pepper
1 tsp cumin
1 tbsp fresh parsley, chopped

Blend together in a mixing bowl.

8 servings

EL – GF – VT – VG

Calories in main ingredients per serving: Avocado 120. Olive oil 15. Corn 10. Total of 145.

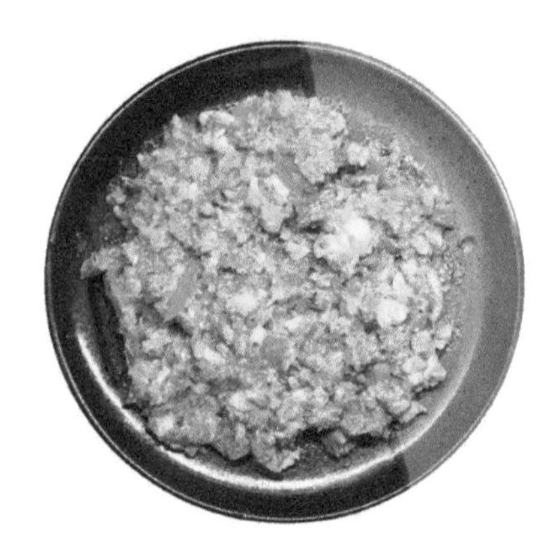

• *Avocados are loaded with nutrients, many of which are lacking in modern diets. They are rich with fiber, powerful antioxidants and monounsaturated fatty acids.*

Pomegranate Pear Relish

½ small red bell pepper, chopped
2 pears, peeled and chopped
1 cup pomegranate seeds
1 tsp orange zest
½ cup fresh mint, chopped
½ tsp black pepper
2 tablespoons extra-virgin olive oil
Juice of ¼ lemon

Place ingredients in a mixing bowl and mix well by hand.

6 servings

EL – GF – VT – VG

Calories for main ingredients in this recipe per serving: Pears 34. Pomegranate seeds 27. Total 61.

• *Nutrients in Pomegranates. They contain large amounts of Vitamins C and K, folate, fiber, potassium and reasonable amounts of protein.*

• *Pears are high on vitamins C, K, and potassium. It has smaller amounts of calcium, iron, magnesium, riboflavin, vitamin B-6, and folate.*

Garlic in Oil

3 cups of peeled garlic cloves. Peel so much garlic is a tedious job. Peeled garlic is available in many markets.
½ cup olive oil
1 tsp red wine vinegar

Place in a food processor and pulse 1 or 2 times. Garlic should be chopped. Place in a small jar, leaving a little space to allow the garlic to expand. Keep it refrigerate at all times and use as needed. The red wine vinegar acts as an extra preservative.

GF – EL – VT – VG

The conversion of ½ tsp should equal one medium garlic clove. However, since garlic gloves vary in size, it is difficult to determine the exact conversion. What do I do? I like to add a bit more garlic – there is no such thing too much garlic, especially when you use garlic in oil. I use fresh garlic or garlic in oil according to the recipe in recipes that are not cooked, like hummus, pesto, etc. I use garlic in oil for a smoother more delicate taste. Also, it takes away the garlicky aftertaste. Using garlic, even if you love it as much as I do, you have to be careful not to overpower your recipe. One thing you never do though, please do not use garlic powder in my recipes or any recipe for that matter. Garlic contains amounts of multiple nutrients, just about almost everything we need. Among these nutrients are, plentiful amounts of vitamin C, vitamin B6 and manganese. It also contains fiber, selenium, and quantities of calcium, copper, potassium, phosphorus, iron and vitamin B1. Additionally, there is a long list of other compounds in garlic.

Feta Pesto

1 ½ cups of fresh basil
3 cloves of roasted garlic
¼ cup of olive oil
1 tbsp Parmesan cheese
¼ cup walnuts
4 oz feta cheese
Mix in a food processor until smooth. Store remaining pesto in a glass jar in your refrigerator. Using a teaspoon, fill the mushroom caps with generous amounts of feta pesto and bake for another 4 to 5 minutes. Refrigerate remaining pesto sauce.

EL – GF – VT

Calories of main ingredients per mushroom: Total at 45.

• *Mushrooms are rich in riboflavin, folate, thiamine, pantothenic acid, and niacin. Mushrooms are also rich in selenium, copper and potassium.*

Sweet and Sour Fruit Relish

1 cup mango, chopped
1 roasted red bell pepper, chopped
1 cup pineapple, chopped
1 tbsp fresh basil, chopped
1 tbsp fresh dill, chopped
1 green onion, chopped
1 clove garlic, minced
1 tsp turmeric
½ tsp white pepper
1 tbsp sesame seeds
1 tbsp juice of a lemon
1 tbsp capers, chopped
1 cup low-fat Greek yogurt
1 tbsp olive oil
Place ingredients in a mixing bowl and mix well by hand.
8 servings

EL – GF – VT

Calories of the main ingredients per serving: Sesame seeds 13. Mango 27. Pineapple 11. Olive oil 20. Greek Yogurt 18. Total at 89.

• *Capers contain fiber, protein, vitamins C, A, K, E, niacin, riboflavin, as well as iron and potassium.*

Gorgonzola Cauliflower Rice

1 medium cauliflower
Place the cauliflower florets in a food processor and pulse 2 to 3 times, until cauliflower resembles rice.
2 tbsp olive oil
Heat in a saute pan on medium heat.
2 green onions, chopped
2 cloves garlic, chopped
1 tsp fresh rosemary, chopped
¼ tsp fennel seeds
The cauliflower rice
Add to the pan. Cook, string frequently, for about 5 to 6 minutes. Until cauliflower is tender.
¼ cup vegetable broth
½ cup raisins
½ cup pecans, chopped
1 tsp black pepper
½ tsp fresh ginger, minced
Juice from ½ lemon
Add to the saute pan and cook for another 6 to 7 minutes.
½ cup Gorgonzola cheese, crumbled
Add to the pan, stir well until the Gorgonzola cheese is melted, about 1 minute.
2 tbsp grated Romano cheese
Turn off heat, add Romano, stir well and serve.

4 servings

GF – VG

Calories of the main ingredients per serving: Blue cheese 40. Pecans 94. Olive oil 119. Cauliflower 36. Raisins 62. Romano 11.Total of 362.

• *Cauliflower contains a high amount of fiber and provides a significant amount of antioxidants. It is high in choline, an essential nutrient for our body, found only in a few foods. Cauliflower, along with broccoli, is one of the best plant-based sources of choline.*

• *Pepper is an excellent source of manganese and vitamin K, an excellent source of copper and dietary fiber, and a good source of iron, chromium and calcium. There is a distinct and undeniable earthiness to the flavor of black pepper. It is packed with a mild heat and depth of flavor. Its aroma is pungent and sharp. It goes well with nearly any dish. White pepper is a bit more spicy from black pepper.*

Sweet Potato Slices

2 long and evenly size sweet potatoes

Bake in a 375-degree oven for about 40 to 45 minutes. Remove, cool and peel. Slice the potatoes into about 1/2 inch rounds.

Place a piece of parchment paper on a baking dish. Layer the potato rounds on top of the parchment paper.

½ cup walnuts, chopped
½ cup crumbled feta cheese
2 green onion, chopped
¼ cup of raisins

On top of each potato round, layer the ingredients in this order: walnut, feta, onions, and raisins. Return pan to the oven and bake for about 5 to 6 minutes. Fresh basil, approximately 24 leaves

Remove from oven and place a basil leaf on top of each slice.

Makes about 24 slices

GF – VT

Calories per slice: Sweet potatoes 11. Walnuts 14. Feta 8. Raisins 5. Total 38.

Walnuts contain good fats. They also contain iron, selenium, calcium, zinc, vitamin E.

• *Besides being calorie-free, basil is a rich source of antioxidants and phenolics, vitamin K, zinc, calcium, magnesium, potassium and dietary fiber. Basil is sweet, highly aromatic with peppery and licorice undertones. Basil shines when fresh or dried. When dried it takes a minty flavor.*

Artichokes Vinaigrette

2 tbsp olive oil

Heat in a saute pan.

8 whole artichoke hearts
3 green onions, chopped
6 cremini mushrooms, cut in halves
1 clove garlic, chopped

Add to the pan and cook on medium heat until artichokes are light brown, about 5 to 6 minutes.

1 tbsp white cooking wine
1 tsp dry oregano
1 tsp dry thyme
1 tsp ground mustard
1 tbsp balsamic vinegar

Add to the pan and cook for 2 to 3 minutes longer.

2 tbsp grated Parmesan cheese

Turn heat off, add Parmesan, stir well and serve.

2 servings

GF – VG

Calories of main ingredients per serving: Olive oil 119. Artichoke hearts 100. Parmesan cheese 22. Mustard vinaigrette 68. Total of 309.

• *Artichokes are a good source of niacin, magnesium, phosphorus, potassium, and copper. Also contains vitamins C, K, folate, and manganese.*

Cauliflower with Sun Dried Tomato Sauce

Preheat oven to 375-degrees

1 small cauliflower, cut into florets
1 tbsp olive oil
Juice of ½ lemon

In a mixing bowl, toss well together. Place mixture in a baking dish and bake in the preheated oven for about 15 minutes, until cauliflower is starting to get light brown. Remove from the oven.

2 tbsp olive oil

Heat in a large saute pan.

½ red onion, chopped
2 cloves garlic, chopped
The baked cauliflower

Add garlic and onion, along with the cauliflower and saute on medium heat for 3 to 4 minutes

2 Roma tomato, chopped
¼ cup sun-dried tomatoes, chopped
¼ cup pine nuts
1 tsp black pepper
1 tsp dry thyme
1 tbsp dry oregano
1 tsp cumin
6 kalamata olives, sliced
1 tbsp capers

Add to the pan and saute for 10 to 12 minutes, until tomatoes are soft.

Remove and serve.

Cauliflower side dish goes well with chicken meat dishes.

4 servings

EL – GF – VT – VG

Calories in the main ingredients per serving: Olive oil 90. Cauliflower 40. Pine nuts 57. Total of 187.

• *Pine nuts contain nutrients that help boost energy, including monounsaturated fat, protein and iron. They are also a good source of magnesium and potassium.*

Double Baked Sweet Potato

2 medium size, round shaped white sweet potatoes

Bake in a 375-degree oven for about 40 to 45 minutes. Remove and cool. Slice potatoes in halves lengthwise. Carefully scoop out the pulp using a small spoon, leaving about a quarter of an inch pulp around the potato skin.

The pulp of sweet potatoes
2 tbsp pumpkin puree
¼ tsp cinnamon
½ tsp orange zest
1 tsp dry thyme
½ tsp cumin
1 clove garlic, minced

Place ingredients in a mixing bowl and with a fork mash the ingredients together.

Place potato skins on a small ceramic baking dish and scoop pulp mixture into the skins.

¼ cup pecans, chopped

Sprinkle pecans on top of potatoes. Return to the oven and bake for about 15 to 18 minutes, until the top of potatoes are lightly golden.

4 servings

GF – EL – VT – VG

Calories of main ingredients per serving: Sweet potatoes 56. Pecans 45. Total of 101.

• *Sweet potatoes are an excellent source of vitamin A and C, manganese, copper, pantothenic acid and vitamin B6. And a good source of potassium, fiber, niacin, vitamin B1, B2 and phosphorus.*

• *Pumpkin is a good source of Vitamin E, Magnesium, Phosphorus, Potassium and Copper, and an excellent source of Dietary Fiber, Vitamin A, Vitamin C, Vitamin K, Iron and Manganese.*

• *Pecans are high in healthy unsaturated fat. They also contain vitamins A, B, and E, folic acid, calcium, magnesium, phosphorus, potassium, and zinc.*

Sweet Potatoes Walnut Mash

Preheat oven to 425-degrees

2 medium-size sweet potatoes

Bake sweet potatoes for 45 to 50 minutes, until they are soft. Cool and peel potatoes.

Place in a mixing bowl and mash it with a potato masher or a fork.

2 cloves garlic, minced
¼ cup walnuts, chopped
1 tbsp lemon juice
2 tbsp olive oil
1 tsp black pepper
1 tsp fresh parsley, chopped
¼ cup low-fat real Greek yogurt

Add the rest of the ingredients and mix well. Serve warm or cold as a side dish.

4 servings

EL – GF – VT

Calories of the main ingredients per serving: Sweet potato 57. Walnuts 33. Greek yogurt 36. Olive oil 96. Total of 222.

• *Sweet potatoes are an excellent source of vitamin A and C, manganese, copper, pantothenic acid and vitamin B6. And a good source of potassium, fiber, niacin, vitamin B1, B2 and phosphorus.*

• *Parsley is a concentrated source of nutrition and antioxidants, and more. It is incredibly high in vitamin K, and vitamin C. Parsley is also a good source of vitamin A, folate and iron. Parsley is grassy, slightly bitter flavor with woody and citrus undertones.*

Gluten Free Bruschetta

1 large sweet potatoes

Bake in 375-degree oven 40 to 45 minutes. Cool and chopped in thick pieces.

½ small red onion finely chopped
¼ cup fresh basil leaves, chopped
½ tsp lemon zest
2 cloves garlic, roasted and chopped
1 ripe tomato, chopped
1 tsp balsamic vinegar
1 tbsp olive oil
¼ tsp black pepper

Mix ingredients in a bowl, refrigerate and use as needed.

To serve the bruschetta use gluten-free bread. Slice the bread into preferred thickness. Place the bread slices on a baking sheet and bake until lightly brown. Spoon the mixture on top of each slice of bread.

GF – EL – VT – VG

Calories for main ingredients in this recipe: Sweet potato 114.

Vegetarian Sweet Potato Skins

Preheat oven to 375-degrees.

4 medium size, round shaped white sweet potatoes. Cut in halves lengthwise.

Scoop out the pulp with a spoon. Save pulp for another use. Place potato shells on a baking pan and bake for about 18 to 20 minutes. Remove from oven.

2 tbsp olive oil

Heat in a saute pan.

1 medium onion, chopped
1 medium red onion, chopped
1 red pepper, chopped
1 large zucchini, chopped
1 clove garlic, chopped

Add to the pan and saute on medium heat for about 6 to 7 minutes.

12 mushrooms, sliced
1 cup artichoke hearts, sliced
4 hearts of palm, sliced
½ cup sliced green olives
½ tsp red wine vinegar
½ tsp black pepper
1 tsp dry oregano
1 tsp dry thyme

Add to the pan and cook for another 3 to 4 minutes longer. Drain liquid, if there is any. Divide filling evenly into the sweet potato shells.

16 slices reduced fat provolone cheese

Place 2 slices on each potato skin. Bake for 7 to 8 minutes.

4 servings

GF – VT

Calories of the main ingredients per potato stuffed skin: Sweet potato 29. Olive oil 30. Hearts of palm 20. Artichoke hears 12. Provolone 100. Total of 191.

• *Mushrooms are rich in riboflavin, folate, thiamine, pantothenic acid, and niacin. Mushrooms are also rich in selenium, copper and potassium.*

• *Artichokes are packed with powerful nutrients. They are low in fat while rich in fiber, vitamins, minerals, and rank among the most antioxidant-rich of all vegetables. Artichokes are particularly high in vitamins C, K and folate. They supply minerals, such as phosphorus, magnesium, potassium, and iron. Artichokes contain an above average plant-based protein.*

Sesame Seed Crackers

Preheat oven to 375-degrees

½ cup almond flour
½ cup brown rice flour
½ cup tapioca flour
2 tbsp sesame seeds
2 tbsp black sesame seeds
2 tbsp chia seeds
1 tsp arrowroot
½ tsp black pepper

Blend ingredients in your mixer.

2 eggs
½ cup almond milk

Add to the mixer and combine in medium speed, until all ingredients blend well.

2 large baking pans
4 sheets of parchment paper cut into the size of large baking pans

Lay two sheet of paper on a working surface and lightly oil them with olive oil.

Divide mixture into two parts, roll each piece into a thick roll and place roll on the center of the parchment paper.

Flattened each dough roll with the palm of your hand and place the other two parchment papers on top of each roll.

Using a rolling pin, roll out the dough to about 1/8 of thickness. Try to roll out the dough into a square shape to avoid waste.

Remove the top parchment papers and with a pizza cutter cut into small squares. With a fork punch holes on top of each square.

Place each of the dough on a baking pan and bake in the preheated 375-degree oven for about 15 to 17 minutes. Remove from oven. Flip parchment paper over in each baking pan, remove the paper and return to oven for about 15 to 16 minutes longer until crackers are lightly brown. Let cool before removing crackers from the pan.

Makes 60 to 65 crackers

GF – VT – These crackers can be made without the eggs. VG

Calories in this recipe per cracker: Almond flour 5. Brown rice flour 5. Eggs 5. Total 15.

Fresh Tomato Bruschetta

3 ripe tomatoes, chopped
1 tbsp capers
3 roasted garlic cloves, chopped
1 tbsp olive oil
1 roasted red pepper, chopped
¼ cup fresh basil, chopped
1 tbsp dry oregano
1 tsp black pepper
1 green onion, chopped. Use the white and light green part only.
Place all ingredients in a mixing bowl and mix well by hand.
8 slices of French banquette, toasted
Place mixture on bread and serve or serve. Refrigerate unused portion.

8 servings

VT – VG

Calories in the main ingredients for the entire recipe: Olive oil 119. Roasted red pepper 31. Total of 150.

• *Capers are low in calories; two tablespoons of capers contain just two or three calories. Apart from its low-calorie benefit, capers are a powerhouse of vitamins A, K, niacin, and riboflavin. They are potent sources of fiber and contain minerals like iron, calcium, and copper. Bottom line, capers are a rich source of antioxidants, phytonutrients, and vitamins essential for our health. If like me, you don't use salt in your cooking, or if you are using limited amounts of salt, capers can give you that salty effect since they contain a good amount of sodium.*

• *Garlic contains multiple nutrients, just about almost everything we need. Among these nutrients are plentiful amounts of vitamin C, vitamin B6, and manganese. It also contains fiber, selenium and small amounts of calcium, copper, potassium, phosphorus, iron and vitamin B1. Additionally, there is a long list of other compounds in garlic.*

Almond Crackers

Preheat oven to 375-degrees.
½ cup almonds, ground
½ cup tapioca flour
1 cup almond flour
1 cup almond meal
½ cup brown rice flour
½ tsp black pepper
1 tsp arrowroot
1 tsp dried thyme

Blend ingredients well in your mixer.

2 eggs
1 cup almond milk

Add to the mixer and combine in medium speed, until all ingredients blend well.

2 large baking pans
4 sheets of parchment paper cut into the size of large baking pans

Lay two sheet of paper on a working surface and lightly oil them with olive oil.

Divide mixture into two parts, roll each piece into a thick roll and place roll on the center of the parchment paper.

Flattened each dough roll with the palm of your hand and place the other two parchment papers on top of each roll.

Using a rolling pin, roll out the dough to about 1/8 of thickness. Try to roll out the dough into a square shape to avoid waste.

Remove the top parchment papers and with a pizza cutter cut into small squares. With a fork punch holes on top of each square.

Place each of the dough on a baking pan and bake in the preheated 375-degree oven for about 15 to 17 minutes. Remove from oven. Flip parchment paper over in each baking pan, remove the paper and return to oven for about 15 to 16 minutes longer until crackers are lightly brown. Let cool before removing crackers from the pan.

Makes 60 to 65 crackers

GF – VT – These crackers can be made without the eggs. VG

Calories in this recipe per cracker: Almonds 14. Sunflower seeds 7. Almond meal 3. Brown rice flour 5. Eggs 5. Total 34.

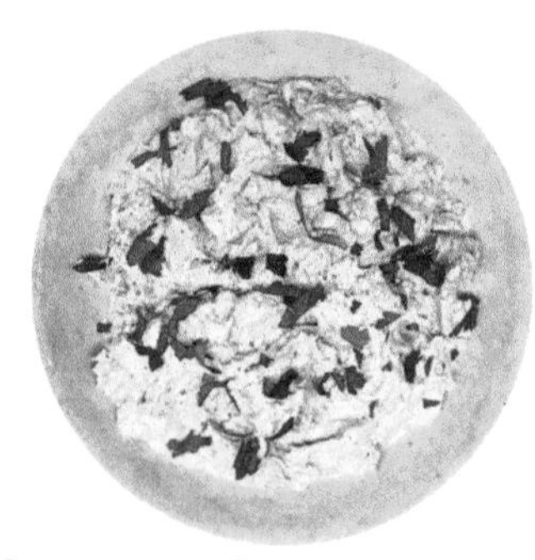

Salmon Spread with Spinach and Artichokes

Preheat your oven to 350-degrees.
1½ lbs salmon
2 tbsp olive oil
1 tsp black pepper
1 tbsp dry thyme
Juice of ½ lime

Place salmon in a baking dish, sprinkle oil, lime and spices on top and bake in the preheated oven for about 20 minutes.

Remove and cool in the refrigeration.

1 tbsp capers
2 tbsp fresh dill
1 clove garlic
2 green onions
3 artichoke hearts
¼ cup sun-dried tomatoes
4 cups baby spinach (about 5 oz)
1 tsp black pepper
2 tbsp grated Parmesan cheese
1 tbsp ground mustard
1 tsp prepared horseradish
1 tsp paprika
1 tsp turmeric

Place all the above ingredients in the food processor and pulse 2 to 3 times.

Remove and place in a large mixing bowl.

8 oz low-fat cream cheese
6 oz low-fat Greek yogurt
Juice of ½ lemon
⅓ of the cooked salmon. Save the rest of the salmon.

Place ingredients in the bowl of your mixer and mix well on low speed.

Remove and add to the mixing bowl with the vegetable mixture. Stir well with a large spoon or a spatula.

The remaining ⅔ cooked salmon

Brake it into pieces, add it to the large mixing bowl and mix gently.

Place it in a serving dish.

2 tbsp fresh Italian parsley, chopped

Sprinkle on top of the spread and serve.

6 servings

VT – VG

Calories in the main ingredients: Salmon 236. Cream cheese 87. Greek yogurt 18. Total of 341.

• *Salmon is an excellent source of omega-3 fatty acids, vitamin B12, D and selenium. It is a good source of niacin, protein, phosphorus and vitamin B6, choline, pantothenic acid, biotin, and potassium. Salmon also provides significant amounts of the antioxidant amino acid taurine.*

Blue cheese

The aroma and taste of blue cheese depend on the intensity of the cure, the climate of the curing cellar and the length of ripening. Blue cheese is excellent crumbled on salads. The main characteristics of all varieties of blue cheese is their bold and sharp taste. However, beyond the common character, the different varieties come with a different tastes. Various blue cheese types are made with either cow's or sheep's milk.

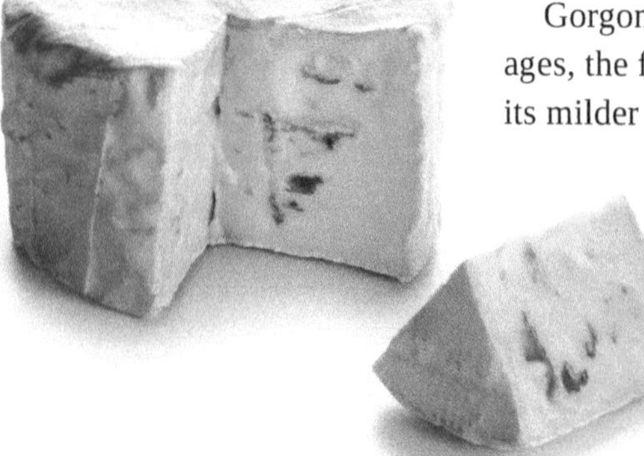

Gorgonzola has a milder flavor. When fresh, it is soft and creamy, but as it ages, the flavor grows stronger and gives a pungent flavor to dishes. Because of its milder and creamy flavor is versatile in the kitchen.

Roquefort is strong and spicy with a sweet undertone. It is, most likely, the strongest blue cheese.

Stilton has a thick crust with creamy interior. Its taste resembles sharp cheddar. Stilton's flavor becomes extremely sharp with age.

The American made blue cheese comes with a stronger flavor with salty undertones. It is more crumbly than other blue cheese. Today there are many excellent blues produced across the United States.

Salads

"Purists rave about Nick Ligidakis' restaurant in Phoenix...a magical blend of Italian and Greek dishes."
Wine Country International

"Ligidakis stresses quality. Because of this he refuses to compromise when it comes to ingredients he uses."
Arizona Republic

Arugula Three Color Quinoa Salad

STEP 1
3 cup water
Bring to a gentle boil.
1 cup three-color quinoa
Add and cook for about 15 to 18 minutes on medium heat. Remove, drain excess liquid and cool.
STEP 2
6 cups arugula
¼ cup sliced almonds, toasted
1 cup blueberries
¼ walnut pieces
1 avocado, sliced
1 pear, sliced
¼ cup raisins
3 hearts of palm, sliced
½ cup pomegranate seeds
Juice of ½ line
¼ cup fresh mint leaves, chopped
2 tbsps olive oil
Place in a large bowl, add the quinoa, toss and serve.

4 servings

GF – EL – VT – VG

Calories of main ingredients per serving: Quinoa 159. Almonds 40. Blueberries 22. Walnuts 40. Avocado 81. Pear 26. Raisins 31. Olive oil 60. Total of 459.

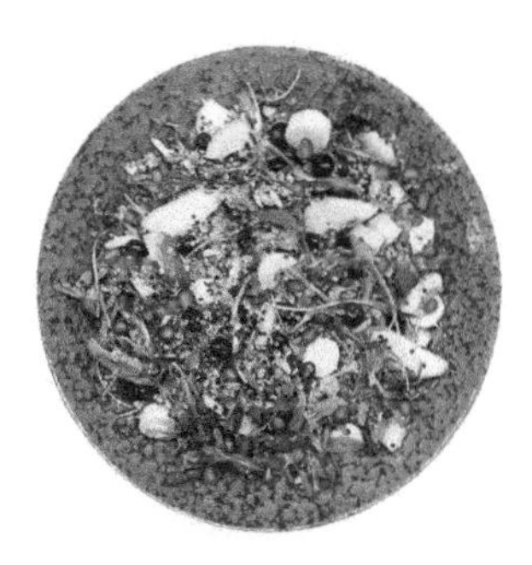

• Arugula is loaded with calcium, potassium, vitamins C, K, a and folate, and it is high in fiber and phytochemicals. Arugula maintains its peppery, spicy taste when its leaves are in the early stages, once the leaves mature arugula loses its character and becomes bitter.

Using heavy dressings in arugula salads is counterproductive. Arugula's distinctive flavor stands on its own merits. Olive oil and balsamic vinegar pairs best with arugula. Arugula pairs well with nuts, especially pecans and pine nuts, and of course tomatoes and avocado.

• *Blueberries: This super-fruit has an impressive nutrition profile. Blueberries have the highest antioxidant content of the most commonly consumed fruits. Flavonoids appear to be the berries' antioxidant with the most significant impact. They contain high amounts of fiber, vitamin C, vitamin K and manganese, and decent amounts of folate, choline, vitamins A and E, and manganese.*

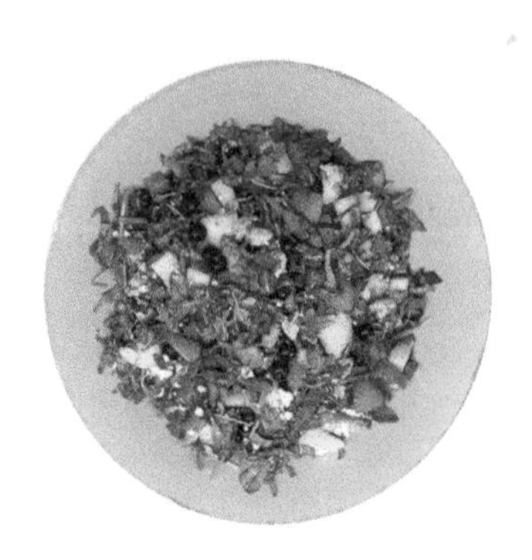

Strawberry and Arugula Fruit Salad with Sun Flower Poppy Seed Dressing

3 cups arugula, break into pieces
1 lb strawberries, sliced
½ small red onion, chopped
1 cup blueberries
1 avocado, sliced
1 mango, sliced
¼ cup pecan pieces
½ cup feta cheese, crumbled
1 tbsp fresh basil, chopped

Toss in a mixing bowl.

Sun Flower Poppy Seed Dressing
½ cup unsalted sun flower seeds

Pulse in a food processor 2 to 3 times. Transfer to a mixing bowl.

¼ cup olive oil
2 tbsp balsamic vinegar
1 tsp Dijon mustard
1 clove garlic, roasted and chopped
¼ tsp black pepper
¼ tsp honey
1 tsp juice from a lemon
1 tbsp poppy seeds

Add to the mixing bowl with the sunflower seeds and mix well.

4 servings

GF – EL

Calories in per serving in salad's main ingredients: Strawberries 38. Blueberries 22. Avocado 80. Mango 50. Pecans 47. Feta 50. Total of 287.

Calories in dressing per serving: Sun flower seeds 93. Olive oil 119. Total of 212.

• *Strawberries contain iron, copper, magnesium, phosphorus, vitamin B6, vitamin K and vitamin E. Strawberries are a good source of vitamin C, manganese, folate and potassium. Strawberries are the most cultivated berry in the United States. Most commercial strawberries in the United States are grown in California or Florida, where the climate helps to extend the strawberry growing season. The best strawberries are brightly colored, plump and have fresh green caps attached. Strawberries do not ripen after being picked, so if you buy the partly white ones, it means that they were not ripe when picked.*

Brown Rice and Sweet Potato Salad

Preheat oven to 375-degrees.

STEP 1

2 cups of water
2 cups

Bring to a gentle boil in a stockpot.

1 cup of brown rice.

Add to the pot and cook for 35 to 40 minutes over medium heat, until rice is tender. Drain, cool the rice and place in a large salad bowl.

STEP 2

1 medium-size sweet potato

While rice is being cooked, baked potato in the preheated oven for about 40 to 45 minutes. Cool cut into pieces and add them to the salad bowl.

STEP 3

2 green onions, chopped
2 roasted cloves garlic, chopped
½ tsp fresh ginger, minced
½ cup dried cranberries
¼ cup walnut pieces
1 pear, peeled and sliced
3 cups arugula
1 tbsp juice from a lime
2 tbsp olive oil
½ tsp cumin
½ tsp black pepper
1 tsp dry thyme

Add to the salad bowl, toss and serve.

2 servings

GF – EL – VT – VG

Calories in main ingredients per serving: Brown rice 171. Sweet potato 62. Cranberries 83 Walnuts 80. Pear 51. Olive oil 119. Total of 566.

• *Brown rice is an excellent source of plant-based protein and fabler.*

Vitamins A, c, D, E, K, B6, B12, thiamin, and folate. Minerals – calcium, iron, phosphorus, manganese, magnesium., selenium, potassium, and zinc.

• Cumin contains excellent amounts of iron and a good source of calcium, manganese, magnesium, phosphorus and vitamin B1. Cumin has a bitter taste with earth and nutty undertones. Cumin has a very distinct smoky and earthy flavor with hints of lemon and nutty and spicy undertones. Cumin seeds are significantly underrated, they are packed with the same flavors and when roasted they have a warm aroma. Ginger is a superspice; it is an excellent natural source of vitamin C, magnesium, potassium, copper, and manganese. Ginger is fierce and peppery with lemon/citrus aroma undertones. When cooked has a mild sweetness with warm flavor. Its complex flavor makes ginger versatile for both baking and cooking.

Grilled Seafood and Spinach Salad

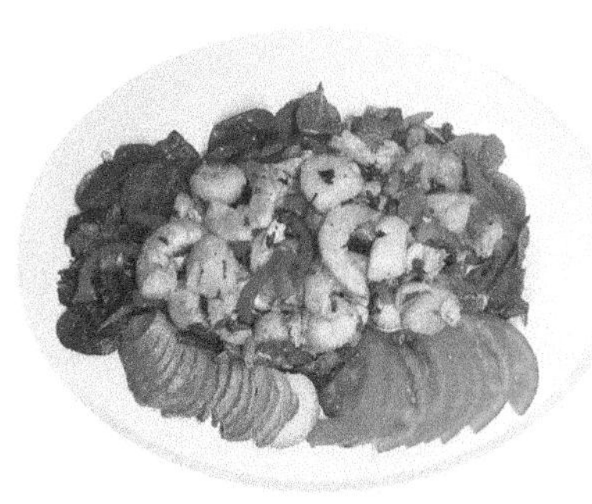

STEP 1

Dressing

4 tbsp olive oil
4 tsp red wine vinegar
1 small clove garlic, chopped
1 tsp fresh basil, chopped
½ tsp black pepper
1 tsp dry oregano
1 tsp dry thyme
1 tbsp ground mustard

Place in a small mixing bowl and blend ingredients well.

Salad

6 cups baby spinach
2 tbsp grated Parmesan cheese
8 snow pea pods, pull off strings and sliced
4 green onions, chopped
1 tbsp fresh dill, chopped
1 tbsp capers

Toss ingredients in a separated large mixing bowl. Pour half of the dressing into the mixing bowl with the salad, toss well and place salad in a serving platter.

Save the other half of the dressing.

STEP 2

Seafood

3 tbsp olive oil

Turn the heat of a flat grill to medium. When grill is hot, pour olive oil on it.

1 red bell pepper, sliced

Add to the grill and cook for 2 to 3 minutes

8 large sea scallops
10 jumbo shrimp, peeled
6 oz mahi-mahi, large cut

Add to the grill and cook with red peppers for about 4 to 5 minutes, until seafood is cooked.

¼ lemon

Squeeze lemon on top of seafood.

Transfer the grilled items into a mixing bowl, add the remaining dressing, toss well and arrange seafood and red pepper on top of the salad.

1 tbsp fresh Italian parsley, chopped

Sprinkle on top of the seafood and red pepper.

1 Avocado, sliced
1 tomato, sliced

Place on the side of the platter and serve.

4 servings

GF – EL

Calories in the main ingredients per serving: Olive oil 90. Scallops 40. Shrimp 30. Mahi-mahi 60. Total of 220.

Calories in dressing per serving: 80.

Spinach and Arugula Salad

4 cups arugula
4 cups baby spinach
¼ cup walnut pieces
¼ cup sliced almonds, toasted
1 red apple, peeled and sliced
1 cup grapes
1 cup raisins
1 tbsp fresh mint leaves, chopped
1 tbsp fresh basil leaves, chopped.

Mix in a large ball. Add Mustard vinaigrette dressing and serve.

2 servings

GF – EL – VT – VG

Calories per serving 253.

Black Beans with Roasted Garlic and Avocado

1 cup black beans. Use the canned black beans for this quick recipe. Drain well.
1 avocado, peeled and sliced
1 large tomato, large cut
3 roasted cloves garlic, chopped
1 yellow bell pepper, sliced
¼ red onion, sliced
Juice of ½ lime
¼ cup of olive oil
½ tsp black pepper
1 tsp of dry oregano
1 tbsp of fresh mint, chopped

Add to the salad bowl along with the black beans, toss and serve.

4 servings

GF – EL – VT – VG

Calories of main ingredients per serving: Black beans 170. Avocado 57. Olive oil 119. Total of 346.Black beans are rich in protein and fiber, extremely high in potassium, phosphorus, magnesium, folate, copper, manganese, iron and vitamin B1.

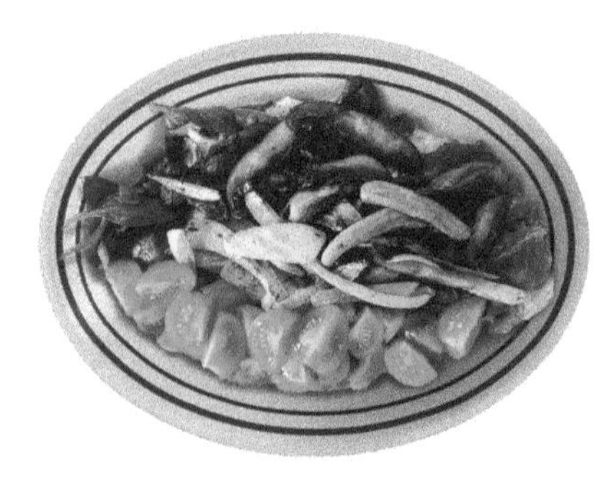

Grilled Fennel and Portobello Mushroom Salad

STEP 1

1 tbsp olive oil
Juice of ½ lemon
1 tsp black pepper

Place ingredients in a mixing bowl and mix well by hand.

2 fennel bulbs

Slice the fennel lengthwise, save the stalks and fronds for other use. Brush fennel with the olive oil mixture and cook on a flat grill until slightly brown, about 7 to 8 minutes. Set aside.

2 large portobello mushrooms, sliced

On the same grill sprinkle a bit of olive oil and grill mushrooms until soft 2 to 3 minutes.

STEP 2

8 large cherry tomatoes, cut in halves
2 cups baby spinach
1 tbsp capers
1 pear, peeled and sliced.
1 tbsp sliced almonds
1 tbsp fresh mint, chopped
1 tbsp fresh dill, chopped
Juice of ¼ lemon
1 tsp olive oil

Place ingredients in a mixing bowl, mix well and place them on a large serving platter.

Top the salad with grilled fennel, mushrooms.

4 servings.

EL – GF – EL – VG

Calories of the main ingredients per serving: Sorghum 79. Olive oil 60. Fennel bulb 14. Almonds 13. Total of 166.

• *Fennel is unique in a sense that has two different characteristics; the bulb is crunchy and citrusy, while the seed is aromatic and extremely licorice. Both bulb and seeds of the fennel plant are highly nutritious. All parts of the fennel plant are rich in powerful antioxidants and are packed with nutrients and are low in calories; fiber, vitamin C, calcium, iron, magnesium, potassium, and manganese. However, the most impressive benefits of all parts of fennel come from the antioxidants and potent plant compounds that they contain.these vegetables from absorbed oil is nearly impossible. It is here that the olive oil shines as the healthiest fat on the planet. Some studies have shown that olive oil unlocks the full nutritional benefits of the vegetables.*

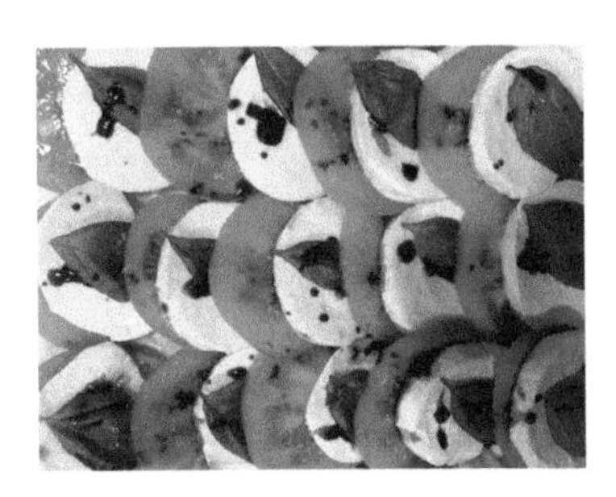

Caprese Salad with Avocado, Cantaloupe and Garlic Balsamic Glaze

4 large ripe tomatoes, sliced lengthwise
1 lb fresh mozzarella, sliced to about ¼ inch thick
¼ cup fresh basil
¼ cup fresh mint, chopped
1 avocado, sliced
½ cantaloupe, sliced

In a large serving platter, arrange tomatoes, mozzarella and basil leaves, alternating and overlapping at the edges. Place cantaloupe and avocado on the side of the platter and sprinkle all ingredients with the mint.

Garlic Balsamic Glaze

2 cups balsamic vinegar
1 tbsp honey
2 cloves garlic, crushed
1 tsp thyme
½ tsp pepper

Add ingredients in a saute pan and bring to boil. Reduce heat and simmer for about 12 to 15 minutes until liquid thickens.

1 tsp olive oil

Add to the pan, stir well and remove from heat.

Sprinkle glaze on top of the salad ingredients.

8 servings

GF – VT

Calories in main ingredients per serving: Mozzarella 138. Avocado 40. Cantaloupe 8. Total of 186.

• *Mozzarella is high in fat. Rich in protein and calcium.*

• *Basil: Besides being calorie-free, in addition to antioxidant vitamins and phenolics, is a rich source of vitamin K, zinc, calcium, magnesium, potassium and dietary fiber. Basil is sweet, highly aromatic with a peppery and licorice undertones. Basil shines when fresh or dried. When dried it takes a minty flavor.*

• *Mint contains potassium, magnesium, calcium, phosphorus, vitamin C, iron and vitamin A. Mint is sweet with an intense refreshing flavor and grassy, bitter undertones. It is surprisingly versatile for such an intensely flavored herb.*

Quinoa Fruit Salad with Yogurt

½ cup three-color quinoa
2 cups of water

Heat water in a small pot on medium heat. Add quinoa and cook for 15 to 18 minutes. Drain excess water. Cool.

1 ½ cups fresh pineapple, large cut
1 cup blueberries
6 kiwi, large cut
1 mango, large cut
½ cup raisins
2 green onions, chopped
1 tsp lime juice
1 tsp sesame seeds
1 tbsp sunflower seeds
½ cup low-fat real Greek yogurt
1 tsp honey
½ tsp nutmeg
The cooked quinoa

Mix gently by hand all ingredients in a mixing bowl.

2 tbsp fresh mint, chopped

Sprinkle on top of the salad and serve

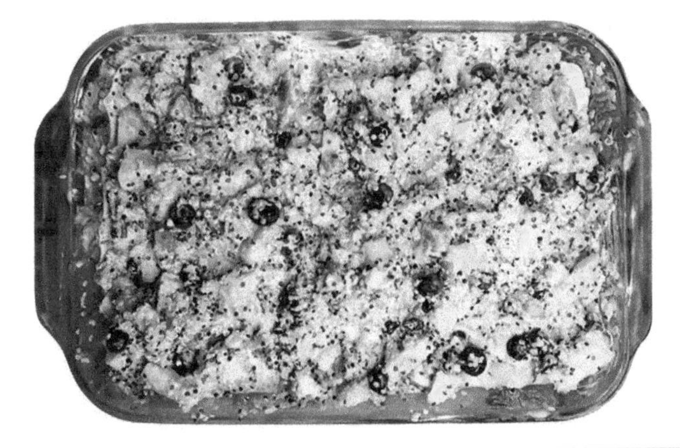

4 servings

EL – GF – VT

Calories of the main ingredients per serving: Quinoa 85. Pineapple 30. Blueberries 22. Kiwi 42. Mango 50. Raisins 31. Greek yogurt 22. Total of 282.

• *Kiwi contains a significant amount of fiber and antioxidants. It's also full of nutrients like vitamin C, vitamin K, vitamin E, folate, and potassium.*

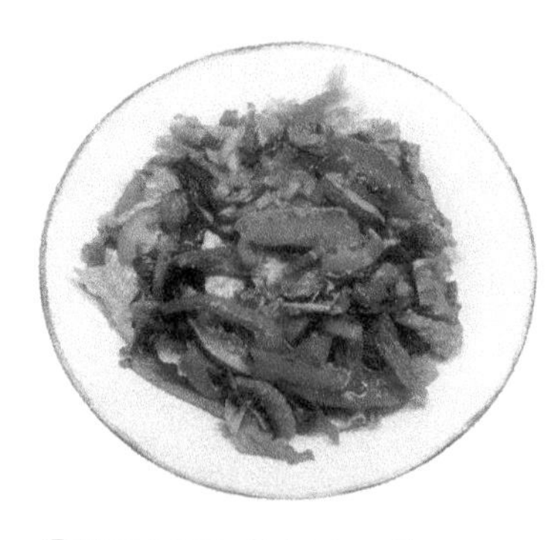

Grilled Lamb Salad

STEP 1

3 tbsp olive oil

Turn the heat of a flat grill to medium. When grill is hot, pour olive oil on it.

4 lamb chops; you could either use rib or loin chops.

Add to the grill and cook for about 5 to 6 minutes on each side. Remove debone and slice. Set aside.

1 large eggplant, sliced lengthwise
1 large red bell pepper, sliced

Place on the grill and cook on all sides until soft. About 6 to 7 minutes. Place vegetables on a paper towel to absorb access oil.

STEP 2

1 cup red cabbage, chopped
1 small green leaf lettuce, large cut
2 green onions, chopped
1 tomato, large cut

Toss in a mixing bowl and place in a serving platter.

STEP 3

Mint Vinaigrette Dressing
2 tbsp olive oil
1 tbsp balsamic vinegar
1 tbsp fresh mint, chopped
1 tbsp fresh basil, chopped
1 tbsp ground mustard
½ tsp black pepper

Blend in a mixing bowl. Add lamb meat, eggplant and red bell pepper, toss and arrange on top of the lettuce mixture.

2 servings

GF – EL

Calories of main ingredients per serving: Lamb chops 320. Eggplant 62. Olive oil 250. Total of 632.

• *Eggplant provides a good amount of fiber, vitamins and minerals in a few calories. They contain Vitamins K, C, B6, thiamin, folate, and minerals like manganese, potassium, magnesium, copper and niacin. Also, eggplants boast a high number of antioxidants. Eggplants are incredibly versatile and can be easily incorporated into your diet. I use them for grilling, salads, soups, or baked. I've heart many tricks to prepare eggplant for cooking; peel the skin, salt the eggplant for several hours, wash and place it between paper towels, and so on. Losing the peel, drenching them with salt or washing them, you lose the essential character of the eggplant – its bitterness, which is the most exciting future. I do none of that – I handle eggplants straight forward. I am careful with the oil used and when I grill them outdoors, I dip them, usually, in a mustard vinaigrette. There are several eggplant recipes in this book; I encourage you to try some of them.*

• *Cabbage is loaded with vitamins and minerals and comes with some surprising health benefits, all backed by science. It is exceptionally high in vitamins K and C and has smaller amounts of vitamins A, B6, folate, and riboflavin. Also, cabbage is high in fiber and powerful antioxidants. It contains manganese, calcium, potassium, and magnesium. Cabbage is versatile in the kitchen; it can be used in salads, soups and stews. Its outstanding nutrient profile, make cabbage an exceptionally healthy food to include in your diet.*

Footnote: Eggplant behaves like a sponge, soaking up large amounts of oil. Some chiefs are suggesting several ways to avoid oil soaking into the eggplant body. I am not sure what works. What works best is to use as less oil as possible. Among the vegetables that could be soaked with oil while grilled or fried are potatoes, bell peppers, zucchini. Preventing these vegetables from absorbed oil is nearly impossible. It is here that the olive oil shines as the healthiest fat on the planet. Some studies have shown that olive oil unlocks the full nutritional benefits of the vegetables.

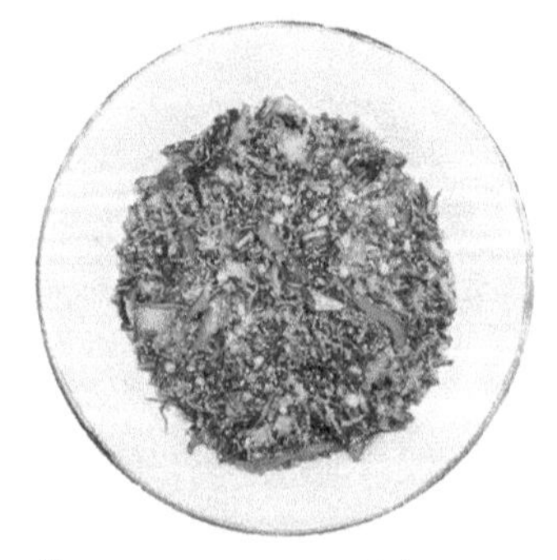

Buckwheat Mung Bean and Corn Salad

Preheat oven to 350-degrees.

STEP 1

3 cups of water

In a stock pot, bring water to a gentle boil.

1 cup mung beans.

Add to the pot and boil on medium heat for about 25 to 30 minutes. Mung Beans cook fast. There is no need to soak them. Remove, drain liquid if any and let it cool.

STEP 2

2½ cups vegetable broth

Bring to a gentle boil in a stock pot

1 cup buckwheat groats

Add to the pot and cook for 15 to 20 minutes. Remove, drain liquid if any and let it cool.

STEP 3

½ cup unsweetened shredded coconut

¼ cup sesame seeds

Place on a baking pan and cook in the preheated oven for 5 to 7 minutes, until coconut is golden brown. Remove and let it cool.

STEP 4

2 cups of frozen organic corn kernels - rinse with cold water to defrost.

2 cups red cabbage, chopped

1 small red bell pepper, sliced

3 green onions, chopped

8 sun-dried tomatoes, large cut

½ mango, peeled and chopped

1 tbsp Italian parsley, chopped

1 tbsp fresh basil leaves, chopped

1 tbsp fresh mint, chopped

1 tsp ground mustard

Add to a salad bowl, along with the mung beans and buckwheat and mix well.

⅛ cup olive oil

Juice from ½ lemon

½ tsp black pepper

Add to the salad bowl, toss well and serve.

4 servings

GF – VT – VG

Calories of main ingredients per serving: Mung beans 60. Buckwheat 47. Corn 40. Mango 18. Olive oil 60. Total of 225.

- *Buckwheat is an excellent source of fiber, rich in minerals, various plant compounds and a great source of fiber.*
- *Corn provides fiber, folate, thiamin, phosphorus, magnesium, and vitamin C.*
- *Mung beans are high in protein, fiber and folate. Reasonable amounts of manganese, magnesium, phosphorus, iron, copper, potassium, zinc, selenium and vitamins B1, B2, B3, B5, B6.*

Watermelon Salad with Basil Vinaigrette

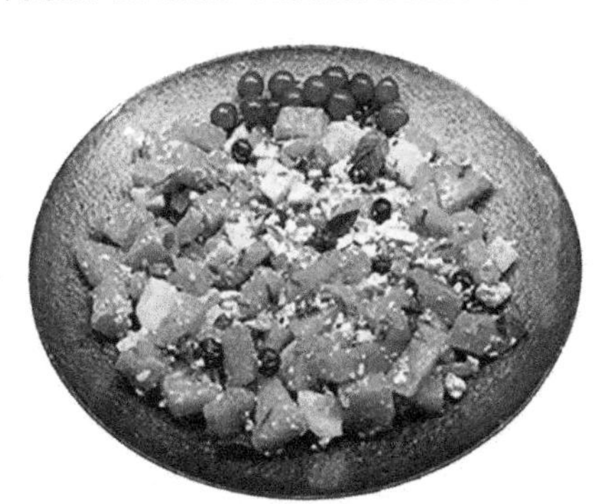

1 - 5 lbs watermelon, large cut.

A 5 lb watermelon will yield about 6 to 7 cups of diced fruit.

Or you could buy an 8 or 9 lb. watermelon and use 7 cups of the fruit and save the rest.

Place watermelon cubes in a colander and let it drain well.

1 cup blueberries

1 large cucumber, peeled and large cut

Place in a large mixing bowl along with the watermelon.

1 cup feta cheese, crumbled

½ cup walnuts pieces

¼ cup mint leaves, chopped

Add to the mixing bowl.

Basil Vinaigrette

2 tbsp fresh basil, chopped

2 tbsp balsamic vinegar

3 tbsp olive oil

½ tsp ground pepper

Mix in a bowl, toss with the watermelon salad and serve.

4 servings

Calories of main ingredients per serving: Watermelon 136. Blueberries 15. Feta 99. Walnuts 85. Olive oil 60. Total of 395.

Greek Peasant Salad

6 tomatoes, large cut
2 cucumbers, peeled and half slice
1 small green peppers, sliced
½ small red onions, sliced
Layer the vegetables in aserving salad plater in the order listed above.
2 cups of crumbled feta cheese.
Top the salad with it.
8 Kalamata olives pitted.
Arrange on top of the salad.
1 tbsp of dry basil
2 tbsp dry oregano
Sprinkle on top along with the basil.
¼ cup olive oil
Pour evenly on top the salad
1 tsp red wine vinegar
Sprinkle on top and serve

4 servings

EL – GF – VT

Calories of the main ingredients per serving: Feta 99. Olive oil 238. Total of 337.

• *Nutrients in tomatoes: They are the primary dietary source of the antioxidant lycopene, the most powerful antioxidant which has been measured in foods, and it has been linked to many health benefits. Other vegetables and fruits with lycopene are guavas, watermelon, papaya, grapefruit, sweet red peppers, asparagus, red cabbage, mango, and carrots. The importance of lycopene in tomatoes is because the general population consumed a higher amount of tomatoes than any other foods which contains the antioxidant lycopene. Tomatoes are also a great source of vitamin C, potassium, folate and vitamin K.*

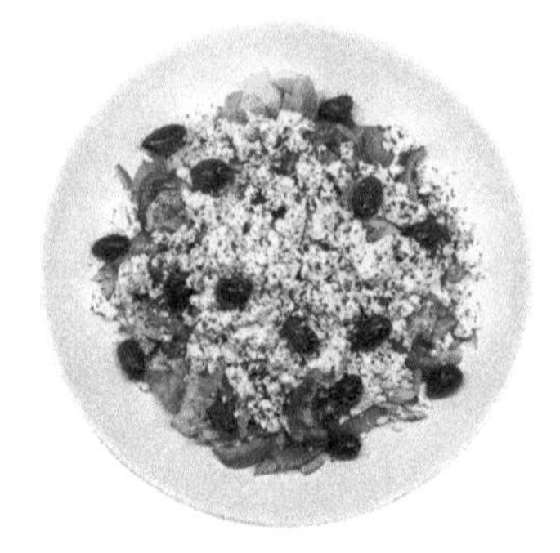

NOTE: This salad is our family's favorite salad and in my humble opinion the best salad ever. It is proof for the belief that some foods which are simple to make taste great. The secret to this salad is the use of fresh and quality ingredients. Use ripe tomatoes, real creamy feta cheese and of course extra virgin olive oil. Arrange the ingredients in order listed. Do not toss and the use of lettuce in this salad is sacrilegious.

Millet Corn Salad

Preheat oven to 400-degrees.

STEP 1

½ cup millet
Place millet in a saute pan and toast on medium heat for about 5 minutes. Stir frequently until millet as lightly golden. This process brings out millet's nutty flavor.
2 cups of water
In a stock pot, bring water to a gentle boil. Add millet and cook on medium heat for about 15 to 18 minutes, until millet is tender. Remove and cool.

STEP 2

1 medium-size sweet potato
While millet is being cooked, baked potato in the preheated oven for about 40 to 45 minutes.
Remove, let it cool, peeled and cubed.

STEP 3

1 cup frozen, organic corn kernels – rinse with cold water to defrost.
2 cups arugula
2 cups baby spinach
1 apple, peeled and large cut
2 green onions, chopped
½ red bell pepper, sliced
½ cucumber, peeled and half sliced
6 cherry tomatoes, cut in halves
1 tsp fresh mint leaves, chopped
1 tsp fresh Italian parsley, chopped
1 tsp fresh dill, chopped
1 tbsp juice from a lemon
1 tbsp olive oil
Place in a salad bowl, add the millet and sweet potato, toss well and serve.

2 servings

EL – GF – VT – VG

Calories of the main ingredients per serving: Millet 189. Olive oil 60. Sweet potato 57. Total of 306. Millet is high in fiber and protein and rich in niacin, B6 and folic acid, phosphorus, manganese.

• *Arugula is a nutrient-dense food that is high in fiber and with several important nutrients. It is loaded with calcium, potassium, vitamins C, K, a and folate, and it is high in fiber and phytochemicals. Arugula maintains its peppery, spicy taste when its leaves are in the early stages, once the leaves mature arugula loses its character and becomes bitter.*

Athenian Potato Salad

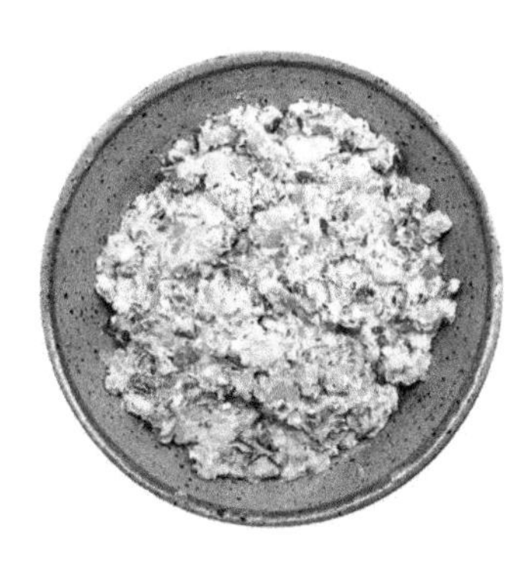

6 medium size potatoes

In a stock pot cover the potatoes with water and boil on medium heat for about 15 to 18 minutes until potatoes are tender. Discard water, cool and remove the skin and dice the potatoes. Place in a large mixing bowl.

1 red onion, chopped
1 celery stalk, chopped
8 cornichons, chopped
1 tbsp dry mustard
¼ cup sliced black olives
¼ cup sliced green olives
1 tsp black pepper
1 tsp prepared horseradish
2 tbsp olive oil
1 tbsp red wine vinegar
1 cup feta cheese, crumbled
2 cloves garlic, minced
1 tbsp dry oregano
1 tbsp dry basil
1 tbsp dry thyme
1 cup olive oil gluten-free mayonnaise

Place all ingredients with the potatoes and mix well with a spatula.

8 servings

EL – GF – VT

Calories of the main ingredients per serving: Potatoes 112. Black olives 8. Green olives 12. Olive oil 34. Feta cheese 55. Mayonnaise 116. Total of 337.

• *Potatoes are a good source of many vitamins and minerals, such as potassium and vitamin C and contain moderate amounts of protein and fiber. The main dietary component of potatoes is carbs. Potatoes lose some of their nutrients during the cooking process, but the reduction of nutrients could be minimized when baked or boiled with the skin on. Here are the vitamins and mineral in potatoes; vitamin C, B6, folate, and potassium. Potatoes are rich in antioxidants that which are responsible for the health benefits of potatoes; however, the potato antioxidants are mostly concentrated in the skin.*

Brown Rice, Black Bean Fruit Salad

3 cups of water
2 cups vegetable broth
Heat in a stock pot.
1 cup brown rice, wash before cooking

Add and cook on medium heat for about 35 to 40 minutes, until rice is tender. Remove, drain extra liquid and cool.

2 cups cooked black beans. Use canned black beans for this salad. Drain well.
1 mango, peeled and chopped
1 apple, peeled and chopped
1 avocado, chopped
½ cup golden raisins
¼ cup walnut pieces
½ red onion, chopped
1 cup artichoke hearts, chopped
½ cup feta, crumbled
1 tbsp capers
1 tbsp fresh parsley, chopped
1 tbsp fresh basil, chopped
1 tsp dry oregano
½ tsp cumin
2 tbsp olive oil
1 tsp red wine vinegar

Place ingredient in a mixing bowl, including brown rice and mix well.

4 servings

GF – EL – VT

Calories of the main ingredients per serving: Brown rice 172. Mango 50. Apple 24. Avocado 80. Golden raisins 31. Walnuts 33. Artichoke hearts 75. Feta 50. Olive oil 60. Total of 517.

• *Black beans are a good source of protein, very high in dietary fiber, magnesium, potassium, phosphorus and folate. Black beans also have high levels of flavonoids, which have antioxidant abilities. They also contain omega-3 fatty acid. They are a great source of folic acid and have incredibly high levels of the rare compound molybdenum, which is very difficult to find in any other food. Black beans have long been a protein-rich staple food of many Latin American cultures. Because of their incredibly high protein content, black beans are great for vegans and vegetarians.*

Tzatziki Sauce

1 large cucumber, peeled and remove seeds
3 cloves garlic

Place into a food processor and pulse 2 or 3 times.
Remove from the food processor and drain the liquid if any.

1 cup low-fat real Greek yogurt
1 tsp white pepper
1 tbsp juice from a lemon
1 tsp white vinegar
1 tbsp olive oil
1 tbsp fresh dill, chopped

Place in a mixing bowl along with cucumber and garlic and mix with a spoon. Refrigerate.

4 servings

EL – GF - VT

Spring Berry Chicken Salad

Preheat oven to 350-degrees
1 cup unsweetened shredded coconut
½ cup sliced almonds

Place in a baking pan and bake for about 4 to 5 minutes until coconut is golden brown. Remove and cool.

2 tbsp olive oil
Heat in a saute pan.
1 - 8 oz chicken breast
2 small yellow squash, half sliced
Add the chicken and saute on medium heat for 4 to 5 minutes. Turn chicken breast and cook for 6 to 8 minutes longer until chicken is done. Remove chicken and add the squash.
Cook for 2 to 3 minutes and remove – slice chicken breast into short strips.
In a large mixing bowl, add the chicken, coconut, almonds, and squash.
1 cup frozen raspberries, defrosted. Discard most of its liquid.
8 cups spring mix lettuce – about 12 oz
8 large strawberries, sliced
1 tbsp sesame seeds
2 tbsp olive oil
1 tbsp balsamic vinegar
Add to the mixing bowl, toss well and serve.

Note: the raspberries, along with the olive oil and balsamic vinegar makes a nice raspberry dressing.

2 servings

EL – GF

Calories of the main ingredients per serving: Coconut 23. Almonds 142. Olive oil 238. Chicken 187. Raspberries 32. Strawberries 24. Total of 646.

• *Strawberries contain iron, copper, magnesium, phosphorus, vitamin B6, vitamin K and vitamin E. Strawberries are a good source of vitamin C, manganese, folate and potassium.*

• *Raspberries are rich in vitamin C and K. Also good amounts vitamin*

E, iron, potassium, manganese and lesser amounts of thiamin, riboflavin, niacin, pantothenic acid, vitamin B-6, calcium.

• *Sesame seeds have beneficial nutrients and are rich in many minerals and vitamins which includes selenium, calcium, phosphorus, zinc, copper, dietary fiber, protein, molybdenum, folate, magnesium, iron, manganese, vitamin B1 and B6.*

Feta Dressing

3 cups feta cheese, crumbled
2 tbsp red wine vinegar
3 tbsp olive
1 tbsp dry oregano
1 tsp black pepper
2 cups low-fat, gluten-free mayonnaise
2 cloves garlic, minced
1 tsp dry thyme
1 tsp dry basil

In a mixing bowl, mix all ingredients well with a spatula. This is by far the most popular dressing I've created.

Use for salad dressing, vegetable dip, in meat sandwiches or eggs. I use this dressing to make the Athenian potato salad – great for BBQ events.

Refrigerate in jars. Good for 2 months. Vinegar and garlic act as natural preservatives

10 servings

GF – VT

Calories of main ingredients per serving: Mayonnaise 116. Feta cheese 120. Olive oil 35. Total of 271.

Sun Flower Poppy Seed Dressing

1 cup unsalted sun flower seeds
Pulse in a food processor 2 to 3 times. Transfer to a mixing bowl.
½ cup olive oil
4 tbsp balsamic vinegar
2 tsp Dijon mustard
2 clove garlic, roasted and chopped
½ tsp black pepper
½ tsp honey
2 tsp juice from a lemon
1 tbsp poppy seeds

Add to the mixing bowl with the sunflower seeds and mix well.

8 servings

GF – EL

Calories in dressing per serving: Sun flower seeds 93. Olive oil 119. Total of 212.

Grilled Eggplant Salad

1 cup red cabbage, sliced
1 romaine lettuce, large cut
2 green onions, chopped
1 tomato, sliced
1 tbsp fresh dill, chopped
1 tbsp fresh basil, chopped

Toss in a mixing bowl and set aside.

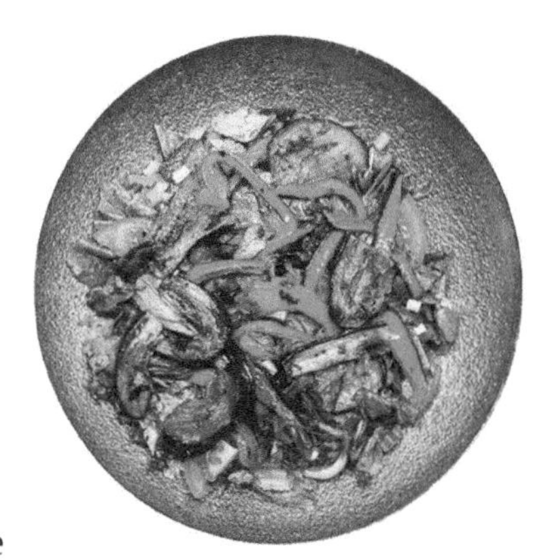

¼ cup olive oil

Pour the olive oil on a flat grill.

1 large eggplant, sliced lengthwise
1 large red bell pepper, sliced

Place on the grill and cook on all sides until soft. About 8 to 10 minutes. Remove from the grill, and set aside. Slice eggplant into large pieces.

Dressing

3 tbsp olive oil
1 tbsp balsamic vinegar
1 tbsp fresh mint, chopped
1 tbsp fresh basil, chopped
1 tsp Dijon mustard
½ tsp black pepper

Place in a mixing bowl and blend well with a fork. Pour half of the dressing into the mixing bowl with the lettuce/cabbage and toss. Place lettuce on a serving platter.

Place the grilled eggplant and red peppers into the bowl with the remaining dressing, gently stir and arrange on top of the lettuce. Ready to serve.

2 servings

GF – EL – VT – VG

Calories of main ingredients per serving: Eggplant 62. Olive oil 250. Total of 312.

The Ultimate Chicken Salad

2 tbsp olive oil
Heat in a saute pan.
1 - 8 oz chicken breast
Add the chicken and saute on medium heat for 4 to 5 minutes. Turn chicken breast and cook for 6 to 8 minutes longer until chicken is done. Remove chicken and slice into small slices.
1 medium size romaine lettuce, cut into large pieces
1 sweet red pepper, sliced
2 hearts of palm, large cut
1 tbsp capers
½ cup quartered artichoke hearts, sliced
4 mushrooms, sliced
1 medium tomato, large cut
1 small cucumber, peeled and half slice
½ cup feta cheese, crumbled
1 tsp fresh dill weed, chopped
1 tbsp fresh basil, chopped
2 tbsp olive oil
1 tbsp red wine vinegar
Add the above ingredients into a large mixing bowl, toss well and place in a salad serving plater. Add the sliced chicken on top and serve.

2 servings

EL – GF

Calories of the main ingredients per serving: Chicken 187. Olive oil 238. Hearts of palm 10. Artichoke hearts 22. Feta cheese 99. Total of 556.

• *Chicken is an excellent source of protein. The different parts of the chicken and are low in fat and low in sodium, making it ideal for people who want to lose weight and maintain muscle. Overall, chicken is an excellent addition to your diet. It is an excellent source of niacin and selenium. And a good source of vitamin B6, and phosphorus, choline, pantothenic acid and vitamin B12.*

Mustard Vinaigrette Dressing

2 ½ cups olive oil
1 cup red wine vinegar
2 cloves garlic, minced
2 tbsp onion, minced
1 tsp dry basil
1 tsp black pepper
1 tsp dry dill weed
1 tbs dry oregano
1 tsp dry thyme
½ tsp dry rosemary
3 tbsp Dijon mustard
Mix well. Refrigerate in a glass jar.

Makes about 32 oz dressing.

EL – GF – VT – VG

Calories of main ingredients per oz: Olive oil 150.

Italian Dressing

2 ½ cups olive oil
1 cup red wine vinegar
2 cloves garlic, minced
1 tbsp onion, minced
1 tbsp grated Romano cheese
1 tbsp dry basil
1 tsp black pepper
1 tsp dry dill weed
1 tbsp dry oregano
1 tsp dry thyme
1 tsp dry parsley
Mix well and refrigerate in glass jars.

Makes about 32 ounces

EL – GF – VT – VG

Calories of main ingredients per oz: Olive oil 150.

Yogurt Dressing

1 cucumber, peeled and cut in pieces
2 green onions, white part only
Place in a food possessor and pulse 2 or 3 times. Move ingredients into a bowl of a mixer.
1½ cups low-fat, gluten-free mayonnaise
1 tbsp Graded Parmesan cheese
1 cup low-fat sour cream
1½ cups Greek yogurt
Juice of 1 lemon
1 tsp Dijon mustard
1 tsp black pepper
Add to the food mixer and mix well. Makes about 4 cups. Refrigerate in a jar. Lemon acts as a natural preservative and will keep sauce fresh for about 60 days in your refrigerator. Use this sauce for salad dressings and vegetable dip as well. Refrigerate in jars and use as needed.

10 servings

GF – VT

Calories of main ingredients per serving: Mayonnaise 87. Sour cream 46. Greek yogurt 16.Total of 149.

When switching to a healthier diet, one of the foods challenging to replace is mayonnaise. If you are looking for food items that taste the same, or even better from the ones you are using, vegenaise is the best substitute for mayonnaise. Vegenaise is lighter and has a pleasant balance of flavors. However, the bonus is in the nutrients. Vegenaise contains no cholesterol, it has, about, one-third saturated fats, and it has no additives or preservatives. Even if you are a mayonnaise connoisseur, on a tasting contest, you won't notice the difference. Once you start to transition into a healthier eating lifestyle and start searching for healthier options, vegenaise should be on the top of your list.

In recipes call for mayonnaise, in this book or any other cookbooks, I recommend to substitute mayonnaise with vegenaise.

What is Wrong with this Picture?

The definition of canning is to preserve processed food sealed in an airtight container. Canning provides a shelf-life ranging from one to five years, and sometimes much longer.

If you are an advocate of fresh food, there is a lot wrong with this picture.

Assuming that the canned foods are safe, the can itself might pose a health-risk. There is no secret that eating canned foods may result in unhealthy eating risks because often the food preservatives used contain high amounts of salt or sugar, both harmful to the body. Personally, I cannot keep up with all the new preservatives. Every so often there is a new friendly-sounding preservative. The name might be different, but the ingredients are pretty much the same. Besides the unhealthy preservatives, the quality of the food in cans tends to be of a lower level. There is the botulism issue, a severe and deadly bacterial infection causing food poisoning. Granted, botulism is an extremely rare possibility, caused by poor and unsanitary processing of packaging canned foods. However, the most worrisome is the plastic contaminants in canned foods, caused by the plastic coating inside the can. The plastic coating (Bisphenol or BPA) was added in order to keep foods fresh. But keeping the foods fresher comes at the expense of harming you because there is good evidence that the inner plastic lining may be toxic. I don't believe that a logical person would suggest that canned foods, especially fruits and vegetables, are better or as good as fresh foods. Fresh foods retain most of their nutrients while items in a can do not. So, why do we keep opening cans of foods? There are many reasons; Convenience, accessibility, long shelf-life, and affordability. To keep BPA out of your body, you must limit the use of canned foods and take these steps:

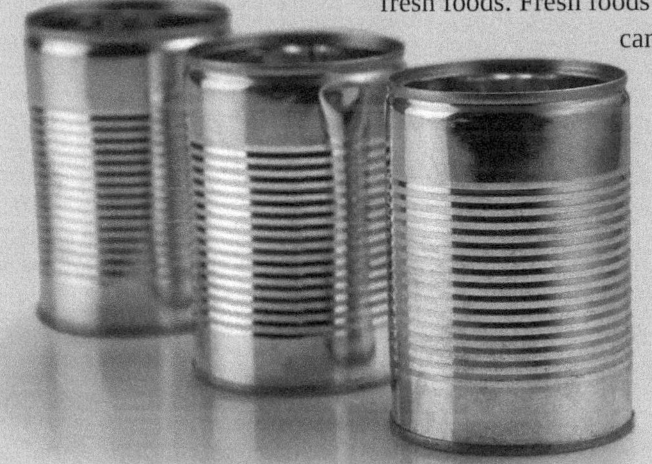

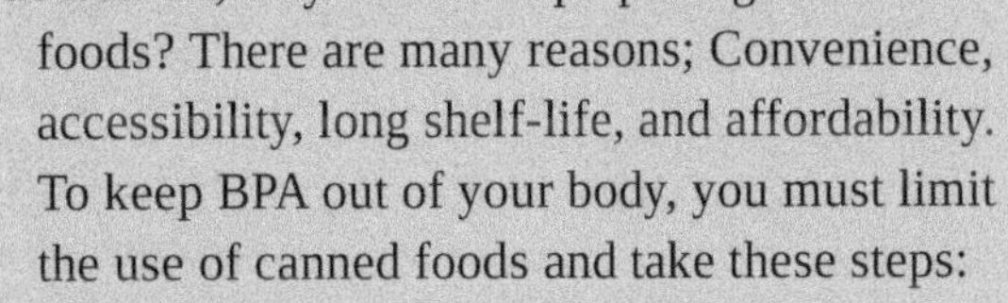

Use fewer canned foods, make sure they are BPA-free. However, BPA-free cans are safer but not completely safe.

If available, it is best to buy foods packed in glass jars.

Soups

"Ligidakis is a legend locally, both for his selfless charitable involvement and his very idiosyncratic restaurant."
Tribune Newspapers

"His fans speak of Nick Ligidakis with the reverence customary reserved for Michealangelo's statue of David."
Phoenix Gazette

Chicken Broth

2 gallons of water
2 lbs chicken parts with bones
1 onion, large cut
4 carrots, large cut
2 celery stalks, large cut
4 garlic cloves, peeled and whole
6 mushrooms, cut in halves
6 bay leaves
8 peppercorns
1 tsp fresh rosemary
1 tbsp dry thyme
1 tbsp fresh parsley
1 tsp ground sage
1 tbsp flaxseed

Add into a large stock pot and simmer on low heat for about 2 to 3 hours. Strain broth and refrigerate in glass jars.

Nutrients: Loaded with protein and fiber. This broth contains lignans and antioxidants, including curcumin and lycopene – plentiful amounts of minerals and vitamins, and omega-3 fatty acids.

Vegetable Broth

2 gallons of water
2 tbsp olive oil
1 onion, peeled and large cut
2 stalks celery, sliced
3 carrots, large cut
4 cloves garlic, peeled, add the whole cloves
2 tsp black pepper
⅛ cup fresh Italian parsley
1 cup of red cabbage, sliced
1 medium tomato, large cut
1 sweet potato, with the skin, large cut
1 cup baby spinach
6 bay leaves
1 tsp dry thyme
1 tsp fresh rosemary
1 tsp dry oregano
½ tsp turmeric
1 small piece of ginger root
1 tbsp flaxseed

Add into a large stock pot and simmer on low heat for about 2 to 3 hours. Strain broth and refrigerate in glass jars.

• *Nutrients: Loaded with plant-based protein and fiber. This broth contains lignans and antioxidants, including curcumin and lycopene – plentiful amounts of minerals and vitamins, and omega-3 fatty acids.*

Roasted Eggplant Soup

½ cup olive oil
1 lg eggplant, large cut
1 lg red bell pepper, large cut
8 baby onions, peeled and sliced in halves

Place in a stock pot and saute on medium heat for about 5 minutes – until eggplant is soft

8 cups vegetable broth
4 cups of water

Add to the stockpot.

1 cup cooked garbanzo beans
½ cup of frozen okra pieces
2 cloves of garlic, chopped
¼ cup sun-dried tomatoes, chopped
6 small ripe tomatoes, chopped
1 tsp fresh rosemary
1 tsp dry thyme
1 tsp cumin
1 tsp black pepper

Add to the pot. Cook on medium heat for 40 to 45 minutes

4 servings

GF – ED – VT – VG

Calories of the main ingredients per serving: Olive oil 15. Garbanzo beans 68. Sun-dried tomatoes 15. Total 98.

Mung Bean Soup with Coconut

4 cups of vegetable broth
6 cups water

Add to a stockpot and bring to a gentle boil.

1 cup dry mung beans.

Add to the pot and start cooking the beans on medium heat.

1 small onion, chopped
2 celery stalks, sliced
2 medium carrots, sliced
2 garlic cloves, chopped.
5 Roma tomatoes, chopped

Place ingredients in a stock pot and continue cooking for about 15 minutes.

1 small zucchini, Julienne sliced
8 asparagus, discard the hard bottom part, sliced
1 cup spinach, chopped
1 tsp ground turmeric
1 tsp black pepper
½ tsp ground ginger
½ tsp ground fennel
1 tbsp red wine vinegar
2 tbsp unsweetened shredded coconut

Add to the pot and cooks for about 15 more minutes. Beans should be tender by now.

If not continue cooking for a few more minutes.

8 servings

GF – EL – VT – VG

Calories of main ingredients per serving: Mung beans 90. Tomatoes 22 Total of 112.

Black Bean Soup

1½ cup black beans

Place them in a stockpot. Cover the beans with water and bring them to a quick boil.

Remove from the heat and let them soak for about 1 hour.

Place the pot back on the stove and turn your heat to medium.

Bring it to a gentle boil.

4 cups vegetable broth
4 cups of water

Add to the pot. Reduce to medium heat.

1 celery stalk, chopped
½ red onion, chopped
2 carrots, sliced
1 yellow bell pepper, chopped
2 bay leaves
3 garlic cloves, chopped
1 tbsp parsley
½ tsp coriander
⅛ cup red wine vinegar
1 tsp cumin
3 small tomatoes, chopped
1 tsp black pepper
1 tsp rosemary
1 tsp thyme

Add all ingredients in the stock pot and cook for about 60 to 65 minutes, until beans are tender.

8 servings

GF – EL – VT – VG

Calories of main ingredients per serving: Black beans 413.

Cranberry Beans and Butternut Squash Soup

STEP 1

1½ cups cranberry beans

Cover the beans with water and bring them to a quick boil. Remove from the heat and let them soak for about 1 hour.

5 cups of water

4 cups vegetable broth

Add to the pot with the beans and bring to a gentle boil. Total cooking time on medium heat 60 to 65 minutes.

In the meantime prepare the ingredients for this recipe.

STEPS 2

1 lg sweet potato, peeled and large cut

1 lg onion, chopped

4 garlic cloves, chopped

6 Roma tomatoes, chopped

At about 30 minutes cooking the beans add to the boiling pot these ingredients in the pot.

1 lg apple, peeled, take off seeds and large cut

1 small butternut squash, peel the skin, large cut

1 cup kale leaves, chopped

2 cups baby spinach

¼ tsp fresh ginger, chopped

2 cinnamon sticks

1 tbsp dry oregano

1 tbsp dry basil

1 tbsp ground cardamom

1 tsp black pepper

¼ tsp ground cloves

1 tbsp ground sage

1 tbsp cumin

Add these ingredients 15 minutes later.

Continue cooking until you reach 60 to 65 total cooking time or until beans are tender.

8 servings

GF – EL – VT – VG

Calories of the main ingredients per serving: Cranberry beans 122. Potato 15. Apple 15. Butternut squash 8. Total of 160.

• *Nutrients in butternut squash: It is a good source of Vitamin E, Magnesium, Phosphorus, Potassium and Copper, and an excellent source of Dietary Fiber, Vitamin A, Vitamin C, Vitamin K, Iron, and Manganese.*

• *Cranberry beans have one of the highest content of the essential nutrients of any plant-based food. They are a rich source of dietary fiber, extremely high in protein, packed with B-complex vitamins, essential minerals and various components of antioxidant properties. This bean is a plant-protein powerhouse.*

Sorghum and Farro, Kale Soup

STEP 1

6 cups vegetable broth

2 cups of water

In a stockpot and bring the liquid to a gentle boil.

½ cup whole grain sorghum.

½ cup farro

Add to the pot and start cooking on medium heat. Total cooking time should be 40 to 45 minutes.

STEP 2

2 tbsp olive oil

As soon as you start cooking the grains, heat the olive oil in a large saute pan.

2 celery stalks, chopped

2 large carrots, sliced

1 small onion, chopped

3 cloves garlic, chopped

Add to the pan and saute for about 5 to 6 minutes.

5 small tomatoes, chopped

Add to the pan and simmer for about 9 to 10 minutes.

Add vegetables to the pot with the grains.

STEP 3

1 cup kale, large cut

½ cup baby spinach

1 tsp black pepper

2 tsp dry thyme

¼ tsp chopped ginger root

1 tsp dry mustard

Add to the pot with the grains and cook until you reach 45 to 50 minutes total cooking time or until the grains are tender.

4 servings

VT – VG

Calories per serving for the main ingredients: Olive oil 60. Sorghum 82. Total of 142.

Potato Spinach and Quinoa Soup

STEP 1

1½ cup water

In a stockpot, bring water to a gentle boil.

½ cup quinoa

Add to the water and cook for about 12 to 15 minutes on medium heat. Set aside.

STEP 2

3 cups vegetable broth
4 cups water
8 medium size potatoes, peeled and large cut

In a separate large stockpot, bring the liquid to a gentle boil, add potatoes and cook on medium heat for about 15 minutes.

4 green onions, chopped, include green part.
2 cups baby spinach
3 garlic cloves, chopped
½ tsp nutmeg
1 tsp white pepper
1 tsp dry thyme
½ tsp cardamom
½ tsp coriander

Add to the pot and continue cooking for another 10 to 15 minutes, until potatoes are tender.

Turn heat to low.

STEP 3

6 eggs
½ lemon

Separated eggs in two mixing bowls. With the wire whisk, beat the egg yolks until smooth then beat the egg whites until foamy. Merge the egg yolks into the egg whites while beating.

1 lemon

In a third bowl, squeeze out the lemon juice. Add the lemon juice slowly to the egg mixture, while mixing with the whisk. With a soup spoon, scoop some of the hot broth from the pot. Slowly add to the egg mixture while whisking. This part is essential. If you add the egg mixture directly to the hot broth, your soup will curl. Turn heat off.

The cooked quinoa
½ cup grated Parmesan cheese.

Once the egg mixture is blended with the rest of the soup, add Parmesan cheese, a little at a time stirring well. Add quinoa, mix well and serve.

Your guest will swear that there is cream in this soup, but you know better. 6 servings

GF – VT

Calories of main ingredients per serving: Quinoa 42. Potato 330. Eggs 175. Parmesan 81. Total of 628.

Lentil Potato Soup

¼ cup olive oil
2 large carrots, sliced
2 celery stalks, sliced
1 small onion, chopped
2 shallots, sliced
10 baby red potatoes, peeled and large cut

Place all ingredients in a stock pot and simmer on medium heat for about 8 minutes.

5 cups vegetable broth
8 cups of water

Bring to a gentle boil.

2 cups lentils
1 tsp black pepper
1 tsp fresh rosemary
1 tsp dry thyme
1 tsp dry oregano
½ tsp cumin
6 bay leaves
½ tsp fresh ginger, chopped
⅓ cup red wine vinegar

Add to the boiling pot, cover and simmer for about 30 to 35 minutes, until lentils are tender.

8 servings

GF – EL – VT – VG

Calories of main ingredients per serving: Vegetable broth 7, Lentils 172. Baby potatoes 25. Total of 204.

It is also a great source of plant-based protein and fiber.

Cranberry Beans with Lamb Meatballs

STEP 1

1½ cups cranberry beans
4 cups vegetable broth
4 cups of water

Place the beans in a stock pot. Cover the beans with water and bring them to a quick boil. Remove from the heat and let them soak for about 1 hour. Place the pot back on the stove and turn your heat to medium. Bring it to a gentle boil. Total cooking time on medium heat 60 to 65 minutes. In the meantime prepare the ingredients for this recipe.

STEP 2

1 large onion, chopped
10 baby carrots
3 celery stalks, chopped
4 small tomatoes, chopped
3 cloves garlic, chopped
¼ cup fresh basil, chopped
¼ cup fresh Italian parsley, chopped
1 tbsp rosemary
1 tsp black pepper
1 tsp dried thyme
1 tsp dried oregano
1 tbsp cumin
4 bay leaves
½ tsp ground cloves
½ tsp fresh ginger, chopped
1 tbsp apple cider vinegar

Add to the pot when 30 minutes in the boiling process. Continue cooking for another 30 to 35 minutes, until beans are tender. Total cooking time 60 to 65 minutes.

While beans are being cooked, prepare the meatballs.

STEP 3

Lamb Meatballs
1 lb ground lamb
2 garlic cloves, minced
¼ onion, minced
½ tsp white pepper
1 tsp thyme
1 tsp oregano
1 tsp cumin
1 tsp mint
1 tbsp juice of a lemon
2 tbsps walnuts, grind in a food processor

Place all ingredients in a mixing bowl and mix well by hand. Shape the mixture into small firm balls. Place on a baking pan, lightly greased with olive oil and bake in a 350-degree oven for about 15 minutes. Makes 10 to 12 meatballs. Add the meatballs to the stock pot when beans are done the cooking.

8 servings

GF – EL

Calories of main ingredients per serving: Black beans 29. Lamb 160. Walnuts 15. Total of 214.

• *Nutrients in cranberry beans: Cranberry beans have one of the highest content of the essential nutrients of any plant-based food. They are a rich source of dietary fiber, extremely high in protein, packed with B-complex vitamins, essential minerals and various components of antioxidant properties. This bean is a plant-protein powerhouse.*

Cauliflower, Beet and Sweet Potato Soup

STEP 1

¼ cup unsweetened shredded coconut, toasted in the oven. Cool and save.

STEP 2

2 tbsps olive oil
Heat in a stock pot.
1 small sweet potato, peeled and large cut
3 beets, peeled and large cut
1 small onion, chopped

Add and sauté 10 to 12 minutes on medium heat.

1 cup cauliflower florets
2 cloves garlic, chopped
1 tbsp red wine vinegar
1 tsp fresh dill, chopped
½ tsp black pepper
1 tsp cumin
1 tsp dry thyme
½ cup ground mustard
4 cups vegetable broth

Add to the pot and simmer for about 15 minutes. Remove and let cool for 10 to 15 minutes. Place ingredient in a food processor and puree the mixture. Return to pot and heat. When served, sprinkle top of the soup with the toasted coconut.

4 servings

GF – EL – VT – VG

Calories of the main ingredients per serving: Coconut 52. Olive oil 60. Beets 27. Potato 41. Total of 180.

• *Cauliflower contains a high amount of fiber and provides a significant amount of antioxidants. It is high in choline, an essential nutrient for our body, found only in a few foods. Cauliflower, along with broccoli, is one of the best plant-based sources of choline. Cauliflower contains high amounts of vitamin C, which acts as an antioxidant. It is low in calories but high in fiber and water, perfect for low-fat diets. Besides vitamin C, cauliflower contains vitamins K, B6, folate and pantothenic acid. It also includes several minerals, like potassium, magnesium, manganese and phosphorous.*

• *Beets contain almost all the vitamins and minerals that we need. It is an excellent source of fiber, folate and vitamin C. Beets are a good source of vitamin B6, magnesium, potassium, phosphorous, manganese and iron. Beets are often recommended to be used by athletes. Several studies suggest that its dietary compounds enhance athletic performance. They are low in calories and high in nutrients, which makes beets a great source of a healthy and balanced diet.*

Millet Soup with Sweet Potato Puree

STEP 1

3 small sweet potatoes

Place potatoes in a stock pot, cover them with water and boil for about 20 to 25 minutes. Cool, peel and mash the potatoes in a mixer on slow speed.

STEP 2

1 cup millet

Add millet to a small saute pan and toast for about 5 minutes under medium heat, frequently stirring, until the millet is golden. This brings out millet's nutty fragrance.

STEP 3

2 tbsp olive oil

Heat in a stockpot.

½ onion, chopped
1 celery stalk, chopped
¼ fennel bulb, chopped
2 medium-size carrots, sliced
1 shallot, chopped
2 cloves garlic, chopped

Add to the pot and simmer for 3 to 4 minutes longer.

3 Roma tomatoes, chopped

Add to the pot and simmer for about 10 minutes, until tomatoes are soft.

4 cups vegetable broth
5 cups of water

Add to the pot and heat for about 5 minutes.

The toasted millet
½ tsp ground coriander
1 tsp cumin
Juice of ½ lemon
1 tsp dry thyme
1 cup baby spinach
½ tsp fresh rosemary
¼ tsp ginger root, minced
1 tsp black pepper
The sweet potato puree

Add to the pot and cook for 15 to 20 minutes on medium heat or until millet is tender.

4 servings

GF – EL – VT – VG

Calories of main ingredients per serving: Sweet potatoes 90. Millet 259. Olive oil 60. Total of 409. Nutrients in sweet potato: Sweet potato is rich in potassium and vitamin B6.

• *Millet is high in fiber and protein and rich in niacin, B6 and folic acid, phosphorus, manganese.*

• *Fennel is an excellent source of vitamin C, calcium, pantothenic acid, magnesium, iron and niacin. It contains reasonable amounts of dietary fiber, potassium, molybdenum, manganese, copper, phosphorus and folate.*

• *Ginger is an excellent natural source of vitamin C, magnesium, potassium, copper, and manganese. Ginger is fierce and peppery with lemon/citrus aroma undertones. When cooked has a mild sweetness with warm flavor. Its complex flavor makes ginger versatile for both baking and cooking.*

Avgolemono Soup

STEP 1

8 cups vegetable broth
1 tbsp black pepper
Heat in a stock pot on medium heat.

6 oz of chicken, large cut
Add and cook for about 4 to 5 minutes

½ cup white basmati rice
Add and cook for about 15 to 20 minutes, until rice is cooked.

STEP 2

While rice is being cooked, prepare the eggs.

8 eggs, separated in two mixing bowls
With the wire whisk, beat the egg yolks until smooth. Beat the egg whites until foamy.
Slowly add the egg yolks into the egg whites while beating.

2 lemons
In a separate bowl, squeeze out their juice. Add the liquid slowly to the egg mixture, mixing with the whisk.

STEP 3

After the rice is cooked, turn heat to low. With a soup spoon, scoop some of the hot broth from the pot. Slowly add to the egg mixture while whisking. This part is very important. If you add the egg mixture directly to the, your soup will curl. Once the egg mixture is blended with the rest of the soup. Remove and serve.

This soup is known as the Greek Penicillin. Whenever someone has a cold in our home, I am called upon to make this soup.

Not sure about the healing properties of this amazing soup but somehow it works.

4 servings

GF

Calories of main ingredients per serving: Eggs 108. Chicken 71. Basmati rice 160. Total of 339.

• *Nutrients in chicken is an excellent source of protein. The different parts of the chicken and are low in fat and low in sodium, making it ideal for people who want to lose weight and maintain muscle. Overall, chicken is an excellent addition to your diet. It is an excellent source of niacin and selenium. And a good source of vitamin B6, and phosphorus, choline, pantothenic acid and vitamin B12.*

• *Eggs, the egg whites contain high-quality protein, riboflavin and selenium. However, while the whole egg provides you with a massive amount of nutrients the majority of the egg's nutrients is found in the yolks: Vitamin D, E, K, A, B6, B12, calcium, iron, phosphorous, manganese, folate and selenium. By not using the egg yolk you are throwing a massive amount of multivitamins away. I suggest doing your research about the myth of the egg yolk. Also, eggs are one of the only foods that naturally contain vitamin D.*

Main Dishes

"Seems only newcomers and visitors to the Valley are unfamiliar,
and then only briefly, with the food of Nick Ligidakis.
Dazzling Phoenix dinners since the 80's."

Phoenix Downtown

"Like saguaros, Camelback mountain and red-tile roofs. Nick Ligidakis
seems to be a permanent part of our desert landscape."

New Times

Ancient Grain Pilaf

STEP 1

4 cups vegetable broth
4 cups of water
  In a stockpot and bring the liquid to a gentle boil.
1 cup barley
1 cup farro
  Add to the pot and start cooking on medium heat. Total cooking time should be 40 to 45 minutes. Discard liquid if any and set aside.

STEP 2

1 ½ cups water
  In a separate stockpot, bring the water to a gentle boil.
½ cup quinoa
  Add to the water and cook for about 15 to 18 minutes. Discard liquid if any and set aside.

STEP 3

1 medium size sweet potatoes
  Boil for about 15 to 18 minutes. It should be tender on the outside and slightly resistance to a fork. Remove and cool. Discard the skin and large cut. Set aside.

STEP 4

¼ cup olive oil
  Heat in a large saute pan.
½ red onion, chopped
1 large carrot, chopped
1 red apple, sliced
1 cup broccoli florets, large cut
4 cloves garlic, chopped
2 Portobello mushrooms, sliced
  Add to the pan and saute on medium heat for about 10 minutes.
¼ cup pecan pieces
1 avocado, peeled and sliced
1 tbsp fresh rosemary, chopped
1 tsp dry thyme
1 tsp dry oregano
½ tsp pepper
½ tsp cumin
½ tsp fresh ginger, minced
1 tsp ground mustard
The cooked sweet potato
1/4 cup of white cooking wine
  Add to the pan and cook for about 5 minutes longer.
The cooked farro
The cooked barley
The cooked Quinoa
  Add to the pan and frequently stirring, cook for 1 to 2 minutes.
  Suggestion: Serve with Mango Relish – see the index to find the recipe.

4 servings

VT – VG

Calories of main ingredients per serving: Farro 207. Barley 176. Quinoa 43. Pecans 47. Avocado 80. Sweet potato 62. Vegetable broth 10. Olive oil 119. Total of 743.

• *Farro is wheat. Therefore, it naturally contains gluten. The level of gluten in farro is lower than any modern wheat. However, farro is a healthy and nutritious ancient grain. It provides more fiber than most other grains and a wide range of healthy antioxidants. It is a good source of protein, fiber, and nutrients like magnesium, zinc and some B vitamins.*

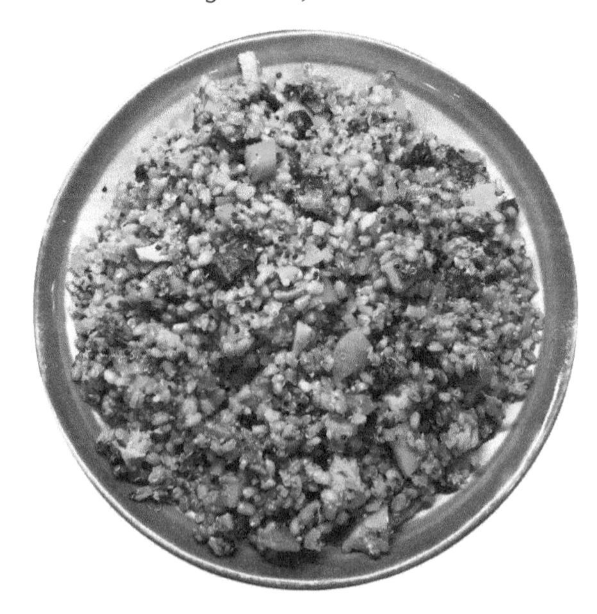

Tomato Pesto Millet

STEP 1

2 cups millet

Add millet to a small saute pan and toast for about 5 minutes over medium heat, frequently stirring, until the millet is golden. This brings out millet's nutty fragrance.

STEP 2

7 cups of water

Bring water to a gentle boil in a stockpot, add millet and boil on medium heat for about 15 to 18 minutes. Drain access water if any.

2 tbsp olive oil
½ onion, chopped
2 shallots, chopped

Saute in a large pan on medium heat for 2 to 3 minutes.

2 tbsp white cooking wine
1 clove garlic, chopped
6 Roma tomatoes, chopped

Add to the pan and cook for 8 to 10 minutes.

1 cup vegetable broth
⅓ cup capers
1 cup baby spinach
1 tbsp dry thyme
½ tsp black pepper

Add to the pan and cook for another 3 to 4 minutes. Turn heat off – do not remove the pan from the stove-top.

STEP 3

½ cup fresh basil
3 cloves garlic, roasted
2 tbsp olive oil
1 tsp grated Parmesan
¼ cup walnuts
2 tbsp feta cheese, crumbled

Place in a food processor and pulse 2 to 3 times. Add to the saute pan.

The cooked millet

Add to the saute pan, turn the heat on to low, stir for a minute or two, remove and serve.

Suggestion: Serve with **Lemony Artichokes** – see the index to find the recipe.

2 servings

GF – VT – omit Parmesan for EL, VG.

Calories of main ingredients per serving: Millet 368. Olive oil 190. Total of 560.

Baked Vegetables

Preheat oven to 375-degrees

In a large baking pan, arrange the following items:

1 large sweet potato, peeled and large cut
8 assorted color baby potatoes, peeled
12 mixed color baby carrots
1 zucchini, large cut
1 yellow squash, large cut
I green red bell pepper, large cut
1 red bell pepper, large cut
10 cremini mushrooms
4 shallots, peeled and half sliced
4 cloves garlic, peeled and half sliced
½ tsp fresh ginger, chopped

Add 1 cup of water into the pan.

In a mixing bowl add the following ingredients:

½ cup olive oil
Juice of 1 lemon
1 clove garlic, chopped
1 tbsp dry basil
1 tbsp dry oregano
1 tbsp dry thyme
1 tsp pepper

Mix well and pour over vegetable – Bake in the preheated oven for about 1 hour.

Periodically baste the vegetables using a large serving spoon.

Suggestion: Serve with **Black Bean Garlic, Avocado Salad** – see index for the recipe.

4 servings

GF – EL – VT – VG

Calories in main ingredients per serving: Sweet potato 31. Baby potatoes 20. Olive oil 238. Total of 289.

• *Carrots are particularly good source of beta-carotene, fiber, vitamin K, potassium and antioxidants.*

• *Zucchini is a good source of protein, vitamins A, C, K, B6, folate, magnesium, potassium, manganese, thiamin, niacin, copper and phosphorus*

• *Mushrooms are rich in riboflavin, folate, thiamine, pantothenic acid, and niacin. Mushrooms are also rich in selenium, copper, and potassium.*

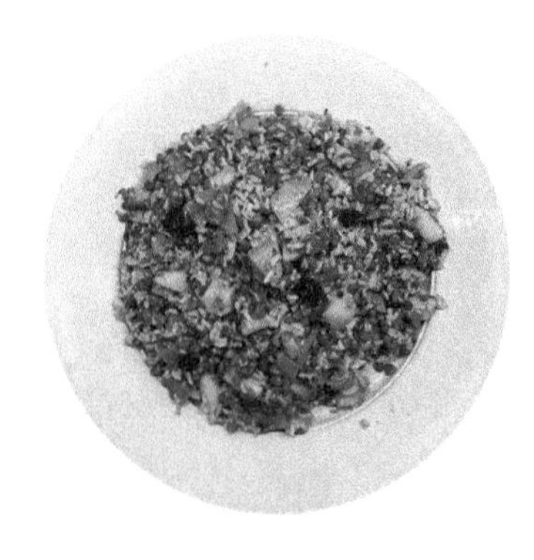

Brown Rice and Lentil Vegetarian Stew

3 cups vegetable broth
4 cups of water
Bring to boil in a large stockpot.
1 cup brown rice
Add to the pot and start cooking on medium heat.
1 cup lentils
Fifteen minutes into the cooking process of the brown rice, add lentils into the stockpot.
Continue cooking for another 18 to 20 minutes until rice and lentils are tender.
Turn heat off, drain any extra liquid.
2 tbsp olive oil
Heat in a large saute pan.
1 large sweet potato, peeled and large cut
1 large carrot, half cut
Add to the pan and saute on medium heat for 8 minutes.
½ onion, chopped
2 cloves garlic, chopp ed
1 cup kale, chopped
4 Roma tomatoes, chopped
½ cup frozen sweet peas
1red apple, peeled and sliced
½ tsp fresh ginger, chopped
½ tsp black pepper
1 tsp cumin
½ tsp turmeric
1 tsp dry oregano
1 tsp dry thyme
½ tsp ground cloves.
½ cup vegetable broth
Add to the pan and saute on medium heat for 8 to 10 minutes.
The cooked rice and lentils
Add to the pan and cook for another 4 to 5 minutes, until liquid from the vegetable broth is absorbed.

4 servings

EL – GF – VT – VG

Calories of main ingredients per serving: Brown Rice 160. Lentils 172. Sweet potato 29. Apple 24. Total of 385.

• *Like brown rice, black rice has similar nutrient levels, but it contains higher amounts of antioxidants, protein, and fiber. Black rice has substantial mineral content including potassium, iron and copper, and high levels of vitamin E and zinc. Lentils are packed with both soluble and insoluble fiber. They are extremely high in manganese, magnesium, thiamin, folate and vitamin B6 and have good amounts of phosphorus, iron, and potassium.*

Eggplant Ragout

4 tbsp olive oil
Heat in a medium-sized stockpot.
2 large eggplants, large cut
2 red bell peppers, large cut
4 shallots, large cut
3 celery stalks, large cut
4 cloves garlic, chopped
Add to the pot and saute, string frequently for about 8 to 10 minutes.
6 Roma tomatoes, chopped
Add to the pot, stir well and continue cooking for 3 to 4 minutes.
1 cups vegetable broth
1 tbsp pine nuts
1 tbsp fresh mint, chopped
1 tbsp fresh Italian parsley, chopped
½ tsp cinnamon
¼ cup golden raisins
1 tbsp capers
1 tbsp balsamic vinegar
1 tsp cumin
1 tsp dry thyme
1 tsp dry oregano
1 tsp black pepper
Add to the pot and continue cooking on medium heat for another 10 to 12 minutes.
Ready to serve.

EL – GF – VT – VG

4 servings

Calories of main ingredients per serving: Olive oil 119. Eggplant 68. Pine nuts 15. Raisins 33. Total of 235.

• *Eggplant contains an impressive array of vitamins and minerals, such as significant amounts of fiber, folate, potassium, and manganese, as well as vitamins C, K, and B6, phosphorus, copper, thiamin, niacin, and magnesium. Bell peppers are loaded with vitamins and minerals and are extremely rich in vitamin C. They also contain vitamins B6, K1, E, A and folate and reasonable amounts of potassium. Bell peppers are rich in various antioxidants, especially carotenoids.*

Grilled Vegetable Mousaka

STEP 1

2 tbsp olive oil

Heat in a saute pan.

1 small onion, chopped

2 cloves garlic, chopped

Add and saute on medium heat for 3 to 4 minutes.

8 Roma tomatoes, chopped

½ tsp cinnamon

½ tsp nutmeg

1 tsp dry oregano

½ tsp black pepper

¼ tsp ground ginger

1 tbsp fresh Italian parsley, chopped

½ cup vegetable broth

Add to the pan and simmer for about 15 to 16 minutes.

1 tbsp grated Romano cheese

Add to the pan, stir well and remove from the heat.

STEP 2

⅓ cup olive oil

1 large eggplant, sliced lengthwise

2 medium size potatoes, peeled and sliced lengthwise

2 small zucchini, cut the tough ends and slice lengthwise

Pour olive oil on a flat grill and grill the vegetables on both sides. Eggplant should be soft, potatoes and zucchini light golden. Remove and set aside.

STEP 3

4 cremini mushrooms, sliced

¾ cup low-fat ricotta cheese

In a large ceramic rectangular baking dish (about 9"x13") first layer half of the eggplant.

Next layer half of the potatoes, half of the zucchini and half of the mushrooms.

Pour half of the sauce over the vegetables.

Spread the ricotta evenly on top of the sauce.

Layer the rest of the vegetables, starting with the eggplant.

Pour the rest of the sauce.

1 cup shredded mozzarella

Layer on top and bake in a preheated 375-degree oven for about 35 to 40 minutes, until the top is light brown.

Suggestion: Serve with **Greek Peasant Salad** – see the index to find the recipe.

2 large servings

GF – VT

Calories of main ingredients per serving: Olive oil 200. Potato 82. Mozzarella 186. Ricotta 60. Total of 525.

• *Tomatoes are the primary dietary source of the antioxidant lycopene, the most potent antioxidant which has been measured in foods, and it has been linked to many health benefits. Other vegetables and fruits with lycopene are guavas, watermelon, papaya, grapefruit, sweet red peppers, asparagus, red cabbage, mango, and carrots. The importance of lycopene in tomatoes is because the general population consumed a higher amount of tomatoes than any other foods which contains the antioxidant lycopene. Tomatoes are also a great source of vitamin C, potassium, folate and vitamin K.*

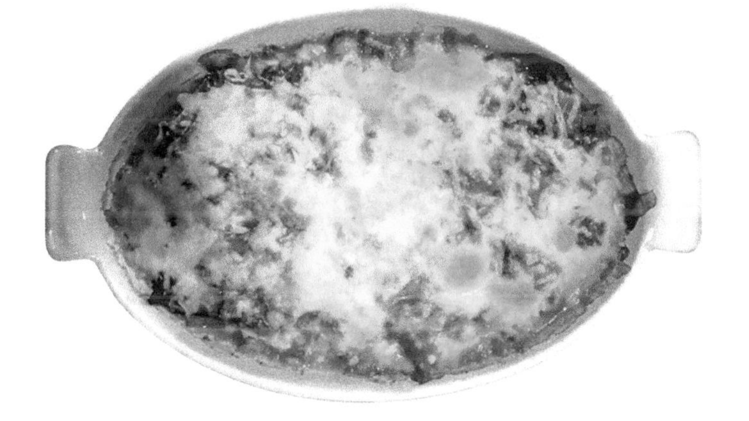

Vegetables Brochettes with Raisin Buckwheat

STEP 1

Vegetable Brochettes

4 long stainless steel or bamboo skewers
2 yellow squash zucchini, sliced into 1/2″ rings
12 mini red bell peppers, or a mix of red and yellow peppers
12 white baby onions, peeled – choose the largest sizes
12 cremini mushrooms – choose the largest sizes
12 baby white potatoes, peeled

Thread the above items in the skewers in the order you like, mixing vegetables and colors. Refrigerate.

STEP 2

Marinate

2 tbsp olive oil
juice of 1 lemon
1 tsp dry oregano
1 tsp dry thyme
½ tsp cumin
1 tsp fresh mint, chopped
½ tsp black pepper
1 clove garlic, minced

Place in a small mixing bowl and set aside.

STEP 3

Raisin and Cashew Buckwheat

2 tbsp olive oil

Heat in a medium-sized stockpot.

½ onion, chopped
½ red bell pepper, chopped
2 cloves garlic, chopped

Add to the pot and cook on medium heat for 4 to 5 minutes.

2 ½ cups vegetable broth

Add to the pot and heat for 2 to 3 minutes

1 cup buckwheat groats
½ tsp cumin
½ tsp ground cardamom
1 tsp ground mustard
½ tsp turmeric
½ tsp black pepper
1 tsp fresh Italian parsley, chopped
¼ cup golden raisins
¼ cup cashews, chopped

Add to the pot and cook for 13 to 15 minutes longer. Remove from the heat.

GF – EL – VT – VG

STEP 4

Grilled Sweet Potatoes

4 tbsp olive oil

Place on a large saute pan.

2 medium-size sweet potatoes, peeled and sliced

Heat the oil on medium heat and add the potatoes. Saute for 2 to 3 minutes.

1 large red pepper, sliced
½ red onion, sliced

Add and saute for 4 to 5 minutes.

½ lime
1 tsp cumin
2 tsp thyme

Squeeze lime juice and sprinkle thyme and cumin on the vegetables and cook for another 2 to 3 minutes until potatoes are cooked.

Set aside.

GF – EL – VT – VG

STEP 5

Grill the prepared brochettes on the outdoor charcoal. Occasionally brushing them with the marinade.

Place buckwheat on a large serving platter. Arrange the brochettes on top of buckwheat and the grilled vegetables on the side.

4 servings

Calories in this recipe for marinade per serving: Olive oil 60.

Calories in this recipe for brochettes per serving: Potatoes 78.

Calories in this recipe for sweet potatoes per serving: Olive oil 119. Sweet potatoes 52. Total of 171.

Calories in this recipe for raisin cashew buckwheat pilaf per serving: Olive oil 60. Buckwheat 142. Raisins 28. Cashews 40. Total of 270.

• *Onions are high in vitamin C, fiber, and folic acid. They also contain calcium and iron. Buckwheat is a rich source of protein and dietary fiber. It has high amounts of potassium, manganese, phosphorus, magnesium and reasonable amounts of zinc, copper, selenium, and iron. It contains decent amounts of folate, riboflavin, niacin, and pantothenic acid vitamins. Buckwheat is a rich source of protein and dietary fiber. It has high amounts of potassium, manganese, phosphorus, magnesium and reasonable amounts of zinc, copper, selenium, and iron. It contains decent amounts of folate, riboflavin, niacin, and pantothenic acid vitamins.*

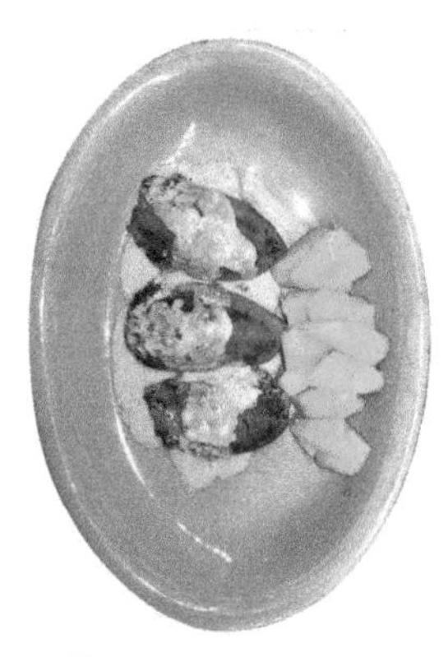

Gorgonzola Roasted Peppers

STEP 1

¼ cup baby spinach, chopped
½ cup feta cheese, crumbled
¼ cup low-fat ricotta cheese
¼ cup low-fat mozzarella cheese, shredded
2 green onions, chopped
1 tsp fresh dill, chopped
1 tsp black pepper
½ tsp cinnamon
1 tsp fresh mint leaves, chopped
1 tbsp pine nuts

Mix all ingredients in a bowl.

2 large size roasted red peppers. *See the index for – How to roast red peppers.*

Being careful not to break the red peppers, stuffed them with the spinach stuffing.

2 tbsp olive oil

Heat in a saute pan and saute the stuffed peppers for 5 to 6 minutes on each side.

Once done, place peppers in a serving dish.

STEP 2

1 tbsp almond milk
½ cup Gorgonzola cheese

Heat gently in a small pan, stirring until cheese is melted.

Pour over peppers and serve.

Suggestion: Serve with **Sautéed** Asparagus – see the index to find the recipe.

2 servings

GF – VT

Calories of main ingredients per serving: Feta 99. Ricotta 107. Olive oil 119. Mozzarella 70. Total of 395.

• *Some of the many nutrients of spinach are folate, vitamin C, niacin, riboflavin, and potassium. However when spinach is cooked there are higher levels of vitamins A and E, protein, fiber, calcium, zinc, thiamin and iron.*

• *Asparagus is an excellent source of fiber, folate, vitamins A, C, E and K, as well as chromium.*

• *Bell peppers are low in calories and exceptionally rich in vitamin C and other antioxidants. Bell peppers come in various colors; green, red, yellow, and orange. The green bell pepper has a slightly bitter flavor than the other three. All bell peppers have similar nutrients. Bell peppers are mainly made up of water and carbs and are an excellent fiber source. Bell peppers are loaded with vitamins and minerals and are extremely rich in vitamin C. They also contain vitamins B6, K1, E, A and folate and moderate amounts of potassium. Bell peppers are rich in various antioxidants, especially carotenoids.*

Brussels Sprouts with Almond, Date Sauce

Preheat oven to 375-degrees.

1 lb Brussels sprouts, trim bottom and cut in halves from top to bottom
Juice of 1 lime
12 pearl onions, peeled
2 shallots, peeled and large cut
2 tbsp olive oil

In a mixing bowl, toss well together. Place mixture in a baking dish and bake in the preheated oven for about 20 to 22 minutes, until sprouts are starting to be light brown. Remove from the oven.

1 tbsp olive oil

Heat in a large saute pan.

2 cloves garlic, chopped

Add the garlic along with the sprout mixture and saute for 2 to 3 minutes on medium heat.

¼ cup golden raisins
6 seedless, dry dates, large cut
1 tbsp fresh dill, chopped
1 tbsp fresh parsley, chopped
1 tbsp fresh mint, chopped
1 tsp dry thyme
1 tsp black pepper
¼ cup slivered almonds
1 tbsp sesame seeds

Add to the pan and continue cooking on medium heat for about 6 to 7 minutes.

Turn heat to low.

1 cup unsweetened almond milk
1 tbsp ground mustard

Add to the pan and stir well for 1 minute. Turn off heat

⅓ cup grated Romano cheese

Add to the pan, stir well and serve.

Suggestion: Serve with **Spinach and Arugula Salad** – see the index to find the recipe.

2 servings

GF – VT

Calories for main ingredients in this recipe per serving: Olive oil 119. Brussels sprouts 98. Romano cheese 70. Golden raisins 55. Dates 69. Almonds 66. Total of 477.

• *Brussels sprouts are high in fiber, vitamin K and vitamin C. They also contain vitamin B6, potassium, iron, thiamine, magnesium, and phosphorus.*

• *Basil is calorie-free, in addition to antioxidant vitamins and phenolics, is a rich source of vitamin K, zinc, calcium, magnesium, potassium and dietary fiber. Basil is sweet, highly aromatic with a peppery and licorice undertones. Basil shines when fresh or dried. When dried it takes a minty flavor.*

• *Dill contains excellent amounts of fiber, niacin, phosphorus, copper, riboflavin, vitamin B6, magnesium, and potassium. Dill is a light herb with sweet, grassy and anise undertones.*

Mung Beans and Barley with Kale

STEP 1.

4 cups of water

In a stockpot bring water to a gentle boil.

1 cup barley

Add to the water and cook on medium heat for about 45 to 50 minutes, until barley is tender. Discard the access liquid.

STEP 2.

3 cups vegetable broth

4 cups water

Bring to a gentle boil. Reduce to medium heat.

1 cup mung beans

1 onion, large cut

1 large carrot, half sliced

1 medium sweet potatoes, peeled and large cut

3 small tomatoes, chopped

3 cloves garlic, chopped

Add to the pot and cook for 15 minutes.

½ cup baby spinach

1 cup kale, large cut

1 tsp coriander

1 tsp dry thyme

1 tsp fresh ginger, chopped

1 tsp turmeric

Add to the pot and cook for another 10 to 12 minutes, until beans are fully cooked.

The cooked barley

Add the cooked barley to the pot, stir well and simmer for another 2 minutes.

Suggestion: Serve with **Feta Pesto Mushrooms** – see the index to find the recipe.

4 SERVINGS

EL – VT – VG

Calories of main ingredients per serving: Mug beans 180. Barley 176. Total of 356. *Mung beans are high in protein, fiber and folate. Reasonable amounts of manganese, magnesium, phosphorus, iron, copper, potassium, zinc, selenium and vitamins B1, B2, B3, B5, B6.*

• *Kale is extremely high in vitamin C, in fact, one cup of kale contains more vitamin C than an orange. Kale is one of the world's best sources of vitamin K, a cup of kale containing almost seven times the recommended daily amount. Kale is also loaded with vitamins A, and many powerful antioxidants are found in kale. It also provides moderate amounts of vitamin B6, thiamin, riboflavin, niacin. Kale is high in minerals; it is an excellent plant-based source of calcium and magnesium. Other minerals like manganese, copper, potassium, iron and phosphorous are found in kale.*

Mediterranean Barley and Artichoke Risotto

STEP 1

6 cups of water

Place in a stockpot and bring water to a gentle boil.

1 cup barley

Add to the pot and cook for 40 to 45 minutes, until barley is tender.

Discard liquid.

While barley is being cooked, prepare the rest of the recipe.

STEP 2.

2 tbsp olive oil

Heat in a large saute pan.

½ onion, chopped
2 cloves garlic, chopped
1 tbsp capers

Add to the pan and saute for 5 to 6 minutes.

5 small tomatoes, chopped
1 tbsp fresh Italian parsley, chopped
6 artichoke hearts, sliced
6 mushrooms, sliced
8 pitted Kalamata olives, sliced

Add to the pan and saute for 7 to 8 minutes.

½ tsp black pepper
1 tsp dry thyme
1 tsp dry oregano
1 tsp dry basil
¾ cup of vegetable broth

Add to the pan, turn heat to low and simmer for 7 to 8 minutes. If barley is not cooked by now, turn off the heat.

The cooked barley
½ cup grated Romano cheese

Add to the pan, stir well on low heat for a minute and serve.

Suggestion: Serve with Sun-Dried Tomato Hummus – see the index to find the recipe.

2 servings

VT

Calories of the main ingredients per serving: Barley 352. Olive oil 119. Romano cheese 28. Artichoke hearts 180. Kalamata olives 25. Total of 704.

• *Artichoke hearts is one of my favorite vegetables, not only for its unique taste but I can use it for just about any foods. What's not to love about this one. Low in fat, high in potassium and a good source of protein, unique fiber, vitamin C, folate, magnesium and dietary fiber. And one of the top vegetables in term of antioxidants.*

Crabmeat Portobello with Blue Cheese and Pear Relish

Preheat oven to 375-degrees

16 oz crabmeat
½ cup blue cheese, crumbled
3 green onions, chopped
2 cloves garlic, roasted and chopped
1 tbsp fresh Italian parsley, chopped
1 tbsp fresh basil, chopped
1 tsp dry thyme
1 tsp dry mustard
1 tsp white pepper
1 tbsp olive oil
½ cup grated Parmesan cheese

Place all ingredients in a mixing bowl and mix well by hand

8 large portobello mushrooms
Remove stem.

Place mushrooms on a baking pan.

½ cup low-fat ricotta cheese

Place the ricotta evenly in the six cavities of the mushrooms.

⅓ cup sun-dried tomatoes, chopped

Divide into six parts and top the ricotta with.

Divide crabmeat mixture into six parts, place each part on the top of the sun-dried tomatoes and press gently to fill the mushroom cavities.

Bake in the preheated oven for 30 to 32 minutes.

Pear and Apple Relish

1 pear, peeled and chopped
1 apple, peeled and chopped
½ small red onion, chopped
1/3 cup golden raisins, chopped
½ cup frozen corn kernels, defrosted
1 tbsp olive oil
1 tsp fresh mint, chopped
1 tsp fresh rosemary, chopped
1 tbsp lemon juice
¼ tsp white pepper
1 tbsp sesame seeds
¼ tsp fresh ginger, minced

Mix all ingredients well.

Lemony Artichoke Hearts

2 tbsp olive oil

Heat in a saute pan.

2 cups artichoke hearts, quartered
½ red onion, sliced
1 clove garlic, chopped

Add to the pan and saute on medium heat for 6 to 7 minutes.

Juice of ½ lemon
1 tbsp fresh rosemary, chopped
1 tbsp fresh Italian parsley, chopped
1 tsp dry thyme
1 tsp dry oregano
½ tsp black pepper

Add and cook for another 3 to 4 minutes.

¼ cup grated Parmesan cheese
Turn heat off, add Parmesan into the pan, steer well.
Serve crab cakes with pear-apple relish and artichokes as a side dish.

4 servings

GF – VT

Calories in the main ingredients of the crabmeat mixture per serving: Crab meat 55. Blue cheese 51. Parmesan cheese 36. Ricotta 30. Sun dried tomatoes 59.Total of 231.

Calories in portobello mushrooms per serving: Total of 30.

Calories in the main ingredients of the pear relish per serving: Pear 26. Apple 24. Corn 20. Total of 68.

Calories in the main ingredients of the lemony artichokes: Artichoke hearts 35. Olive oil 96. Parmesan cheese 27. Total of 158.

• *Crabmeat is a good source of vitamin C, folate and magnesium, and an excellent source of protein, vitamin B12, phosphorus, zinc, Copper and selenium.*

• *Capers contain fiber, protein, vitamins C, A, K, E, niacin, riboflavin, as well as iron and potassium.*

• *Mushrooms are rich in B vitamins such as riboflavin, folate, thiamine, pantothenic acid, and niacin.*

Sorghum Chicken Pilaf

STEP 1

3 cups of vegetable broth
3 cups water
Add to a stockpot, turn your heat to medium and bring the liquid to a gentle boil.

1 cup sorghum
Add sorghum and begin the cooking process: total cooking time, 50 to 55 minutes.

STEP 2

Begin this step right after start cooking the sorghum:

2 tbsp olive oil
Heat in a large saute pan.

8 oz chicken breast, large cut
juice of ½ lemon
Add chicken to the pan, sprinkle with lemon and saute for 5 to 6 minutes.

1 onion, chopped
1 shallot, chopped
1 small zucchini, half sliced
3 cloves garlic, chopped
6 mushrooms, sliced
½ tsp fresh ginger, chopped
Add to the pan and saute on medium heat for about 4 to 5 minutes.

4 Roma tomatoes, chopped
4 asparagus, large cut
1 tsp black pepper
1 tbsp pine nuts
1 tbsp fresh Italian parsley, chopped
1 tbsp dry thyme
1 tsp dry tarragon leaves
⅛ tsp cinnamon
Add to the pan and continue to simmer for about 5 more minutes.

Add the chicken and vegetable mixture to the stockpot with the sorghum – at about 30 to 35 minutes in the cooking process of the sorghum – and continue cooking until you reach the final cooking time of 50 to 55 minutes, until sorghum is tender.

All liquid should be absorbed by now. If needed add a bit more hot water.

Suggestion: Serve with **Arugula Fruit Salad** – see the index to find the recipe.

4 servings.

GF – EL

Calories of main ingredients per serving: Sorghum 194. Olive oil 60. Pine nuts 15. Chicken 93. Total of 362.

• *Sorghum is a powerhouse regarding nutrients. It provides large amounts of protein, vitamins B6, niacin riboflavin, and thiamin. High levels of iron, calcium, magnesium, copper, phosphorus and potassium and a significant amount of fiber. Sorghum contains a wide variety of beneficial phytochemicals that act as antioxidants in the body, significantly higher amounts than plums, blueberries and strawberries.*

Lentil Ragout

2 tbs of olive oil
  Heat in a medium-sized stockpot.
1 red onion, large cut
1 green pepper, large cut
1 stalk of celery, chopped
1 large carrot, half sliced
3 Roma tomatoes, chopped
  Add to the pot and saute on medium heat for 5 minutes.
¼ cup of white cooking wine
4 cups vegetable broth
  Add to the stockpot and heat for 2 minutes.
1 cup lentils
  Add to the stockpot and continue cooking for another 10 minutes.
  Once you add the lentils to the stockpot, prepare the following ingredients.
1 small zucchini, half sliced
1 small yellow squash, half sliced
4 cloves garlic, chopped
¼ cup sun-dried tomatoes, chopped
1 tbsp dry thyme
1 tbsp dry oregano
1 tsp cumin
1 tsp black pepper
  Add to the stockpot (10 minutes in to the cooking process of the lentils) and cook for about 10 to 12 minutes, until lentils are tender and liquid is absorbed.

Suggestion: Serve with **Gluten Free Bruschetta** – see the index to find the recipe.

2 Servings

GF – EL – VT – VG

Calories of main ingredients per serving: lentils 345. Vegetable broth 13. olive oil 119. Total of 477.

• *People throughout the decades ate celery because of its low-calorie content. But, celery is an excellent source of antioxidants and contains flavonoids, beta carotene and vitamin C. In fact, there are several kinds of antioxidants found in a single stalk of celery. Celery has a generous amount of dietary fiber as well. It also contains vitamins K and C, folate and minerals like potassium, magnesium and iron. Once celery loses its crunchy, crispy effect, some of these nutrients are lost.*

White Meatballs with Tomato Sauce

STEP 1.

Preheat oven to 325 degrees.
1 lb ground turkey
1 lb ground chicken
½ small onion, chopped
2 cloves garlic, minced
¼ cup grated Parmesan cheese
1 tbsp dry oregano
1 tbsp dry basil
1 tbsp fresh parsley, chopped
½ tsp ground sage
½ tsp white pepper
¼ tsp cinnamon
¼ tsp nutmeg
  Blend all ingredients well in a mixer. Using an ice cream scoop, form round balls, about 2 to 3 oz each. Press meatball by hand to make them firm. You should have about 20 meatballs.
  Layer a baking pan with parchment paper, place meatballs on the pan and bake for about 15 minutes. Remove from oven.

STEP 2.

Tomato Sauce
2 tbsp olive oil
  Heat in a large saute pan on medium heat
½ onion, chopped
4 mushrooms, chopped
2 garlic cloves, chopped
  Add and saute for 4 to 5 minutes
6 Roma tomatoes, chopped
½ red bell pepper, chopped
1 large carrot, shredded
2 tsp dry oregano
2 tsp dry thyme
2 tsp fresh basil, chopped
1 tsp black pepper
  Add to the saute pan and simmer for about 10 to 12 minutes.
  Add the meatballs into the pan with the tomato sauce and continue cooking for another 4 to 5 minutes longer.
2 tbsp grated Romano cheese
  Turn heat off. Remove meatballs from the pot. Add the Romano cheese a little at a time, mix well and serve.
  Suggestion: Serve with **Avocado Feta Hummus** – see the index to find the recipe.

4 servings

GF – omit Parmesan and Romano cheese for EL.

Calories of the main ingredients per meatball: Turkey 33. Chicken 26. Parmesan 5. Total of 64.Calories in tomato sauce per serving: Olive oil 60. Tomatoes 8. Romano cheese 11. Total of 79.

• *Turkey is high-protein, low-carb food. Turkey without the skin is low in fat and high in protein. It is a good source of iron, zinc, phosphorus, potassium and B vitamins.*

• *Chicken is an excellent source of protein. The different parts of the chicken and are low in fat and low in sodium, making it ideal for people who want to lose weight and maintain muscle. Overall, chicken is an excellent addition to your diet. It is an excellent source of niacin and selenium. And a good source of vitamin B6, and phosphorus, choline, pantothenic acid and vitamin B12.*

Tomato Cinnamon Chicken

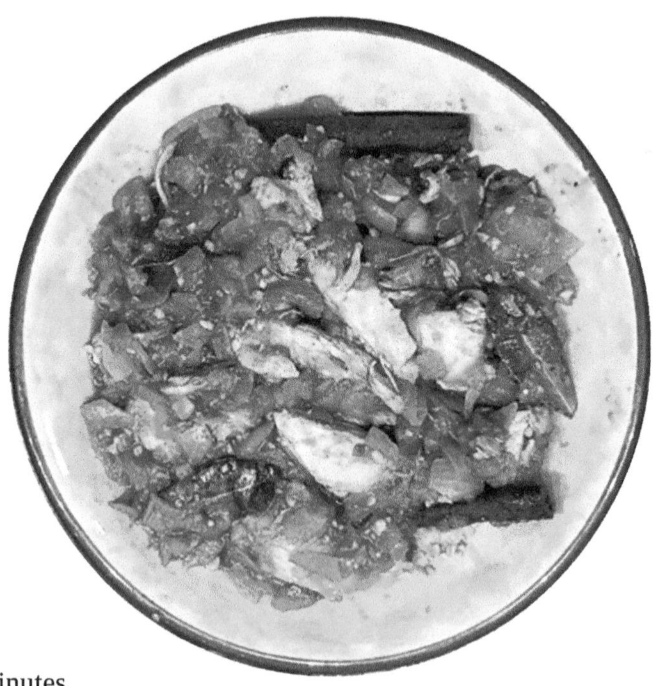

¼ cup olive oil
  Heat gently in a saute pan.
12 chicken breasts, sliced in thick strips
  Add to the pan and lightly brown on all sides, about 5 minutes.
½ onions, chopped
2 cloves of garlic, chopped
  Add onions and garlic and continue cooking on medium heat for another 2 minutes.
2 tbsp of red cooking wine
4 Roma tomatoes, chopped
1 tsp black pepper
2 cinnamon sticks
6 whole cloves
½ tsp of rosemary
3 bay leaves
½ tsp ground cinnamon and cloves
½ tsp ground cloves
  Add to the pan and simmer for about 9 to 10 minutes.
  Suggestion: Serve with Brown Rice Pilaf –See the index.

2 servings

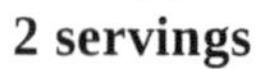

Calories of the main ingredients per serving: Chicken 281. Olive oil 158. Tomatoes 70. Total of 509.

• *Cinnamon is another good healing superspice that contains large amounts of highly potent polyphenol antioxidants. It is so powerful that cinnamon can be used as a natural food preservative. Cinnamon also includes a small amount of vitamin E, niacin, vitamin B6, magnesium, potassium, zinc, and copper.*

• *Cloves contain fiber, vitamins and minerals. Among them vitamin K and C, calcium, magnesium and potassium. Cloves have a bitter, intense aroma and fruity, woody undertones. Cloves contain high consternation of oil which during cooking or baking time releases a sweet, warm flavor.*

Chicken with Black Bean and Almond Pesto

½ cup fresh basil
2 cloves garlic, roasted
1 tbsp olive oil
1 tbsp Parmesan cheese
⅛ cup almonds
Place in a food processor and pulse 2 or 3 times. Set the almond pesto aside.
¼ cup olive oil
Heat gently in a large saute pan.
2 - 6 oz chicken breasts, sliced
Add to the pan and lightly brown on one side, about 4 minutes.
¼ onion, chopped
½ zucchini, half sliced
½ green pepper, sliced
2 cloves garlic, chopped
Turn chicken to the other side and add the vegetables. Continue cooking for another 2 minutes.
2 tbsp of white cooking wine
Pour the wine into the pan.
3 Roma tomatoes, chopped
6 sun-dried tomatoes, large cut
1 tsp dry oregano
½ tsp black pepper
½ tsp of cumin
1½ cup cooked black beans
Add to the pan and simmer for about 9 to 10 minutes.
The almond pesto
Add to the pan, mix well and serve.
Suggestion: Serve with Arborio Rice Pilaf – See the index.

2 servings

GF

Calories of the main ingredients per serving: Chicken 281. Black beans 170. Olive oil 158. Pesto 164. Tomatoes 53. Total of 826.

• *I believe beans are some of the most underrated foods. Black beans are a good source of protein, very high in dietary fiber, magnesium, potassium, phosphorus, and folate. Black beans also have high levels of flavonoids, which have antioxidant abilities. They also contain omega-3 fatty acid. They are a great source of folic acid and have an extremely high level of the rare compound molybdenum, which is very difficult to find in any other food.*

• *Almonds deliver a massive amount of nutrients: Fiber, manganese, magnesium, vitamin E, copper, riboflavin and phosphorus.*

Farro with Sun-Dried Tomatoes and Hearts of Palm

STEP 1

6 cups of water
Place a stockpot and bring it to a gentle boil.
1 cup farro
Add the farro, turn heat to medium and 40 to 45 minutes until farro is tender.
Discard the liquid, if any.
While farro is cooking, prepare the rest of the ingredients for this recipe.

STEP 2

2 tbsp olive oil
Heat in a large saute pan on medium heat.
1 small onion, chopped
2 cloves garlic, chopped
1 shallot, chopped
1 red bell pepper, sliced
Add to the pan and saute for 4 to 5 minutes.
½ cup sun-dried tomatoes, chopped
½ cup hearts of palm, sliced – usually, 3 hearts of palm equals ½ cup.
Add and saute for 3 to 4 minutes.
1 cup vegetable broth
1 tbsp pine nuts
1 tsp dry oregano
1 tsp dry thyme
1 tsp black pepper
Add, turn heat to low and simmer for 5 to 6 minutes. If farro is not cooked by now, turn off the heat.
The cooked farro
Add to the pan, stir well on low heat for a minute and serve.
Serve with **Greek Peasant Salad** – See the index.

2 servings

VT - VG

Calories of the main ingredients per serving: Faro 404. Olive oil 129. Sun-dried tomatoes 20. Hearts of Palm 80. Total of 633.

• *Sun-dried tomatoes are loaded with antioxidants, vitamins, minerals. Most important, sun-dried tomatoes savory flavor bring another dimension to the art of cooking.*

• *Heart of palm is harvested from the inner core of certain palm trees. The main supplying countries are Costa Rica and Brazil, but they grow in several countries in South America.*

Harts of palm is one of my favorite vegetables. I loved its mild, delicate and crisp taste and been using for as long as I remember for salads, appetizers or in main dishes. Heart of palm is low in calories and high in carbohydrates. It a good source of potassium and a good source of protein, dietary fiber, vitamin C, folate, calcium, iron, magnesium, phosphorus and manganese. It also contains zinc, copper and riboflavin. hearts of palm are high in sodium.

Chicken Stuffed with Basil and Garlic

STEP 1

2 - 8 oz boneless chicken breast
Place the breasts on a cutting board and gently flattened them with a meat mallet, or any heavy, clean item.

STEP 2

¼ cup fresh basil, chopped
4 cloves garlic, roasted and chopped
1 tsp olive oil
⅛ cup walnuts, chopped
1 tbsp grated Romano cheese
Mix ingredients in a bowl. Divide the mixture into two parts and place each part at the edge of each breast. Secure the basil mixture inside by rolling the breasts tightly.
¼ cup gluten-free baking flour
Roll the breasts in the flour.
3 tbsp olive oil
Heat in a saute pan. Add the breasts to the pan, with the seam of the stuffed breast down. Saute for about 4 minutes, turn and cook another 4 minutes until chicken is lightly brown. Place stuffed breasts, seam down in a ceramic baking dish. Set aside

STEP 3

2 tbsp olive oil
Heat in a saute pan on medium heat.
¼ onion, chopped
2 cloves of garlic, chopped.
Add to the pan and saute for 2 to 3 minutes.
5 Roma tomatoes, chopped
1 tsp dried oregano
1 tsp dry basil
1 tsp dry thyme
⅛ cup vegetable broth
Add and simmer for about 9 to 10 minutes. Remove from heat. Pour the tomato sauce over stuffed chicken and bake in a 350-degree oven for about 15 to 18 minutes.
Suggestion: Serve with **Millet Pecan Risotto** – See the index.

2 servings

GF

Calories of main ingredients per serving: Chicken 374. Olive oil 178. Walnuts 50. Tomatoes 88. Total of 690.

• *Garlic is the ultimate superfood. Garlic contains amounts of multiple nutrients, just about almost everything we need. Among these nutrients are plentiful amounts of vitamin C, vitamin B6, and manganese. It also contains fiber, selenium, and amounts of calcium, copper, potassium, phosphorus, iron and vitamin B1. Additionally, there is a long list of other compounds in garlic.*

• *Basil contains antioxidant vitamins and phenolics. It is a rich source of vitamin K, zinc, calcium, magnesium, potassium and dietary fiber.*

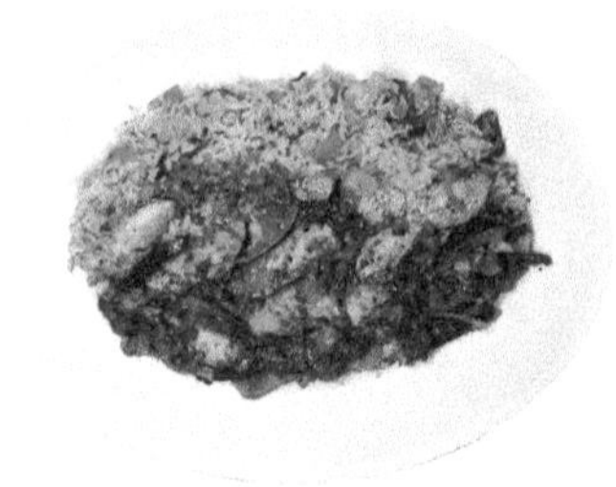

Sun Dried Chicken

4 tbsp olive oil
Heat in a saute pan.
2 - 6 oz chicken breast
Add to the pan and lightly brown on one side on medium heat, about 4 minutes.
2 tbsp capers
10 sun-dried tomatoes, packed in oil, chopped
1 clove garlic, chopped
Turn chicken to the other side, add the above ingredients and continue cooking on medium heat for another 2 minutes.
1 tbsp red cooking wine
2 Roma tomatoes, chopped
½ tsp black pepper
1 tsp dry oregano
1 tbsp fresh basil, chopped
1 tsp dry thyme
¼ tsp fresh rosemary, chopped
Simmer for about 9 to 10 minutes.
Suggestion: Serve with **Basmati White Rice Pilaf** – See the index.

2 servings

GF – EL

Calories of the main ingredients per serving: Chicken 281. Olive oil 178. Tomatoes 35. Sun-dried tomatoes 30. Total of 524.

Mushroom Lemon Chicken

4 tbsp olive oil
Heat gently in a saute pan.
2 - 6 oz chicken breasts
Add to the pan and lightly brown on one side on medium heat, about 4 minutes.
Turn chicken and saute for another 2 minutes.
Juice of ½ lemon
1 small zucchini, sliced
8 mushrooms, sliced
½ tsp black pepper
Add to the pan and continue cooking for another 6 minutes.
2 tbsp white cooking wine
Add and cook for 3 to 4 minutes longer.
Suggestion: Serve with Brown **Rice Pilaf** – See the index.

2 servings

GF – EL

Calories of the main ingredients per serving: Chicken 281. Olive oil 178. Total of 459.

• *Mushrooms are rich in B vitamins such as riboflavin, folate, thiamine, pantothenic acid, and niacin. The minerals in mushrooms are copper, iron, phosphorous, selenium and potassium. Mushrooms are naturally low in sodium, fat, calories, and are high in fiber and protein content. Mushrooms are composed of mostly water.*

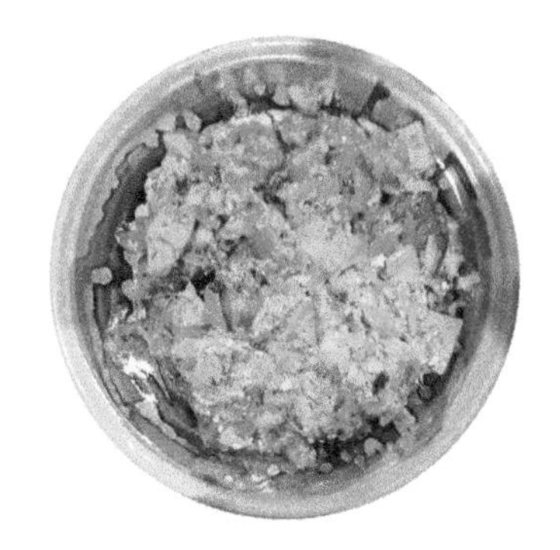

Artichoke Lamb

¼ cup of olive oil
Heat in a large saute pan.
6 lamb loin chops
Add and saute on medium heat for about 6 to 7 minutes. Turn lamb chops.
2 tbsp of red cooking wine
Add to the pan.
½ red onion, chopped
2 cloves garlic, chopped
Add and saute on medium heat 2 to 3 minutes.
6 artichokes hearts, chopped
1 small tomato, chopped
1 tsp dry oregano
1 tsp fresh rosemary, chopped
1 tsp dry thyme
1 tsp fresh mint, chopped
1 tsp black pepper
Add to the pan and cook for about 8 to 10 more minutes.
4 oz feta cheese
Add to the pan and stir until cheese is melted.
Suggestion: Serve with Millet **Pecan Pesto** – See the index.

Makes 3 servings

GF

Calories of the main ingredients per serving: Lamb 418. Artichokes hearts 30. Feta 100. Olive oil 119. Total of 667.

• *Lamb meat has more iron than other protein sources like chicken or fish. It is also a good source of B12 and loaded with other essential B vitamins, including B6, niacin, riboflavin and pantothenic acid. Lamb is also packed with immune-boosting zinc. Lamb does contain fat. However, a large portion of that fat is anti-inflammatory omega 3 fatty acids – much more than beef. The primary nutrition component of lamb is the high-quality protein, a rich source of many vitamins and minerals. Moderate consumption of lean lamb is likely both safe and healthy.*

Cornish Hens with Apricots and Ginger

Preheat oven to 375-degrees
2 Cornish hens, wash well and set aside.

STEP 1

2 apricots, chopped
¼ cup dried dates, chopped
2 cloves garlic, chopped
4 mushrooms, sliced
½ cup kale leaves, finely chopped
½ tsp fresh ginger, chopped
3 green onions, chopped
1 tbsp olive oil
½ tsp black pepper
½ tsp dry sage
1 tsp dry thyme
1 tsp fresh basil
1 tsp fresh Italian parsley
Place all ingredients in a mixing bowl and mix well. Spoon stuffing into the hens. Place hens, their back down, in a baking pan.

STEP 2

2 medium-size sweet potatoes, peeled and large cut
12 baby carrots
2 medium-size yellow squash, large cut

Arrange vegetables around the hens.

2 tbsp olive oil
Juice of 1 lemon
1 tsp dry thyme
1 tsp fresh rosemary, chopped
½ tsp ground mustard
¼ tsp ground ginger

Brush hens and vegetables with and bake for 40 to 45 minutes, occasionally basting, until hens are light brown.

4 servings

Calories of main ingredients per serving: Cornish hen 333. Dates 34. Olive oil 90. Sweet potatoes 57. Yellow squash 16. Total at 530.

• *Apricot is an excellent source of vitamins A and C, copper, fiber and potassium.*

• *Ginger is an excellent natural source of vitamin C, magnesium, potassium, copper, and manganese. Kale is among the most nutrient foods: Loaded with vitamins A, K and C. It contains fiber, antioxidants, vitamin B6, calcium, copper, potassium and a healthy amount of manganese.*

• *Carrots are a particularly good source of beta-carotene, fiber, vitamin K, potassium and antioxidants.*

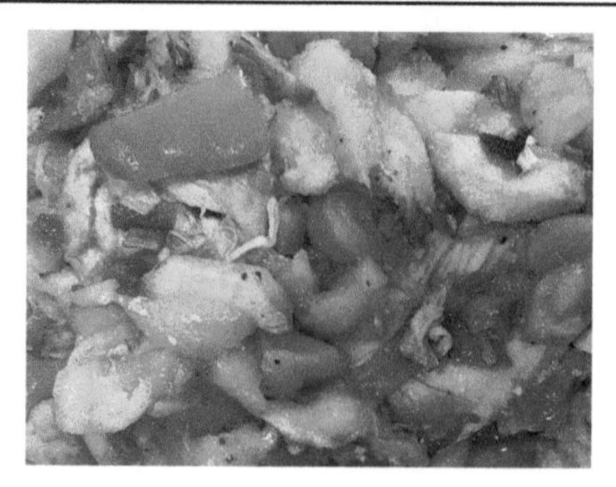

Chicken with Apples and Mango

Preheat over to 350-degrees

4 tbsp olive oil

Heat gently in a saute pan.

2 - 6oz chicken breasts

Add to the pan and lightly brown on one side, about 3 minutes.

½ onions, sliced
½ red bell pepper, sliced
2 cloves of garlic, chopped
½ tsp fresh ginger, chopped

Turn chicken to the other side, add the vegetables and continue cooking on medium heat for another 3 minutes. Place ingredients, chicken first, in a deep ceramic or glass baking dish.

1 small mango, peeled and chopped
1 apple, peeled and chopped
3 green onions, chopped
½ tsp white pepper
1 tsp cumin
¼ tsp nutmeg
½ tsp ground coriander
¼ tsp turmeric
½ tsp ground mustard

Combine all ingredients in a mixing bowl and pour on top of the chicken.
Bake in the preheated oven for 16 to 18 minutes.
Suggestion: Serve with **Arborio Rice Pilaf.** See index.

2 servings

GF – EL

Calories of main ingredients per serving: Chicken 281. Olive oil 178. Mango 50. Apple 26. Total of 535.

• *Mango is high on vitamins C and A. It contains reasonable amounts of vitamins B6, K, and folate. Proper amounts of potassium, calcium, copper, and iron, as well as antioxidants and beta-carotene, and small amounts of protein.You might want to re-think before removing the skin from the apple. The skin of the apple contains large amounts of vitamin C, potassium, calcium and fiber. The skin of many other fruits and vegetables also contain various nutrients. The problem with the skin of fresh produce is the pesticide. It is one of the many reasons that many fruits and vegetables we eat should be organic. Apples are a good source of fibers and several antioxidants.*

Cornish Hens with Spinach and Feta

Preheat oven to 375-degrees

2 Cornish hens, wash and set aside.

STEP 1

¼ cup millet

Place millet in a small saute pan and toss for about 5 minutes under medium heat, frequently stirring, until the millet is lightly golden. This brings out the millet's nutty flavor.

1 cup vegetable broth

1 cup of water

Heat in a stock pot, bring to a gentle boil.

¼ cup millet

Turn heat to medium and add the millet. Cook for about 12 to 14 minutes, until millet is tender. Remove from heat and drain excess liquid, if any. While millet is being cooked prepare for the rest of the recipe.

STEP 2

12 baby potatoes, peeled

12 baby onions, peeled

4 shallots, peeled and cut in halves

Set aside.

STEP 3

2 tbsp olive oil

Heat in a saute pan.

1 small onion, chopped

2 cloves garlic, chopped

Add to the pan and saute for about 5 minutes.

2 tbsp white cooking wine

½ tsp black pepper

1 tsp dry thyme

1 cup spinach, chopped

Add to the pan, stir for a minute. Remove and place the mixture in a mixing bowl.

½ cup feta cheese, crumbled

The cooked millet

Add to the bowl and mix well. Spoon mixture into hens cavities and place hens, their back down, in a baking pan. Arrange potatoes, onions and shallots around the Cornish hens.

1 tsp black pepper

1 tsp dry oregano

2 tbsp olive oil

Juice of 1 lemon

Mix in a small bowl and brush vegetables and hens with.

1 cup of water

Add to the pan.

Bake for 40 to 45 minutes, occasionally basting, until Cornish hens are light brown.

4 servings

Calories of main ingredients per serving: Cornish hen 333. Millet 48. Potatoes 69. Olive oil 119. Feta 50. Total at 619.

• *Cornish hens, are rich in protein and fiber.*

• *Millet is high in antioxidants, iron, magnesium, zinc and calcium. A good source of protein, fiber and vitamins B.*

• *Some of the many nutrients of spinach are folate, vitamin C, niacin, riboflavin, and potassium. However when spinach is cooked there are higher levels of vitamins A and E, protein, fiber, calcium, zinc, thiamin and iron.*

White Burgers with Avocado Pesto and Mango Relish

STEP 1

1 lb ground turkey

1 lb ground chicken

½ small onion, minced

3 mushrooms, chopped

2 cloves garlic, minced

1 tbsp dry oregano

1 tbsp dry basil

1 tsp ground mustard

1 tsp cumin

½ tsp ground sage

½ tsp white pepper

¼ tsp cinnamon

¼ tsp nutmeg

Juice of ½ lemon

Blend all ingredients well in a mixer. Divide into six parts and form six round patties.

2 tbsp olive oil

Pour on a flat grill and cook the white burger patties 3 to 4 minutes on each side.

6 servings

GF – EL

Calories of main ingredients per serving for white burgers: Turkey 154. Chicken 167. Olive Oil 40. Total of 361.

STEP 2

Avocado Pesto

2 avocado, peeled

1 tbsp fresh mint

2 cloves garlic, roasted

Juice of ¼ lemon

1 tbsp chopped almonds

Place ingredients in a food processor and pulse 2 or 3 times.

GF – EL – VT – VG

Calories of main ingredients per serving for Avocado pesto: Avocado 80. Almonds 9. Total 89.

STEP 3

Mango Relish

2 mangoes, chopped
1 red pepper, roasted and chopped
½ medium red onion, chopped
1 cup fresh pineapple, chopped
1 tbsp fresh basil, chopped
Juice of ¼ lemon
1 tsp olive oil

Place ingredients in a mixing bowl and blend well using a spatula.

To serve: Place white burgers in a large oblong plater, scoop the pesto on top of burgers and arrange relish on the side of the plater.

GF – EL – VT – VG

Calories of the main ingredients per serving for relish. Mango 67. Pineapple 14. Olive oil 7. Total 88.

• *Avocados are loaded with nutrients, many of which are lacking in modern diets. They are rich with fiber, powerful antioxidants and monounsaturated fatty acids.*

• *Pineapple is a superfood. Loaded with vitamin C. It is a source of other essential vitamins and minerals: Vitamins A, B6, folate, thiamin, pantothenic acid and riboflavin. It contains calcium, magnesium, manganese, potassium, and antioxidants. Fresh pineapple is the only known source of an enzyme called bromelain, which might play a role in a range of different health benefits.*

Ground Lamb with Artichoke Buckwheat

STEP 1

1 cup of water
2 cups of vegetable broth

Heat in a stock pot, bring to a gentle boil.

1 cup buckwheat

Add to the pot and cook for about 15 to 18 minutes, until buckwheat is tender.

STEP 2

Prepare the ground lamb.

¼ cup of olive oil

Heat in a large saute pan

8 oz ground lamb

Add to the pan and saute until light brown

½ onion, sliced
½ red onion, sliced
2 shallots, large cut
6 mushrooms, sliced
2 cloves garlic, chopped
2 small ripe tomatoes, chopped
½ cup of artichoke hearts, sliced

Add to the pan and cook until onions are soft, about 5 to 6 minutes

1 tbsp pine nuts
1 tbsp capers
1 tbsp lemon juice
1 tsp grated lemon peel
6 Kalamata olives, cut in halves
1 tbsp raisins
1 tsp dry basil
1 tsp black pepper
1 tsp dry mint
1 tsp fresh rosemary, chopped
1 tsp dry oregano

Add to the pan and simmer for 4 to 5 minutes

The cooked buckwheat

Add to the pan, stir for a minute, remove from heat and serve.

3 servings

GF – EL

Calories of the main ingredients per serving: Buckwheat 74. Olive oil 161. Pine nuts 20. Raisins 160. Ground lamb 253. Total of 646.

• *Artichokes are packed with powerful nutrients. They are low in fat while rich in fiber, vitamins, minerals, and rank among the most antioxidant-rich of all vegetables. Artichokes are particularly high in vitamins C, K and folate. They supply minerals, such as phosphorus, magnesium, potassium, and iron. Artichokes contain an above average plant-based protein. The earthy flavor of the artichoke is unique and diverse. Its flavor profile changes according to the way the artichoke is cooked. I used the non-marinated artichoke hearts extensively in my cooking. The fact is that artichokes are unique in flavor are challenging to be substituted by any other vegetable.*

Turkey Fingers with Pumpkin Seed Walnut Pesto

STEP 1

Pumpkin Walnut Pesto

1 cup green pumpkin seeds, unsalted
½ cup walnut pieces
½ cup sun-dried tomatoes
½ cup kale leaves
1 cup fresh basil
2 tbsp olive oil
1 tbsp lemon juice
3 cloves garlic, roasted
½ tsp black pepper
1 tbsp grated Romano cheese
¼ cup low-fat Greek yogurt

Place all ingredients in a food processor and pulse 2 to 3 times making a smooth paste.

STEP 2

Caper Lemon Sauce

2 tbsp olive oil
1 tbsp capers, chopped
1 tbsp fresh dill, chopped
2 tbsp lemon juice
½ tsp black pepper
1 green onion, chopped
½ tsp fresh ginger, minced

Place in the mixing bowl and mix well by hand.
Transfer into a serving dish.

STEP 3

Turkey Fingers

1 medium-size sweet potato

Place in a small stockpot, cover with water and cook for about 12 minutes until soft.
Potato does not have to be cooked all the way.
Remove and cool.
Preheat oven to 350-degrees

½ onion, chopped
1 lb ground turkey
2 cloves garlic, chopped
¼ cup ground flaxseed
¼ cup fresh Italian parsley, chopped
1 egg beaten
1 tsp white pepper
½ tsp nutmeg
1 tsp orange zest
1 tsp grated Parmesan cheese
1 tsp ground sage
½ tsp turmeric
The cooked sweet potato

Blend all above ingredients with a mixer on slow speed.
Scoop out mixer with an ice cream scoop and form oblong patties. Makes about 16 patties.
Brush a baking pan lightly with olive oil and bake in the preheated oven for 12 to 15 minutes, until lightly brown.
Remove and place on a large serving platter.
Arrange the pumpkin walnut pesto in the platter and serve along with the caper lemon sauce.

4 servings

GF

Calories for main ingredients per serving in turkey patties: Sweet potatoes 28. Turkey 164. Olive oil 60. Egg 20. Total of 300.

Calories for main ingredients per serving in pesto: Olive oil 96. Pumpkin seeds 72. Walnuts 66. Grated Romano 28. Total of 262.

• *Sweet potatoes are an excellent source of vitamin A and C, manganese, copper, pantothenic acid and vitamin B6. And a good source of potassium, fiber, niacin, vitamin B1, B2 and phosphorus.*

• *Walnuts are high in healthy unsaturated fat. They also contain vitamins A, B, and E, folic acid, calcium, magnesium, phosphorus, potassium, and zinc.*

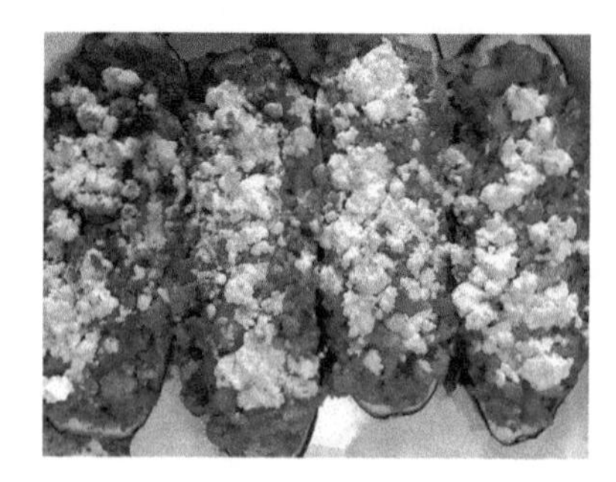

Stuffed Zucchini with Ground Turkey

Preheat oven to 375-degrees

4 thick Italian zucchini,

Slice the zucchini lengthwise and scoop out the seeds and pulp. Zucchini shell should be about ½ inch thick. Brush lightly with olive oil a class or ceramic medium size baking dish.

Bake zucchini shells in the preheated oven for about 10 minutes.

3 tbsp olive oil

Heat in a saute pan.

1 small onion, chopped
2 cloves garlic, chopped

Add to the pan and saute on medium heat 2 to 3 minutes.

16 oz ground turkey

Add to the pan and cook for 5 to 6 minutes.

1 tbsp white cooking wine
2 Roma tomatoes, finely chopped
4 artichoke heart, chopped
1 tbsp dry oregano
1 tsp black pepper
1 tsp fresh dill, chopped
½ tsp ground ginger

Add to the pan and cook for another 5 to 6 minutes. Turn off the heat.

1 cup cooked garbanzo beans
8 Kalamata olives, pitted

Place in a food processor and pulse 2 or 3 times. Add to the pan with the rest of the mixture. Do not turn heat back on.

2 tbsp grated Parmesan cheese

Add to the mixture and stir to mix well. Scoop the mixture evenly into the zucchini shells.

1½ cup feta cheese, crumbled

Top stuffed zucchini with the feta.

Bake 20 to 25 minutes, until feta is light brown.

Romaine salad
1 romaine lettuce, large cut
1 large tomato, large cut
1 cucumber, half sliced
¼ red onion, sliced
2 tbsp olive oil
1 tbsp balsamic vinegar

Toss ingredients in a salad bowl and serve with the baked zucchini.

4 servings

Calories of main ingredients per serving: Turkey 231. Garbanzo 68. Feta 148. Olive oil 119. Zucchini 54. Total at 620.

Nutrients in turkey: Turkey is a rich source of protein. It also contains vitamins B12 and B6, Choline, niacin, selenium, and zinc.

• *Zucchini is a good source of protein, fiber, vitamins A, C, K, B6, folate, magnesium, potassium, manganese, thiamin, niacin, copper, and phosphorus. Most of the water zucchini contains is found in its flesh. Since the skin is a more concentrated source of nutrients, by discarding the flesh you are not missing many nutrients. My main reasons for not using the flesh is because it does not blend well with the stuffing I chose for this recipe. Also, since it contains much water, which breaks down the flavors and texture of my stuffing. The zucchini skin is high in vitamin C and K, potassium and healthy fiber. The skin is also a rich source of antioxidants and beta-carotene. And I believe that most of the flavor is on the skin.*

Basmati Seafood

3 tbsp. olive oil
Heat in a medium-size stockpot.
½ onion, sliced
3 cloves garlic, chopped
2 artichoke hearts, sliced
4 green onions, chopped
8 mushrooms, sliced
6 asparagus, large cut
½ red pepper, sliced
⅛ cup capers
Add to the stockpot and cook on medium heat for about 5 minutes.
4 Roma tomatoes, chopped
¼ cup parsley, chopped
1 tbsp fresh rosemary
Add and simmer for about 4 minutes.
½ lb medium-size shrimp, peeled
½ lb bay scallops – bay scallops are the smaller size scallops.
1 tsp black pepper
1 tsp dry basil
1 tsp dry thyme
Add and simmer for 3 minutes longer.
3 cups vegetable broth
½ cup white cooking wine
½ cup of water
½ cup basmati rice
Add and cook for about 20 minutes, until rice is cooked.

4 servings

GF

Calories of main ingredients per serving: Olive oil 89. Shrimp 34. Scallops 44. Halibut 32. Cod 24. Basmati rice 80.Total of 303.

• *Nutrients in shrimp includes a good amount of selenium, vitamin B12, iron, phosphorus, niacin and zinc. Scallops contain selenium, phosphorus, vitamin B12 and choline.*

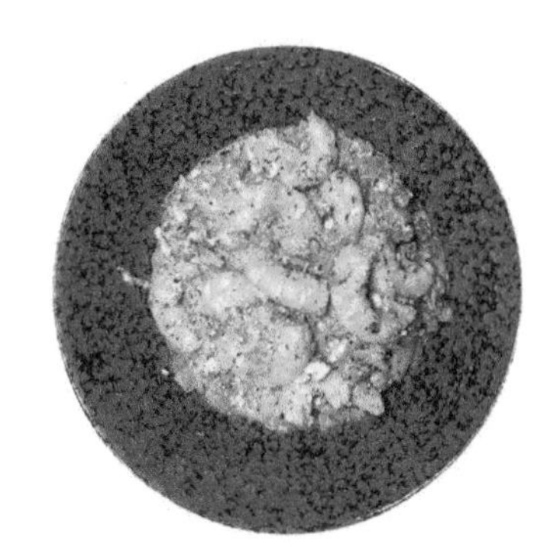

Feta Shrimp

2 tbsp olive oil
Head in a large saute pan. Turn heat to medium.
½ onion, chopped
2 garlic cloves, chopped
Add to the pan and saute for 5 minutes.
¼ cup white wine
4 Roma tomatoes, chopped
½ tsp black pepper
1 tsp dry oregano
1 tsp dry thyme
1 tsp fresh basil
Add to the pan and simmer for about 6 minutes.
12 jumbo shrimp, peeled
Add and cook 7 to 8 minutes longer, until shrimp is cooked.
½ cup feta cheese, crumbled
Add and stir until feta is melted.

Serves 2

GF

Suggestion: Serve with Basmati White Rice Pilaf – see the index.

Calories of the main ingredients per serving: Olive oil 119. Shrimp 63. Feta 99. Total of 281.

• *Shrimp contains a good amount of selenium, vitamin B12, iron, phosphorus, niacin and zinc.*

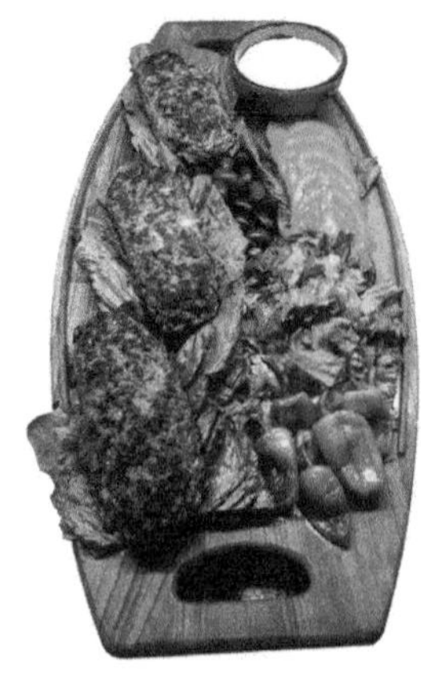

Mediterranean Lamburger with Feta Sauce

STEP 1

Feta Sauce

¼ cup feta, crumbled
1 tbsp red wine vinegar
1 tsp dried oregano
½ tsp black pepper
¼ cup low-fat olive oil mayonnaise
1 tsp dry thyme
1 tsp dry basil
1 clove garlic, chopped

Place all ingredients in a mixing bowl, mix well with a spatula. Set aside.

STEP 2

Grilled Sweet Potatoes

3 tbsp olive oil

Place on a flat grill on medium heat.

2 sweet potatoes

Peel and half sliced. Grill for about 6 to 7 minutes on each side.

1 large red pepper, sliced
½ red onion, sliced

Add to the grill when potatoes are halfway cooked.

½ lime
1 tsp cumin
1 tbsp dry thyme

Squeeze lime juice and sprinkle thyme and cumin as potatoes are beings cooked, about 8 minutes into the cooking process.

STEP 3

Mediterranean Lamburgers

12 oz grass fed ground beef
1 lb ground lamb
½ onion, finely chopped
1 clove garlic, chopped
1 egg
1 tsp dry basil
1 tsp black pepper
2 tsp dry oregano
1 tsp fresh mint leaves
2 tsp dry thyme
1 tsp cumin
2 tsp ground mustard

Blend well in a mixer. Divide into 4 equal parts. Place on a working surface, press each meat with the palm of your hand to flatten them. Shape meat into a rectangular shape.

6 sun-dried tomatoes in oil, chopped
2 tbsp capers
2 tbsp feta cheese, crumbled

Place in a mixing bowl, mix well by hand and divide the mixture into four parts.
Spread the mixture in the center of each lamburger and fold the meat around the mixture.
Press well to make the patties firm and oblong.

2 tbsp olive oil

Grill lamburgers on a flat grill or saute in a saute pan, about 5 or 6 minutes on each side.
Arrange lamburgers on a serving plater, serve with the feta sauce and grilled sweet potatoes.

GF – EL

NOTE: you can prepare the lamburgers first and grill them at the same time with the sweet potatoes.

4 servings

Calories per serving in the main ingredients: Ground beef 282. Ground lamb 213. Sun-dried tomatoes 10 Feta 13. Olive oil 60. Total of 578.
Calories in sweet potatoes per serving: Sweet potatoes 98. Olive oil 144. Total of 242.
Calories in sauce per serving: Feta 25. Mayonnaise 25.
Total 50.

• *Grass-fed beef comes from cows which have grazed in pasture year-round. Rather than being fed a processed diet for much of their life. Anyone who plans to include beef in their healthy diet, grass-fed beef is the only option. Grass-fed beef is richer in omega-3 fats, high in protein, and beta carotene, vitamin E, B12, B3, B6. It contains reasonable amounts of selenium, zinc, phosphorus, choline and pantothenic acid.*

Keftedakia with Sun-Dried Tomatoes and Yogurt Sauce

STEP 1

1 lb grass fed ground beef
1 lb ground lamb
½ onion, minced
1 clove garlic, minced
1 egg
1 tsp dry basil
1 tsp black pepper
2 tsp dry oregano
1 tsp fresh mint leaves, chopped
2 tsp dry thyme
1 tsp cumin
2 tsp ground mustard
1 tbsp fresh parsley, chopped
½ cup sun-dried, chopped

Blend well in a mixer on slow speed. Scoop out the mixture with an ice cream scoop and make small patties. Each. Makes about 20 patties.

4 tbsp olive oil

In a large saute pan on medium heat, saute the keftedakia, a few at a time, about 3 to 4 minutes on each side.

GF

STEP 2

Yogurt Sauce

1 cucumber, peeled and minced
2 green onions, minced
1 cup light sour cream
1 cup low-fat Greek yogurt
Juice of 1 lemon
1 tbsp grated Parmesan cheese
1 tsp ground mustard
1 tsp white pepper

Place ingredients in a mixing ball and mix well with a wooden spoon.

Place keftedakia on a rectangular serving platter and arrange sauce on the side of the platter.

Suggestion: Serve with **Greek Peasant Salad.**

2 servings

GF

Calories in the main ingredients for each patty: Ground beef 48. Ground lamb 64. Olive oil 24. Sun-dried tomatoes 6. Sour cream 16. Yogurt 8. Total of 134.

• *About Greek yogurt: There is a hype about this superfood for a reason. Greek yogurt is a nutrition powerhouse. It provides about twice as much protein as regular yogurt, about half as many carbs and less sugar than regular yogurt. Bottom line Greek yogurt packs more of a variety of health benefits: Extra protein, fewer carbohydrates, lower in lactose sodium, rich in probiotics. Greek yogurt is made by adding healthy bacteria to milk which causes it to ferment. Fermentation transforms lactose into lactic acid. As a result, yogurt is given the creamy texture and tart flavor. Furthermore, the Greek yogurt is strained through a cheesecloth more times than the regular yogurt to get its thicker consistency. For someone who grew up consumed Greek yogurt and honey on a daily bases, I found the best Greek yogurt out there is Fage Greek Yogurt. This company has been making yogurt for nearly 100 years and has remained true to the flavor and consistency of the yogurt I grew up with. In this cookbook, I use Greek yogurt to substituted other ingredients such as sour cream, heavy cream, mayonnaise and cream cheese. Because of its thicker consistency and unique flavor, it gives an extra dimension to the flavor and body of my recipes.*

Veggie Burger with Avocado Pomegranate Sauce

½ cup brown rice

In a stock pot boil 3 cups of water. Reduce heat to medium add rice and simmer for about 40 minutes. Drain water and cool. Place in a large bowl.

2 large size red beets
4 cups of water

Boil for about 40 to 50 minutes. After cooling, take the skin of the beets and run them through the shredder of a food processor. Add beets to the bowl with the rice.

½ cup oat

Grind in the food processor. Add to the mixing bowl.

1 tbsp olive oil

Heat in a saute pan.

1 small onion, chopped
3 cloves garlic, chopped

Add to the pan and saute for 3 to 4 minutes.

4 large mushrooms, chopped

Add to the pan, saute for a couple more minutes. Cool and add to the mixing bowl.

1½ cups cooked black beans, drained well.

Place in a small bowl and break beans with a fork. Add to the bowl with the rest of the mixture.

2 tbsp chopped walnuts
½ cup baby spinach, chopped
½ cup fresh basil, chopped
1 tbsp fresh mint, chopped
2 tsp ground mustard
1 tsp dry thyme
1 tsp black pepper
½ tsp paprika
½ tsp chili powder

1 tsp cumin
Add to the mixing bowl. Mix well by hand. Refrigerate for a couple of hours.
Divide mixture into 4 parts and form round patties.
Grill on a flat grill with olive oil. Serve with the avocado pomegranate sauce.
Makes 4 veggie burgers.

GF – EL – VT – VG

Avocado Pomegranate Sauce

2 avocados, peeled
¼ red bell pepper
1 tbsp olive oil
2 cloves garlic
¼ cup fresh basil
1 tbsp fresh parsley
juice of ¼ lime
1 tbsp dry mustard
½ tsp white pepper
2 tbsp real Greek yogurt
Add all ingredients in the food processor and pulse 2 or 3 times.
Remove and place the mixture in a bowl.
½ cup pomegranate seeds
Add to the bowl and mix well with a spatula.

Note: You can precook the brown rice and beets and refrigerate them until ready to use.

GF – VT

Calories of main ingredients veggie burger: Brown rice 46. Beets 15. Oats 38. Olive oil 30. Black beans 113. Walnuts 25. Total of 267.

Calories of main ingredients in avocado pomegranate sauce per serving: Avocados 161. Pomegranate 24 Olive oil 30. Total 215.

• colors of its seeds have a similar taste, I believe that the common deep red ones are the ones with the most complex taste. They are sweet with a sour and tart undertone.

Artichoke Sole with Cranberry Quinoa

STEP 1

2½ cups of water
Heat in a stock pot, bring to a gentle boil.
½ cup quinoa.
2 tbsps dried cranberries
Juice of ½ lemon
2 green onions, chopped
1 tbsp fresh mint leaves, chopped
½ tsp black pepper
Add and cook on medium, heat for about 18 to to 20 minutes. Drain liquid if any and set aside.

STEP 2

4 tbsp olive oil
Heat in a saute pan.
12 or 14 oz fillets of sole
1 egg, beaten
¼ cup almond flour
Dip sole in the egg batter and roll it in the flour. Place in the saute pan and saute for 3 to 4 minutes and turn the fish.
3 mushrooms, sliced
4 artichoke hearts, sliced
3 green onions, chopped
Add to the pan cook for another 3 to 4 minutes.
Place cooked quinoa in a serving plater, remove the sole only from the pan and place it on top of the quinoa. Leave the vegetables in the saute pan.
⅛ cup white cooking wine
Juice of ¼ lemon
¼ tsp black pepper
Add to the pan and heat for 2 to 3 minutes. Turn heat to low.

STEP 3

½ cup unsweetened almond milk
Add to the pan.
1 egg yolk, beat lightly in a bowl.
Add to the pan while stirring with a fork. In about 1 minute the sauce will thicken
Remove and pour the sauce over the sole and serve.

2 servings

GF – EL

Calories of main ingredients per serving: Sole 125. Quinoa 170. Cranberries 24. Eggs 38. Almond flour 75. Artichoke hearts 89. Olive oil 60. Total of 581.

• Sole is high in selenium, phosphorus and magnesium. It contains reasonable amounts of Vitamins B12 and B6 and protein.

Sun-Dried Mahi Mahi

STEP 1

2 cups of water

1 cup vegetable broth

Heat in a stock pot.

½ cup quinoa

Juice of a ¼ lemon

1 tsp lemon zest

1 tbsp fresh parsley, chopped

2 cloves roasted garlic, chopped

1 tsp fresh basil, chopped

Add to the pot and cook for about 13 to 15 minutes.

While quinoa is being cooked, prepare the mahi-mahi.

STEP 2

4 tbs olive oil

Heat in a medium-size saute pan.

2 - 6 oz mahi-mahi steaks

Add to the pan and cook in about 3 to 4 minutes.

1 tbsp white cooking wine

Turn mahi-mahi and add the wine. Cook for another 4 to 5 minutes, until the fish is cooked. Remove the fish and set aside.

1 small tomato, chopped

8 sun-dried tomatoes, chopped

1 tbsp capers

1 clove garlic, chopped

½ tsp of black pepper

½ tsp fresh rosemary, chopped

1 tsp dry basil

Add to the same saute pan and cook ingredients for about 7 to 8 minutes, until tomatoes are cooked.

In the meantime, discard any liquid from quinoa. Place quinoa on a serving plater and arrange the mahi-mahi over quinoa. When sauce is done, pour over the mahi-mahi and serve.

2 servings

GF – EL

Calories of the main ingredients per serving: Mahi-mahi 210. Olive oil 119. Sun-dried tomatoes 40. Quinoa 159. Total of 528. Nutrients in mahi-mahi: Most of the fats in mahi-mahi are unsaturated fats.

• Mahi-mahi contains omega-3 fatty acids, a good amounts of protein and several minerals like calcium, magnesium, phosphorus and potassium. It is hight in vitamin A and has amounts of folate, niacin and vitamin B12.

• Capers contain fiber, protein, vitamins C, A, K, E, niacin and riboflavin. It also contains iron, sodium, and potassium.

• Capers are flower buds that thrive across the Mediterranean region. In the early eights, in Phoenix Arizona, my customers unfamiliar with some of the ingredients listed in my menu, like hearts of palm, sun-dried tomatoes, artichoke hearts, capers, feta, asked some unusual questions especially about hearts of palm and capers. The common question was "what is capers?" and the strangest one was "are capers seafood?" The Mediterranean wild capers have been part of local cuisines since the beginning of time. In Greece, capers grow in the rocky cliffs of islands and the mainland. They are pickled in a brine of vinegar, water and a bit of salt. Because of their unique taste, they are versatile in cooking. Capers are used for salads, vegetable dishes, poultry, seafood and meats. Towards the end of the nineteenth century as more chefs began to use unique European ingredients, slowly they gain popularity.

Salmon with Spinach Pesto

STEP 1

Preheat oven to 450-degrees

2 - 6 oz salmon fillets

2 tbsp olive oil

Juice of ½ lemon

1 tbsp rosemary, chopped

In a bowl mix olive oil, lemon and rosemary and brush salmon with on both sides.

Place on a baking dish and bake 12 to 14 minutes.

STEP 2

Spinach Pesto

1 cup baby spinach

2 cloves garlic

Juice of half lemon

1/8 cup of olive oil

¼ cup of fresh basil

¼ cup of almonds
Place in a food processor and pulse 2 or 3 times. Set aside.

STEP 3

Sautéed Asparagus

2 tbsp olive oil
Heat in a saute pan, on medium heat.
12 asparagus, cut off the hard bottom parts
2 portobello mushrooms, sliced
2 cloves of garlic, chopped
Add to the pan and saute for 3 to 4 minutes.
4 Kalamata olives, chopped
½ tsp black pepper
1 tbsp fresh basil, chopped
½ tsp ground mustard
¼ cup sliced almonds
1 tsp lemon juice
Add to the pan and saute for another 4 to 5 minutes.
Place salmon in a serving platter.
In a small saute pan add the spinach pesto, heat gently on low heat and pour over salmon.
Arrange asparagus on the side of the platter and serve.

2 servings

GF – EL

Calories per serving for sautéed asparagus Olive oil 191. 114.
Calories per serving for main salmon ingredients: Salmon 291. Almonds 104. Total of 395.
Calories per serving in Spinach pesto: Almonds 104.

• Salmon provides good amounts of the antioxidant, vitamins B12, D, B6 and selenium. It is a good source of omega-3 fatty acids, niacin, protein and phosphorus. It is also a good source of potassium. choline, pantothenic acid and biotin.

• Asparagus is loaded with essential vitamins, minerals and antioxidants. It is an excellent source of vitamins A, C, E, K, folate and riboflavin. Asparagus also has small amounts of protein, potassium, phosphorous, iron and zinc. Asparagus is popular because of its unique taste and it could be used in a variety of dishes. It is a good source of antioxidants. It is low in calories, high in water and rich in fiber, that makes it a weight loss friendly food.

Mediterranean Calamari with Buckwheat

STEP 1

2 cups vegetable broth
1 cup of water
Heat in a stockpot, bring to a gentle boil.
½ cup buckwheat
2 garlic cloves, chopped
1 tsp cumin
1 tsp ground mustard
½ tsp ground cardamom
Juice of ½ lemon
1 tbsp chopped almonds
Add to the pot and cook for about 15 to 20 minutes, until buckwheat is tender. Drain liquid if any and set aside.

STEP 2

Prepare the calamari

1 lb small calamari tubes – 15 to 16 count
2 eggs beaten, in a mixing bowl
1 cup almond flour, place in a separate bowl
Dip the calamari tubes, a few at a time, into the eggs and rolled them in the almond flour.
1 cup olive oil
Heat on high heat in a large saute pan. Place calamari, a few at a time, in the hot oil and cook until brown, 3 to 4 minutes.

STEP 3

¼ cup of grated mytzithra cheese
In a bowl toss calamari with mytzithra.
Juice of ½ lemon
Squeeze on top of calamari. Set aside.

STEP 4

1 tbsp olive oil
Heat in a large saute pan. Reduce heat to medium.
3 green onions, chopped
1 small red onion, sliced
1 small roasted red pepper, sliced
4 pepperoncinis, chopped
Add saute for about 5 minutes.
2 tbsp white cooking wine
4 Roma tomatoes, chopped
½ tsp black pepper
1 tsp dry basil
1 tsp fresh rosemary, chopped
Add in and simmer about 7 to 8 minutes.
The cooked calamari
Add to the pan stir for 2 to 3 minutes and remove from heat.

STEP 5

Place buckwheat on an oblong serving plater, arrange calamari over it and serve.

2 servings

GF

Calories of main ingredients per serving: Buckwheat 148. Almonds 26. Fried calamari 397. Olive oil 95. Mytzithra cheese 58. Total of 724.

Peppercorn Calamari

STEP 1

½ cup millet

Place millet in a small saute pan and toss for about 5 minutes under medium heat, frequently stirring, until the millet is lightly golden. This brings out the millet's nutty flavor.

STEP 2

1 cups vegetable broth

2 cups of water

Heat in a stockpot, bring to a gentle boil.

Toasted millet

1 clove roasted garlic, chopped

½ tsp nutmeg

1 tbsp fresh parsley, chopped

1 tsp cumin

½ tsp ground cardamom

1 tsp ground fennel

Add to the stockpot and cook for about 16 to 18 minutes, until millet is tender.

STEP 3

Prepare the calamari:

1 lb small calamari tubes – 15 to 16 count

2 eggs beaten, in a mixing bowl

1 cup almond flour, place in a separate bowl

Dip the calamari tubes, a few at a time, into the eggs and rolled them in the almond flour.

1 cup olive oil

Heat on high heat in a large saute pan. Place calamari, a few at a time, in the hot oil and cook until brown, 4 to 5 minutes.

STEP 4

2 tbsps grated Romano cheese

In a bowl toss cooked calamari with Romano.

½ lemon

Squeeze on top of calamari. Set aside.

STEP 5

1 tbsp olive oil

Heat in a large saute pan. Reduce heat to medium.

4 green onions, chopped.

8 medium mushrooms, sliced

4 Roma tomatoes, chopped

8 black peppercorns

6 whole cloves

½ tsp black pepper

1 tsp dry basil

1 tsp fresh rosemary

1 tbsp dry oregano

Add to the pan and simmer for about 10 minutes.

STEP 5

The cooked calamari

Add the calamari to the pan and continue cooking for another 2 to 3 minutes.

Place cooked millet on a rectangular serving platter and the peppercorn calamari over millet and serve.

2 servings

GF

Calories of the main ingredients per serving: Millet 130. Fried calamari 397. Romano cheese 21. Olive oil 95. Total of 643.

• *Calamari is rich in protein and contains high amounts of vitamin B12, copper, potassium and phosphorus.*

• *Cardamom contains calcium, potassium and vitamins B and C. It also contains small amounts of protein, fiber, and fatty acids. Cardamom has a sweet and light lemony flavor, with a robust fruity, aroma.*

• *Cumin has an excellent amount of iron and a good source of calcium, manganese, magnesium, phosphorus and vitamin B1. Cumin has a bitter taste with earth and nutty undertones. Cumin has a very distinct smoky and earthy flavor with hints of lemon and nutty and spicy undertones.*

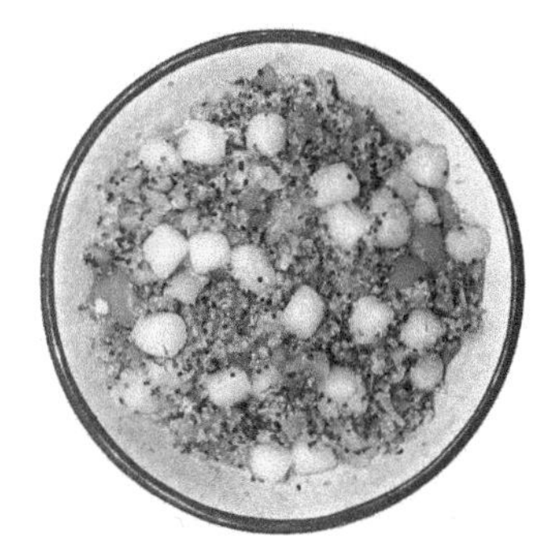

Scallops with Pine Nuts and Three Color Quinoa

STEP 1

2 cups vegetable broth

1 cup water

Heat liquid in a stock pot, bring to a gentle boil.

½ cup three-color quinoa

Add to the pot and cook on medium heat for about 15 to 18 minutes.

STEP 2

While quinoa is being cooked prepare the rest of the recipe.

4 tbsp olive oil

Heat in a large saute pan on medium heat.

½ small onion, sliced

½ red bell pepper, sliced

1 clove garlic, chopped

½ medium carrot, half sliced

1 shallot, chopped

Add to the pan and saute for about 5 minutes.

2 Roma tomatoes, chopped
½ cup vegetable broth
¼ cup pine nuts
¼ cup raisins
Add to the pan and cook for 6 to 7 minutes.
Juice of ¼ lemon
½ tsp black pepper
1 tsp fresh mint, chopped
1 tsp Italian parsley, chopped
1 tsp fresh basil, chopped
1 tsp dry thyme
½ tsp fresh rosemary, chopped
Add to the pan and stir well.
1 lb bay scallops
Add to the pan and cook for about 5 to 6 minutes longer, until scallops are tender.
The cooked quinoa
Place on a large serving platter. Arrange scallops on top and serve.

2 healthy servings

GF – EL

Calories of main ingredients per serving: Olive oil 119. Scallops 200. Total of 319.

• *Quinoa is gluten-free and one of a few plant foods that are considered a complete protein, and it is high in fiber content compared with other grains. Among the gluten-free diet plants, quinoa provides the highest amounts of antioxidants. Quinoa also offers large quantities of manganese, calcium, fiber, iron and magnesium, as well as vitamins B and E. Bottom line; It is difficult to ignore the powerful nutrient in the tiny grain; higher in nutrients and quality protein than most other grains. High amounts of vitamins, minerals and plant compounds and exceptionally high in antioxidants*

White BBQ Grouper

STEP 1

6 cups vegetable broth
2 cups of water
In a stockpot and bring the liquid to a gentle boil.
1 cup whole grain sorghum.
Add to the pot and start cooking on medium heat. Total cooking time should be 45 to 50 minutes. Drain excess liquid if any.

STEP 2

4 tbsp olive oil
Heat in a large saute pan on medium heat.
2 - 8 oz grouper fillets
1 egg, beaten
¼ cup almond flour
Dip grouper in the egg and roll it in the flour. Place in the saute pan, saute for 4 minutes and turn the fish once.
Juice of ½ lemon
½ red onion, sliced
½ red bell pepper, sliced
1 clove garlic, chopped
½ tsp fresh ginger, minced
1 tsp fresh rosemary, chopped
1 tsp dry thyme
½ tsp white pepper
Add in and simmer 7 to 8 minutes. Remove grouper only and set aside.

STEP 3

½ cup unsweetened coconut milk
1 tsp dry mustard
1 tsp curry powder
1 tsp paprika
1 tbsp grated Romano cheese
Turn heat to low, add to the rest of the ingredients into the saute pan, stir well for about a minute and remove from the heat.
Place cooked sorghum on a serving plater, arrange grouper on top and pour sauce over grouper and serve.

2 servings

GF

Calories of main ingredients per serving: Sorghum 193. Olive oil 120. Grouper 165. Egg 38. Almond flour 150. Unsweetened coconut milk 45. Romano cheese 11. Total of 602.

• *Grouper has a good amount of protein and potassium. Also it has good amounts of phosphorus, vitamins A, B6, as well as thiamin and calcium.*

• *Ginger is an excellent natural source of vitamin C, magnesium, potassium, copper, and manganese. Ginger is fierce and peppery with lemon/citrus aroma undertones. When cooked has a mild sweetness with warm flavor. Its complex flavor makes ginger versatile for both baking and cooking. Rosemary provides a bit more of everything: fiber, iron, calcium, vitamin C, and vitamin A.*

• *Rosemary is most likely the most complex flavor of all herbs. It has strong lemon-pine flavor and a distinct minty one. There is a noticeable peppery taste with hints of eucalyptus. Rosemary isn't a shy herb when it comes to the aroma – it is strong. It is extraordinary that this incredibly unique flavor profile is something works extremely well with a vast array of various dishes.*

Coconut Fried Shrimp and Bananas with Pineapple with Cocktail Sauce

STEP 1

Sauce

1 cup organic cocktail sauce
¼ cup pineapple, chopped
medium peach, peeled and chopped
1 tsp juice of a lime
½ tsp prepared horseradish

Mix all ingredients well by hand. Refrigerate while preparing the shrimp and bananas.

EL – GF – VT – VG

STEP 2

12 jumbo shrimp – 12 to 16 count.

Remove the shells without removing the tail Butterfly the shrimp. To butterfly shrimp, slice the top of the shrimp halfway and opened it flat.

1 cup gluten-free flour
4 eggs beaten well
3 cups unsweetened shredded coconut

Place ingredients in 3 separate bowls. Deep the shrimp, one at the time into flour, then into the eggs and coat them with coconut, pressing coconut firmly against the shrimp. Repeat the process with all shrimp. You might need a bit more flour or eggs, depends on the size of the shrimp. Refrigerate while preparing the rest of the ingredients. The breading process could be a bit messy. Make sure you are near a water faucet to wash your hands often.

2 bananas, peeled and cut into about 1 inch pieces. You should have 12 banana pieces.

Repeat the shrimp's breading process: Egg – Flour – Egg – Coconut. Once you bread the banana pieces, roll them between your palms into a round shape and press to flaten into a thick patties.

You might have to add more flour, eggs or coconut to complete the banana coating.

1 cup olive oil

Heat in a large saute pan on medium heat. When the oil is hot start cooking the shrimp, a few at a time, on both sides, 2 to 3 minutes on each side or when coconut turns to golden brown. Once the shrimps are cooked, repeat the process with the bananas. You might have to add more olive oil to the pan to finish cooking the bananas.

STEP 3

3 cups of spring mix lettuce
1 cucumber, chopped
½ tsp olive oil
½ tsp balsamic vinegar

Arrange in a serving platter and lay the shrimp on top. Serve with the pineapple cocktail sauce.

3 servings

EL – GF

Calories in coconut fried shrimp per serving: Coconut fried shrimp 252. Coconut fried bananas 132. Total of 384.

- *Coconut is rich in fiber, vitamins C, E, B1, B3, B5 and B6 and minerals including iron, selenium, sodium, calcium, magnesium and phosphorous.*
- *Bananas contain vitamins B6, C, A, as well folate, riboflavin, niacin, manganese, potassium, magnesium, iron, protein and fiber.*

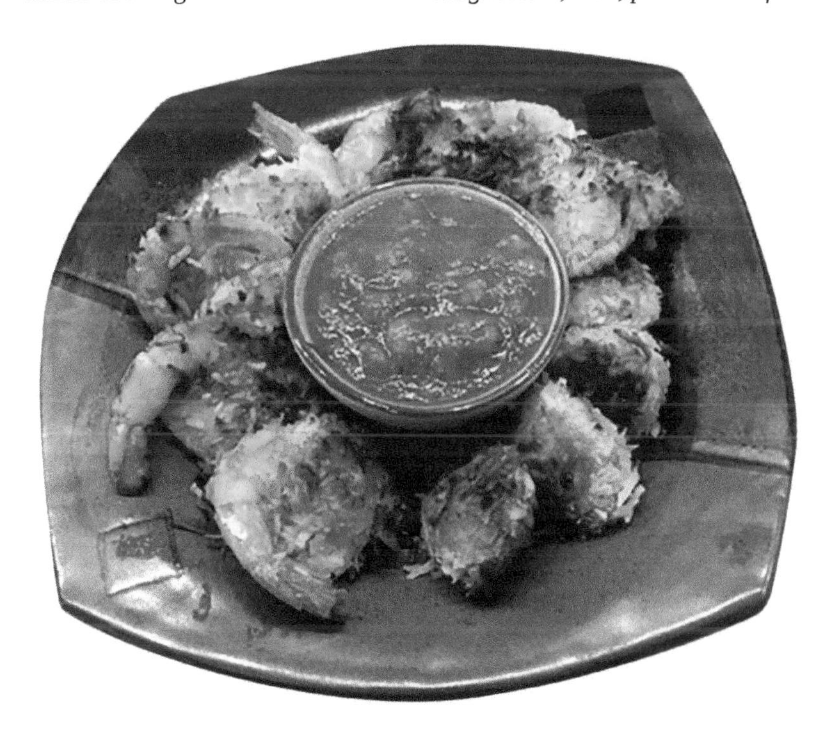

Salmon Burgers

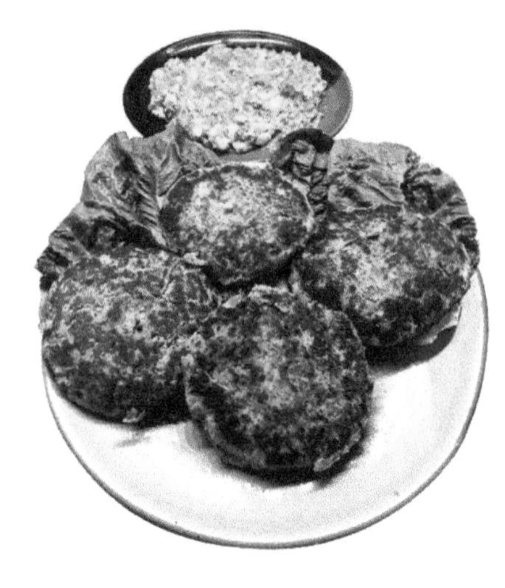

Preheat the oven to 425-degrees.
1 ½ lbs salmon
1 tsp olive oil
½ tsp black pepper
Drizzle the salmon with the olive oil and black pepper. Bake for 10 to 12 minutes. Remove, refrigerate and let it cool. If you are using salmon with the skin on, remove the skin.
1 red bell pepper, large cut
½ onion, large cut
2 cloves garlic, chopped
Place in the food processor and pulse 2 times. Remove and place in a mixing bowl.
2 eggs, beaten
1 tbs low-fat Greek yogurt
1 tbsp cup fresh Italian parsley, chopped
1 tsp fresh rosemary, chopped
1 tsp fresh dill, chopped
¼ tsp black pepper
1 tsp ground mustard
1 tsp ground ginger
juice from ½ lime
½ cup coconut flour
¼ cup almond meal
Add all ingredients in the mixing bowl with the pepper and onion and blend well using a wooden spoon or a spatula.
The cooked salmon
Place in a separate mixing bowl and flake salmon with a fork. Add to the bowl with the rest of the ingredient and mix well. Separate mixture into four parts and press to form the salmon patties.
4 tbsp olive oil
Heat on a flat grill or a large saute pan. Cook salmon patties about 3 to 4 minutes on each side.
Serve with the avocado relish on a gluten free bun or with lettuce wrap.
4 servings
GF

Avocado relish
½ red bell pepper, large cut
¼ red onion, large cut
Place in the food processor and pulse 1 time. Remove, drain well and place in a mixing bowl.
1 lg avocado, peeled and diced
Add to the mixing bowl and toss with the pepper and onion.
1 tbs olive oil
1 tsp red wine vinegar
juice of ¼ lemon
1 small Roma tomato, chopped
1 clove garlic, chopped
1 tsp ground mustard
¼ tsp ground cumin
1 tsp fresh parsley, chopped
¼ tsp white pepper
Add to the mixing bowl and blend well.
GF – VT
Calories in salmon burger per serving: Salmon 249. Almond meal 41. Egg 40. Olive oil 90. Coconut flour 60. Total of 480.
Calories in avocado relish per serving: Total of 90.
Suggestion: Serve salmon burger and avocado relish with grilled sweet potatoes.

Grilled Sweet Potatoes

3 tbsp olive oil
Place on a flat grill on medium heat.
2 sweet potatoes
Peel and half sliced. Grill for about 6 to 7 minutes on each side.
1 large red pepper, sliced
½ red onion, sliced
Add to the grill when potatoes are halfway cooked.
½ lime
1 tsp cumin
1 tbsp dry thyme
Squeeze lime juice and sprinkle thyme and cumin as potatoes are beings cooked, about 8 minutes into the cooking process.
Calories in sweet potatoes per serving: Sweet potatoes 98. Olive oil 144. Total of 242.

Farro Risotto with Turkey Meatballs

Preheat oven to 375-degrees

STEP 1

Prepare the turkey meatballs.

12 oz ground turkey
½ small onion, chopped
3 mushrooms, chopped
2 cloves garlic, chopped
½ stalk celery, chopped
1 tbsp fresh basil, chopped
1 tbsp fresh mint, chopped
1 tbsp dry oregano
1 tsp ground mustard
1 tsp cumin
½ tsp ground sage
½ tsp white pepper
¼ tsp cinnamon
¼ tsp nutmeg
1 egg
¼ cup grated Parmesan
Juice of 1/2 lemon
½ cup oats, place in the food processor and pulse for 2 to 3 times.

Place all ingredients in a mixing ball and mix well. Scoop out the mixture and form small balls. You should have, approximately 16 turkey meatballs. Place a piece of parchment paper on a baking pan, arrange turkey meatball on it and bake for about 12 to 14 minutes. Remove and set aside.

STEP 2

6 cups of water

Place a stockpot and bring it to a gentle boil.

1 cup farro

Add the farro to the stockpot, turn heat to medium and start cooking the farro – total cooking time 45 to 50 minutes.

While farro is being cooked , prepare the rest of the ingredients for this recipe.

STEP 3

2 tbsp olive oil

Heat in a saute pan.

1 onion, sliced
2 cloves garlic, chopped
2 shallots, chopped
1 red bell pepper, sliced

Add to the pan and saute on medium heat for about 5 to 6 minutes

¼ cup white cooking wine
1 portobello mushroom, sliced
1 tbsp capers
1 tsp fresh rosemary, chopped
1 tbsp Italian parsley, chopped
1 tsp black pepper

Add to the pan and saute for another 4 to 5 minutes. Remove from heat.

In about 30 minutes into the cooking process of farro, add the vegetables to the pot. Stir well.

Continue cooking for another 10 minutes.

The baked turkey meatballs

Add the meatball into the stockpot. Stir the mixture gently and let it simmer for another 5 to 10 minutes.

You've reached the total cooking time of 45 to 50 minutes. Farro should be tender and the liquid should be absorbed by now.

Remove and serve.

4 servings

Omit turkey meatballs for VT - VG

Calories in Farro risotto per serving: Farro 202. Olive oil 96. Total of 298.

Calories in turkey meatballs per serving: Turkey 31. Egg 20. Oats 21. Total of 72.

• *Farro is loaded with fiber and protein. It is rich in magnesium, zinc and vitamins A, B, C and E. The larger farro is the whole grain variety and packs more nutrients than the other two.*

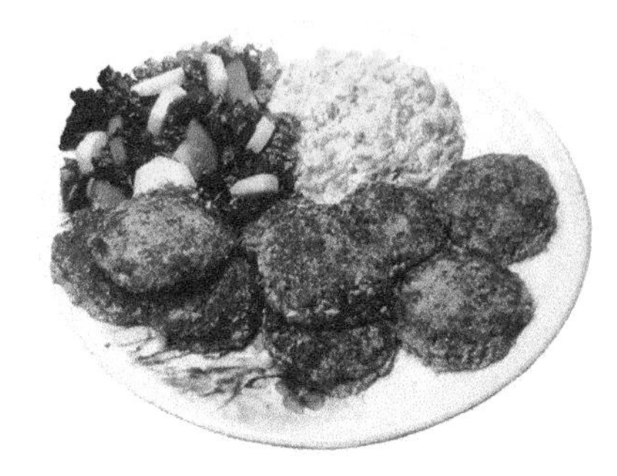

Broccoli Fritters with Sweet and Sour Fruit Relish

STEP 1

Prepare the sauce.

Sweet and Sour Fruit Relish

1 cup mango, chopped
1 red bell pepper, roasted and chopped
1 cup fresh pineapple, chopped
1 tbsp fresh basil, chopped
1 tbsp fresh dill, chopped
1 green onion, chopped
1 clove garlic, chopped
1 tsp turmeric
½ tsp white pepper
1 tbsp sesame seeds
1 tbsp juice of a lemon
1 tbsp capers, chopped
1 cup low-fat real Greek yogurt
1 tbsp olive oil

Place in a large mixing bowl and mix well by hand. Refrigerate until broccoli fritters are done.

EL – GF – VT

8 servings

STEP 2

Prepare the fritters

4 cups broccoli florets
2 cloves garlic
½ large onion
Place in the food processor and pulse 3 or 4 times, until broccoli is minced.
Place mixture in a large mixing bowl.

2 cups reduced fat cheddar cheese, shredded
1 tsp cumin
1 tsp black pepper
2 tbsp almond flour
2 egg
2 tbsp grated Parmesan cheese
Add to the mixing bowl and mix well.
Separate the mixture into 8 parts and make 8 firm balls.

1 cup rolled oats
Place oats in the food processor and pulse 3 or 4 times. Move into a mixing bowl.
Heat the flat grill to medium heat. The broccoli fritters are best cooked on a flat grill, if not available use a large saute pan and cook the broccoli patties a few at a time.
Roll the broccoli balls, one at a time, into oats then press them to make patties, approximately 4 inches round

½ cup olive oil
Pour half of the olive oil on the flat grill and start cooking the broccoli patties.
Let the first side cook well, about 5 to 6 minutes. Turn the patties, add more oil and cook the other side for another 5 to 6 minutes, until golden brown.

4 servings

GF – VT

Calories in per serving in broccoli fritters: Broccoli 31. Cheddar cheese 98. Oats 57. Olive oil 238. Total of 424.
Calories per serving in sweet and sour fruit relish: Sesame seeds 13. Mango 27. Pineapple 11. Olive oil 20. Greek Yogurt 36. Total 89.

• *Broccoli, is a great source of vitamins K and C, a good source of folate, potassium, fiber.*

Complete Meals

"Nick's restaurant has a following so loyal it could be called a cult."
Phoenix Gazette

"Ligidakis talks about cooking like some men talk about courting a beautiful woman...as if each dish were a beloved child."
Echo Magazine

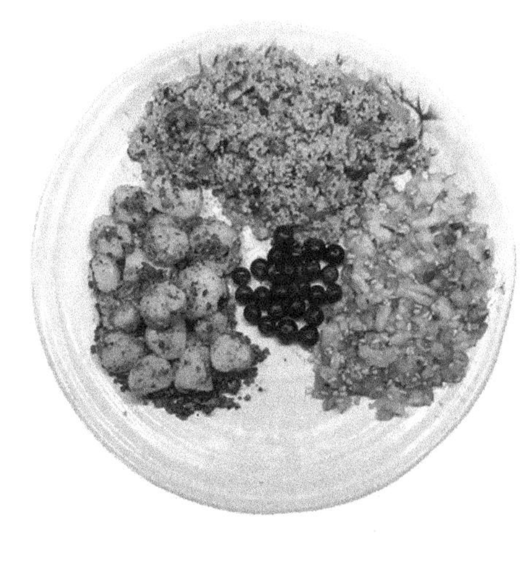

Hazelnut Scallops with Pomegranates and Millet Risotto

STEP 1

Pomegranate Pear Relish

½ small red bell pepper, chopped
2 pears, peeled and chopped
½ cup pineapple, chopped
1 cup pomegranate seeds
1 tsp orange zest
½ cup fresh mint, chopped
½ tsp black pepper
2 tbsp olive oil
Juice of ¼ lemon

Toss ingredients in a mixing bowl and refrigerate.

EL – GF – VT – VG

STEP 2

Millet Pecan Risotto

1 cup millet

Place millet in a small saute pan and toss for about 5 minutes under medium heat, frequently stirring, until the millet is lightly golden. This brings out the millet's nutty flavor.

2 cups vegetable broth
1 cup of water
Heat in a stock pot, bring to a gentle boil. Turn heat to medium and add the millet. Cook for about 18 to 20 minutes, until millet is tender. Remove from heat. Do not discard liquid, if any.
While millet is being cooked prepare the rest of the recipe.
2 tbsp olive oil
Heat in a large saute pan.
½ onion, chopped
Add and saute on medium heat for about 2 to 3 minutes.
2 tbsp white cooking wine
1 portobello mushroom, sliced
2 cloves roasted garlic, chopped
½ cup pecan pieces
½ tsp fresh rosemary, chopped
1 tsp fresh basil leaves, chopped
1 tsp dry thyme
1 tsp black pepper
¼ cup vegetable broth
Add to the pan and cook for about 3 to 4 minutes longer.
The cooked millet.
Add to the pan and cook for 3 to 4 minutes longer, until the liquid is absorbed.

2 servings

EL – GF – VT – VG

STEP 3

Hazelnut Scallops

1 cup hazelnuts, pulse 2 to 3 times in the food processor
1 shallot, chopped
1carlic clove, chopped
½ cup red wine
2 green onions, chopped
Place in a bowl and set aside. Have these ingredients available to finish the scallops.
3 tbsp olive oil
Heat in a large saute pan to medium-high.
16 large sea scallops.
Place scallops between two paper towels and make sure they are dried.
When the oil is hot place scallops in the pan. Saute for about 3 to 4 minutes. Turn scallops over. At this stage scallops are delicate. It is best to use a spatula to flip them over.
½ tsp black pepper
Juice of ¼ lemon
Sprinkle on top of scallops. Cook for another 2 to 3 minutes. At this stage, scallops should be light brown. Remove scallops from the pan.
Pour the hazelnuts mixture into the saute pan.
With your spatula or a large spoon, scrape the pan and continue stirring and scraping for 1 to 2 minutes. Remove and place the hazelnut sauce on a large serving plater.
Place scallops on top of the hazelnut sauce.
Arrange millet risotto and pomegranate relish on the side of the plater and serve.

3 servings

EL – GF

Calories in Pomegranate relish per serving : Pears 68. Pineapple 14. Pomegranate seeds 45. Olive oil 80. Total of 207
Calories in millet risotto per serving : Millet 189. Olive oil 119. Pecans 180. Total of 488.
Calories in hazelnut scallops per serving: Hazelnuts 157. Olive oil 119. Total of 276.

• *Hazelnuts are high in magnesium, calcium and vitamins B and E.*

• *Portobello mushroom is an excellent source of protein, dietary fiber, magnesium, zinc, manganese, thiamin, vitamin B6, folate. It is also a very good source of riboflavin, niacin, pantothenic acid, phosphorus, potassium, copper and selenium.*

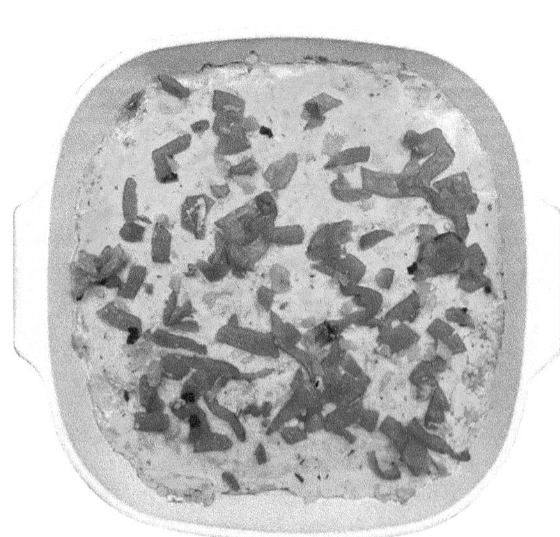

Baked Salmon with Sweet Potato Crust

Page 117

Tomato Shrimp with Pineapple Quinoa

STEP 1

2 cups vegetable stock
2 cups of water
In a stockpot, bring the liquid into a gentle boil.
1 cup three-color quinoa.
¼ red bell pepper, chopped
2 green onions, chopped.
½ cup fresh pineapple, chopped
½ tsp tarragon leaves
1 tbsp fresh parsley, chopped
2 cloves roasted garlic, chopped
1 tsp fresh basil, chopped
½ tsp white pepper
Juice of ½ lemon
Add to the pot and cook for about 18 to 20 minutes, until quinoa is cooked.

STEP 2

In the meantime prepare the shrimp.
4 tbsp olive oil
Head in a large saute pan. Turn heat to medium.
½ onion, chopped
2 garlic cloves, chopped
1 shallot, chopped
Add to the pan and saute for 5 minutes.
⅛ cup white wine
4 Roma tomatoes, chopped
½ tsp black pepper
1 tsp dry oregano
1 tsp dry thyme
½ tsp fresh dill, chopped
Add to the pan and simmer for about 8 minutes.
12 jumbo shrimp, peeled
Add and cook 7 to 8 minutes longer, until shrimp is cooked.
¼ cup feta cheese
Add and stir until feta is melted.

GF

STEP 3

Steamed Ginger Vegetables

1 cup broccoli florets
1 cup cauliflower florets
6 baby carrots
Heat the water in a steamer basket. Add vegetables into the basket and steam for 2 minutes.
1 red bell pepper, sliced lengthwise
1 cup pea pods, remove strings and cut sliced
1 yellow squash, sliced
1 tsp fresh ginger, chopped
Add to the basket and steam for another 2-3 minutes. Remove and place in a mixing bowl.
Juice of ½ lemon
1 tbsp olive oil
1 tbsp fresh Italian parsley, chopped
1 tbsp fresh dill, chopped
1 tbsp sesame seeds
Add to the mixing bowl, toss and serve as a side dish.

EL – GF – VT – VG

2 servings

Calories of the main ingredients per serving: Quinoa 318. Olive oil 119. Shrimp 42. Total of 479.

Baked Salmon with Sweet Potato Crust

Preheat oven to 375-degrees

STEP 1

Sweet Potato Crust

2 medium-size sweet potatoes
Place potatoes in a stock pot, cover with water and boil on medium heat for about 20 to 25 minutes, until potatoes are soft. Drain water, cool and peel.
1 clove garlic, chopped
½ cup slivered almonds
1 tbsp juice of a lemon
1 tbsp olive oil
1 tsp black pepper
1 tsp rosemary, chopped
1 tsp dry thyme
½ cup low-fat real Greek yogurt
Place all ingredients, including sweet potatoes in a mixing bowl of the mixer and mix well.

STEP 2

Baked Salmon

2 lbs skinless salmon fillets.
1 tsp olive oil
Brush with the olive oil the bottom of a large rectangular ceramic or glass baking dish. Spread the sweet potato crust evenly on top of salmon.
1 roasted red pepper, chopped
3 roasted cloves garlic, chopped
Sprinkle on top of the sweet potato crust.
Bake in the preheated oven for about 22 to 25 minutes.
Serve with Mango Relish – see index.

4 servings

Calories for main ingredients in sweet potato crust per serving: Sweet potato 52. Almonds 64. Greek yogurt 12. Total of 188.

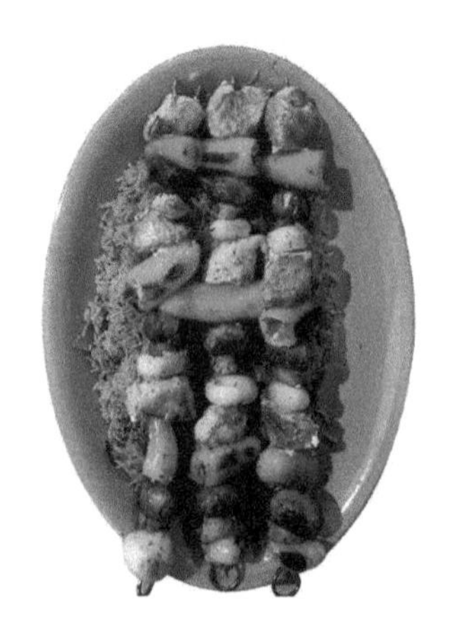

Chicken Brochettes with Tzatziki and Arborio Rice

STEP 1.

Tzatziki Sauce

1 medium cucumber.
Peeled and remove seeds. Place it in a food processor and pulse 2 or 3 times.
Remove from the food processor, drain extra liquid and place in a mixing bowl.

1 cup low-fat real Greek yogurt
2 cloves garlic, minced
1 tsp white pepper
1 tsp lemon juice
1 tsp white vinegar
1 tbsp olive oil
1 tsp fresh dill, chopped
Place in the bowl with the cucumber and mix well with a spoon. Refrigerate.

EL – GF – VT

STEP 2

Marinade

2 tbsp olive oil
juice of ½ lemon
1 tsp dry oregano
1 tsp dry thyme
½ tsp black pepper
1 clove garlic, minced
Place in a small mixing bowl and mix well.

STEP 3

Arborio Rice Pilaf

2 tbs olive oil
Heat in a stockpot.

1 small onion, chopped
8 cremini mushrooms, sliced
2 cloves garlic, chopped
Add to the pot and saute on medium heat for 5 to 6 minutes

¼ cup white cooking wine
1 tsp black pepper
1 tsp fresh parsley, chopped
1 tsp fresh basil, chopped
1 tsp fresh rosemary, chopped
1 tsp dry oregano
1 tsp dry thyme
2 cups vegetable broth
1 cup of water
Add to the pot and cook for 2 to 3 minutes.

1 cup Arborio rice
Add and cook for about 20 to 22 minutes longer, until rice is tender.
While rice is being cooked prepare the brochettes. (It helps if you could prepare the brochettes earlier and refrigerate.)

EL – GF – VT – VG

STEP 4

Chicken Brochettes

4 long iron skewers
24-oz chicken breast meat. Cut into 12 pieces of about 3-inch cubes.
12 medium size cremini mushrooms
12 baby onions, peeled
12 assorted baby sweet pepper
Thread the above items in the skewers in this order: onion, mushroom, pepper, chicken. Repeat threading the food items in the same skewer two more times.
Prepare the other three skewers the same way.

3 tbsp olive oil
Pour on a flat grill or a wide saute pan on medium heat and grill the brochettes well on one side, about 3 minutes. Brush with marinating and turn.
Repeat turning until cooked on all sides, brushing with marinade. Cooking time 12 to 14 minutes.
Place Arborio rice on a large plater, arrange brochettes on top and tzatziki on the side.

EL – GF

4 servings

Calories per serving in tzatziki sauce: Greek yogurt 25. Olive oil 60. Total of 85.
Calories per serving in Arborio rice risotto: Olive oil 60. Arborio Rice 179. Total of 239.
Calories per serving in chicken brochettes: Chicken 280. Mushrooms 57. Olive oil 90. Total of 427.

• *Arborio rice contains a good amount of protein and most of its calories comes from its carbohydrate content. Arborio rice is a better source of fiber from the long-grain rice and it is sodium-free. It contains a small amount of iron and it is packed with vitamins A and C and easy to digest.*

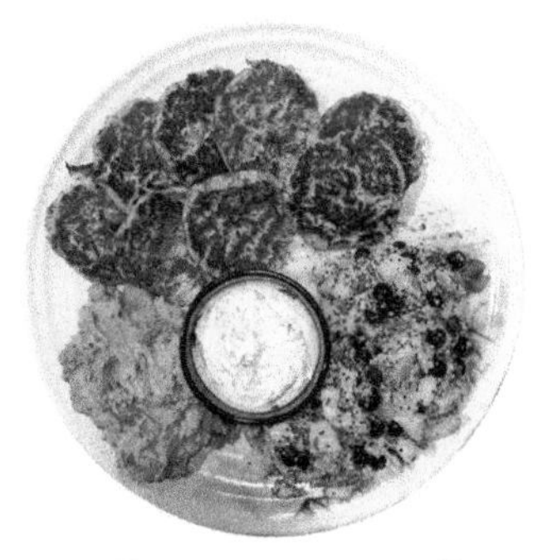

Crab Cakes with Sweet Potatoes Walnut Mash

STEP 1

Crab Cakes

½ small red onion, chopped
½ medium red bell pepper, chopped
2 cups crab meat
½ cup ricotta cheese
1 egg
1 tbsp fresh basil, chopped
1 tbsp fresh mint, chopped
1 tsp fresh dill, chopped
3 cloves garlic, chopped
¼ cup grated Parmesan cheese
3 green onions, chopped
1 tsp white pepper
1 tsp ground mustard

Place all ingredients in the food processor and pulse 1 or 2 times.

Refrigerate for about 1 hour.

GF

STEP 2

Yogurt Quinoa Fruit Salad

½ cup three-color quinoa
2 cups of water

Heat water in a small pot on medium heat. Add quinoa and cook for 15 to 18 minutes. Drain excess water if any. Cool.

1 cup fresh pineapple, chopped
1 cup blueberries, choose the smallest size
2 kiwi, chopped
1 mango, chopped
¼ cup raisins
2 green onions, chopped
¼ tsp fresh ginger, minced
1 tsp fresh mint, chopped
1 tsp lime juice
1 tsp sesame seeds
1 tbsp sunflower seeds
½ cup low-fat real Greek yogurt
1 tsp honey
½ tsp nutmeg

Mix all ingredients in a bowl. Refrigerate until crab cakes are ready to serve.

EL – GF – VT

STEP 3

Caper and Dill Dipping Sauce

1 cup low-fat Greek yogurt
1 tsp prepared horseradish
1 tbsp capers, chopped
1 tbsp lemon juice
1 tbsp dry mustard
1 green onion, minced
1 clove garlic, minced
½ cucumber, minced
½ tsp white pepper
1 tbsp fresh dill, chopped

Place in a mixing bowl and mix well. Refrigerate until ready to serve.

STEP 4

Sweet Potatoes Walnut Mash

2 medium-size sweet potatoes

Peel potatoes and place in a pot, cover with water and boil on medium-high heat for about 20 to 25 minutes, until potatoes are soft. Drain water, peel the potatoes, and place them in a mixing bowl. Mash potatoes with a potato masher.

2 cloves garlic, minced
¼ cup walnuts, chopped
1 tbsp lemon juice
1 tbsp olive oil
1 tsp black pepper
1 tsp fresh parsley, minced
¼ cup low-fat real Greek yogurt

Add the rest of the ingredients and mix well. Serve warm or cold.

EL – GF – VT

STEP 5

Pull the crab meat mixture from the refrigerator. Separate the crab cake mixture to eight balls. Flatten balls to thick patties. You should have eight large patties.

¼ cups almond meal
¼ cup almond flour

Place in a bowl and mix well. Coat the crab cakes lightly with the almond mixture and set aside.

4 tbsp olive oil

Heat the oil on a flat grill. Add the crab cakes and brown the one side well, about 5 to 6 minutes. Flip the cakes and continue cooking for 6 to 7 minutes longer.

Arrange crab cakes, dipping sauce, sweet potatoes and fruit salad in a plater and serve.

4 servings

Calories in main ingredients of crab cakes per serving: Olive oil 30. Ricotta 54. Eggs 39. Parmesan cheese 28. Crab meat 53. Almond meal 40. Almond flour 38. Olive oil for grilling 90. Total of 372.

Calories in main ingredients of sweet potatoes walnut mash per serving : Sweet potato 57. Walnuts 33. Greek yogurt 36. Total of 126.

Calories in main ingredients of yogurt quinoa fruit salad per

serving: Quinoa 85. Pineapple 20. Blueberries 22. Kiwi 21. Mango 50. Raisins 31. Greek yogurt 18. Total of 247.
Calories in caper and dill dipping sauce per serving: Greek yogurt 38.

Stuffed Grapevine Leaves

STEP 1

6 green onions, chopped
1 tbsp fresh parsley, chopped
½ cup raisins
½ cup pine nuts
2 cups white basmati rice
1 tbsp fresh dill, chopped
½ tsp black pepper
1 tbs olive oil

Mix all ingredients in a mixing bowl

1 to 2 large jars of grapevine leaves

Most likely there will be different sizes of grapevine leaves in the jar. Lay a large leaf on a working surface and place a small one at the top end of the large one. Use a teaspoon of the mixture and place it on the bottom center of the large leaf. Fold the edges of the leaf over the rice mixture and roll I as tightly as possible. Repeat this process for the rest of the mixture. You should end up with about 20 rolled grape leaves. Once cooked, refrigerate the extra ones, they are good cold for lunch or appetizer.

Layer tightly the stuffed grape leaves in a stockpot.

Juice of 1 lemon
1 tsp black pepper
1 tbsp olive oil

Sprinkle over the grape-leaves Add a heavy item on top of the grape leaves. I use a couple of plates on top of the stuffed grape leaves to keep them from breaking up.

1 quart vegetable broth
1 quart water

Pour in the pot and simmer over medium heat for about 1 hour. Let cool before removing the grape-leaves from the pot.

5 servings

GF – EL – VT – VG

STEP 2

Yogurt Sauce

1 cucumber, peeled and cut in pieces
2 green onions

Place in a food possessor and pulse 1 or 2 times. Drain access liquid if any.

1 tbsp grated Parmesan cheese
1 and ½ cups light sour cream
1 cup and ½ cups low-fat Greek yogurt
Juice of 1 lemon
1 tsp Dijon mustard
1 tsp black pepper

Place in a mixing bowl of a mixer, add cucumber and green onion and mix well.

Refrigerate leftover sauce in a jar. Lemon acts as a natural preservative and will keep for about 30 days in your refrigerator.

GF – VT

STEP 3

Grecian Grilled Vegetables

12 asparagus
2 red peppers, cut in halves
1 eggplant, sliced lengthwise
2 yellow squash, sliced lengthwise.

Set aside

Dressing
¼ cup olive oil
1/8 cup balsamic vinegar
2 cloves garlic, chopped
1 tsp fresh mint, chopped
1 tbsp dry oregano
1 tsp dry thyme
1 tsp dry basil
1 tsp black pepper
1 tbsp dry mustard

Mix ingredients in a large ball. Heat your outdoor grill, dip vegetables in the dressing and grill well on both sides. Remove vegetables cut into large cuts place in a large serving plate.

Option: Grill vegetables on a flat grill.

1 tbsp fresh mint, chopped

Sprinkle on top of the vegetables.

Serve grape leaves with the yogurt sauce and grilled vegetables.

Calories for main ingredients in grape leaves per serving of four grape leaves: Raisins 42. Basmati rice 60. Pine nuts 76. Olive oil 20. Total of 198.

Calories for main ingredients in yogurt sauce per serving: Sour cream 37. Greek yogurt 62.Total of 99.

- *Raisins include protein and dietary fiber. Raisins, like prunes and apricots, are also high in certain antioxidants, but they are low in vitamin C compared to the fresh grapes. Raisins, like any dried fruit, can be high on sugars.*
- *Pine nuts are found between the*

scales of pine cones. All pine trees yield pine nuts, but only some species have pine nuts large enough to be eaten. It takes a long time for pine nuts to mature, as long as two to three years. It also takes time and a lot of patience to harvest the pine nuts. It is why the pine nuts are very expensive. Pine nuts are high in potassium, magnesium and phosphorus. They also contain fiber, protein, iron, zinc, thiamin, niacin, B12, and vitamins c and K.

Baked Chicken with Baby Vegetables

STEP 1

1 whole chicken, about 4 lbs

Place in a baking dish, with its back down

2 lbs of assorted color baby carrots

2 lbs of assorted color baby potatoes, peeled

10 baby onions, peeled

4 cloves garlic, cut into quarters

4 shallots, peeled and cut into quarters

Place vegetables around the chicken.

STEP 2

4 tbsp olive oil

juice of 1 lemon

1 tbsp fresh rosemary, chopped

1 tsp ground sage

1 tsp black pepper

2 tbsp dry thyme

2 tbsp dry basil

1 tbsp dry oregano

Mix all ingredients in a mixing bowl and pour over chicken and vegetables

Bake in a 375-degree oven for about 70 to 80 minutes, until chicken is golden brown.

EL – GF

STEP 3

Brown Rice, Black Bean, Fruit Salad

3 cups of water

2 cups vegetable broth

Heat in a stockpot.

1 cup of brown rice

Add and cook on medium heat for about 35 to 40 minutes, until rice is tender. Remove, drain extra liquid and cool.

2 cups cooked black beans, drained well.

1 mango, chopped

1 apple, peeled and chopped

1 avocado, chopped

½ cup golden raisins

¼ cup walnut pieces

½ red onion, chopped

1 cup artichoke hearts, sliced

½ cup feta, crumbled

1 tbsp capers

1 tbsp fresh parsley, chopped

1 tbsp fresh basil, chopped

1 tsp dry oregano

½ tsp cumin

2 tbsp olive oil

1 tsp red wine vinegar

The cooked brown rice

Place ingredient in a mixing bowl and mix well.

6 servings

EL – GF – VT

Calories of main ingredients per serving: Chicken 178. Potatoes 224. Onions 28. Carrots 90. Olive oil 60. Total of 580. Brown Rice, Black Bean, Fruit Salad: Brown rice 172. Mango 50. Apple 24. Avocado 80. Golden raisins 31. Walnuts 33. Artichoke hearts 75. Feta 50. Olive oil 60. Total of 517.

Learning to work with leftovers

Leftovers could be an inspiration for new recipes. Working in the restaurant, while preparing, especially desserts, sometimes we had some leftover melted chocolate or cake. Rather than refrigerating the leftover items we used them to create something new. Part of respecting food is that you do not waste it. The other day we had some one-day leftover baked chicken.

I cut the chicken into large pieces, placed it in a small baking ceramic dish, sprinkle some crumbled feta on the chicken and made a quick tomato sauce; Sautéed onions and garlic in olive oil. I added red cooking wine, 5 chopped Roma tomatoes, and vegetable broth. Along with black pepper, oregano, thyme, and basil. I poured the sauce over the chicken and sprinkled it with some grated Parmesan cheese. Topped it with shredded mozzarella and baked it in a 350-degree oven for about 20 minutes. Along with some lettuce salad, we had a nice dinner.

Working with leftovers, it is an excellent chance to practice your skills on measurements and the preparation of your new recipe.

Gluten-Free Flours

Back in the day, when I wrote a recipe containing flour, it meant the use of white flour, unless it was specified to use whole wheat. Occasionally there was rye flour, semolina, durum wheat, and a few other unusual flours but none were gluten-free. Back then, if you looked for a gluten-free flour in the grocery store, there wasn't any. And then, it all changed. The selection of gluten-free flours displayed in the grocery stores is now overwhelming. In general, we use flour to create structure in baked goods or to occasionally thicken soups or sauces. Before the invasion of gluten-free flours, there was no interest in knowing how wheat flour worked. When you work with gluten-free flours, the first challenges is to understand the profile of each gluten-free flour. Thus begins the journey of trial-and-error baking with gluten-free flours. The problem is that not a single gluten-free flour behaves precisely like wheat flour; therefore, you must use a blend of various gluten-free flours to achieve your goal of baking without wheat flour. The various gluten-free flours produce a different consistency and flavor. As it is true with wheat flour, the liquids used in recipes with flours can affect the texture of the mixture. For example, the size of an egg or the origin and type of an oil will affect the consistency, and most likely, alter the result of your recipe. It is essential, in baking, to be familiar with the constancy of various mixtures. Familiarity with the consistency, allows us to add a bit more flour or some more liquid, to bring your mixture to your desired consistency. Wheat flour is known for its texture and taste. It is the taste where gluten-free flours have an advantage – they all have a different flavor; therefore, the tastes you can create with gluten-free flours are endless. The question is, which blend of gluten-free flours is best? It depends on what you want to bake. Some flours have a strong flavor, others are sweet, and some are nutty. When you start the fascinated journey of baking with gluten-free flours, you must be flexible and try as many as you can. The texture is the biggest challenge for gluten-free baking. Even since I began the writing of this book, new flours appeared on the market. Therefore, there is a lot more information about the combinations of flours and additives. Because of its texture and taste, the most common flour used in gluten-free baking is the white rice flour. The white rice flour has a very mild flavor, which allows for other flours to be mixed in to create the various gluten-free baked product. There is no question that baking with gluten-free flours is challenging, but the rewards are many, not only in the taste but most importantly for your health.

Buckwheat flour

Buckwheat flour is bold, rich with earthy flavors. It works best in pancakes and quick breads. The main reason to use buckwheat is for its flavor and to boost the nutrition quality of your gluten-free recipes.

Like all gluten-free flours, buckwheat is difficult when used all on its own, but when combined with other whole-grain flours and ingredients, you can create some unique recipes in your kitchen. Buckwheat seems to concern some people, having the word wheat in its name. However, buckwheat has no relation to wheat. It is entirely gluten-free. It is a pseudo-grain just like quinoa, amaranth and millet. The buckwheat's earthy color gives baked goods a darker brown color effect. The taste depends on what you are combining it with; it could be mild or intense, yet distinctive and delicate. I find it easier to work with than most gluten-free flours.

Buckwheat flour carries some impressive health benefits. It has the highest levels of manganese, magnesium, copper, and zinc from other cereal grains. It also has high levels of potassium, niacin, phosphorus, iron, calcium, and vitamin D. Buckwheat is loaded with soluble fiber and comes with a stellar protein profile, making it an ideal plant-based protein option.

Coconut flour

Coconut flour is another low-carb, gluten-free baking alternative flour. Its superior texture is suitable for baked goods and can even be added to smoothies and soups to increase nutrition. The caution with coconut flour is that a small amount of flour will absorb a considerable amount of liquid; because it is so absorbent, it tends to have a drying effect on baked goods. The fact about glutenous flours is that the ones with higher protein content absorb more liquid. It is the same with gluten-free flours. Coconut flour has a high protein content, therefore, consumes high amounts of liquid. To control the drying effect when baking with coconut flour, use liquid or soft foods that are difficult to be absorbed, like plenty of eggs, honey, Greek yogurt or bananas. The egg whites help to provide structure to baked goods while the yolks offer moisture. It is always a good practice to beat your eggs separately. Separating the eggs improves the structure of many baked goods, mainly when you use coconut flour. Coconut flour is also a good source of fiber, and iron.

Almond Flour and Almond Meal

Almond flour is becoming a popular alternative to wheat flour. The difference between almond flour and almond meal is that almond flour is made from blanched and peeled almonds and almond meal contains the almond skin. Without the skin, almond flour is ideal for lighter texture foods, like cakes and muffins and the coarser almond meal is better suited for denser foods like biscotti, cookies or even pizza crusts. Pure almond flour and almond meal have just one ingredient – almonds. The extra fat in both almond products adds some excess moisture and richness to the recipes. The oil in the almond flour makes it safe to be baked in high temperatures. Almonds don't contain gluten. Therefore, a dough made with it doesn't act like a traditional dough; it will not rise with yeast. Almond flour combines well with mild spices and grated Parmesan cheese.

The drawback with almond flour is that it is expensive. Almond meal is a bit less expensive, but they are worth the high price. Be careful though, if you find an inexpensive almond flour/meal, most likely it is not pure – it contains other flours as fillers.

Brown rice flour

Brown rice flour is one of the best substitutions for wheat flour. Even though brown rice flour contains much oil, it absorbs a lot of moisture. If you are using it for baking to compensate for the lack of gluten and to achieves a smoother consistency, adding additional liquid, like eggs or extra oil, is essential. If you are using a rising agent, like arrowroot powder, with brown rice flour, it tends to rise quickly. Gluten-free flours need to be baked in lower temperatures than recipes that contain wheat flour. It helps to refrigerate the gluten-free dough or batter for about an hour before using it. Although brown rice flour is an excellent replacement in baking, because of its darker color and flavor, it can be used as a thickening agent for sauces and soups. Because the bran of brown flour is milled with the endosperm, brown rice flour has a higher level of fiber, iron, B vitamins than white rice flour. It is also high in protein, as all types of rice flour are.

White rice flour

Most gluten-free flours blend well with white rice flour. This is the reason that the majority of gluten-free baked goods contain rice flour. White rice flour behaves well in combination with other gluten-free flours and combines well with oils and with other starches. It can be used as a thickener for soups and sauces as well. The problem with white rice flour is that its neutral flavor and color gives baked goods a flavorless taste and an unappealing white color. It is another reason that white rice flour must be blended with darker flours such as buckwheat or brown rice flour. White rice flour behaves well in cakes, biscotti, muffins, quick breads and pie crusts.

Garbanzo flour

Beyond the health benefits, garbanzo flour is remarkably versatile and has a subtle flavor. It is excellent for cooking flavorful baking items and sweet desserts. Garbanzo flour is used as a staple in various cuisines all over the world. Besides its taste, garbanzo flour is one of the most nutrient-packed gluten-free flours available. It is packed with healthy protein, fiber, vitamins, and more. This unique flour has it all; nutritional benefits, taste, texture and versatility which makes garbanzo flour an important piece in the gluten-free cooking and baking puzzle. Garbanzo flour has a nutty flavor and grainy texture.

Millet flour

Millet flour has a mild flavor, making it a good flour for sweet baking. In my opinion, millet flour is often overlooked in gluten-free baking, yet it adds a delicate taste and a firm texture to muffins, pancakes, and waffles and it is especially useful in quick breads. This mild and slightly sweet grain is an adaptable grain because it soaks up the tastes of the foods surrounding it. The impressive thing about millet in baking is that it blends in harmony, rather than overpowering other ingredients. Millet contains high levels of essential amino acids and is therefore, a good source of protein and dietary fiber. Millet is also an excellent source of manganese, phosphorus and magnesium.

Sorghum flour

Sorghum flour is a powerhouse of nutrition and adds a superb flavor to gluten-free baking, especially in breads, cakes, and cookies. Sorghum flour soft textured and mild taste is becoming a popular ingredient to use in gluten-free baking. People in India and across the continent of Africa have been using sorghum for generations. I believe that sorghum flour is the closest in texture and taste to traditional wheat flour of any of the gluten-free flours. Sorghum makes a reasonable basis for a decent gluten-free bread. Sorghum is high in fiber, potassium, iron and zinc. It contains a good amount of protein and decent amounts of magnesium, phosphorous and selenium, vitamins E, B6, thiamin, riboflavin, niacin, folate and pantothenic acid.

Oat flour

You can easily make your oat flour by putting dried oats into your food processor and pulse them into a fine powder. Oat flour adds moisture into baked goods. Therefore, it is an excellent choice for making cookies, quick breads, cakes or muffins. The mild flavor and light texture of oats do not overpower your baking items. Oats gives a chewy texture to cookies and moistness to breads, cakes and muffins. Also, it lends thickness to brownies and pancakes. Bottom line, oat flour is a useful flour for gluten-free baking. It is also one of the healthiest flours. Oat flour is high in fiber and many vitamins and minerals. It is high in potassium, phosphorous, magnesium, iron, manganese, calcium and reasonable amounts of calcium, zinc and selenium. And contains decent amounts of protein, vitamins B6, E, K, thiamin, riboflavin, niacin, choline and folate.

Tapioca flour

Tapioca flour is now a staple for the gluten-free diet. Tapioca is low in all types of fats, protein, fiber, and essential vitamins or minerals. It tastes mild and slightly sweet. Tapioca is extracted from cassava roots, and even though will not provide the essential nutrients using tapioca makes it possible to recreate recipes without the use of all-purpose flour. Tapioca's presence in gluten-free diets is to be a thickening food agent. Tapioca has decent amounts of calcium, potassium and phosphorus. It contains low amounts of iron, magnesium and selenium.

Arrowroot flour

Arrowroot flour is made from a starchy substance extracted from a tropical plant known as Maranta arundinacea. It is a versatile flour and can be used as a thickener or mixed with other flours for gluten-free baking. Arrowroot gives a crispy texture to baking products. Because it is a starch-based flour it can be a good thickener for creamy soups and sauces. It could also be used to thicken the fillings for fruit pies. Arrowroot is a rich source of vitamin B9, calcium, potassium, magnesium, and phosphorus. It also contains low amounts of zinc and iron, as well as vitamins B1 and B6.

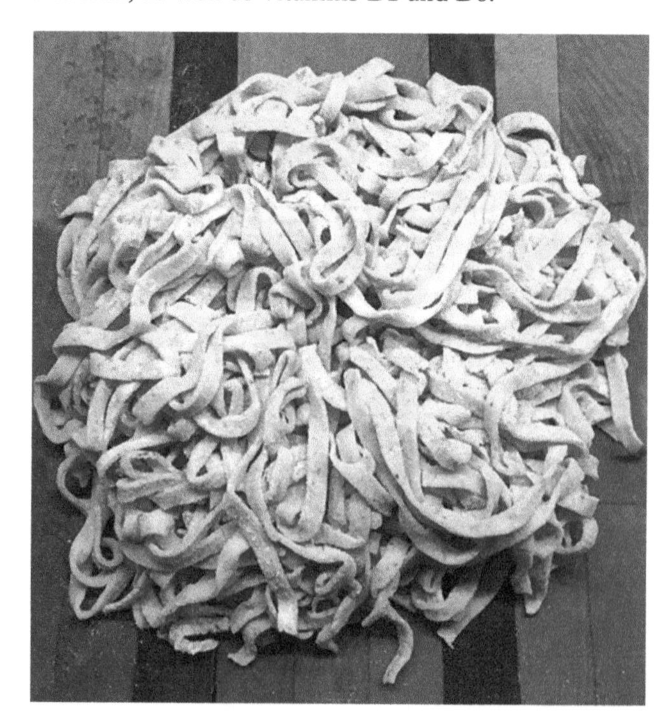

Pizza and Pasta

"One of the most special parts about Nick is that he continually experiments to come up with complex original recipes to add to his already stunning selections of hundreds of recipes."
Western Express

"Nick is a man who marches to his own culinary drummer."
Best of Phoenix Restaurant Guide

PIZZA

Usually, I don't have a difficult time creating recipes. I've been doing it for decades but working with gluten-free flours is a different experience. The gluten-free pizza dough recipe gave me a headache for a couple of days. With wheat flour, I was used to a particular texture, taste and technique but working with gluten-free flours is an entirely different process. The point is that if you are used to making a regular pizza, forget everything you knew. There is no long process of dough-rising or pizza round flour-rolling mess. In this new recipe, there were some flours that I was attracted to use which I wasn't familiar with how they would perform in pizza dough making, and in high temperature baking. Creating recipes with ingredients of unfamiliar behavior can be challenging at best. The texture and flavor wasn't my only concern, I wanted to include as many nutrients as possible. I did my research and tried a couple of things to study the texture and flavor of different blends and I believe that my gluten-free pizza dough recipe is pretty close to what I had conceived in my head. Once you are done blending all the ingredients the texture of the dough is completely different from the traditional pizza dough. It is like thick yogurt. After ninety or so minutes of rest, the batter will thicken a bit. The good news is that there is no rolling pins or flour all over the table to roll your dough. Here is what I've learned: The making of gluten-free pizza is pretty simple and can be fun to make. Don't pay attention to the lengthy explanations in most recipes out there – it is not that complicated. Use the following pizza crust and sauce recipes and create your toppings. You must be careful not to put too many toppings on these crusts. If you are using vegetables for pizza toppings, make sure you sauté the vegetables for 3 to 4 minutes.

Gluten Free Pizza Dough

Preheat oven to 400-degrees

1 tsp quick-rise dry yeast

2 and ½ cups lukewarm water.

Place in a bowl, let it sit for about 10 minutes.

1 cups white rice flour

½ cup buckwheat flour

¾ cup sorghum flour

¼ cup potato starch

½ cup tapioca flour

½ cup almond flour

1 tbsp xanthan gum

1 tbs psyllium husk powder

2 tsp baking powder

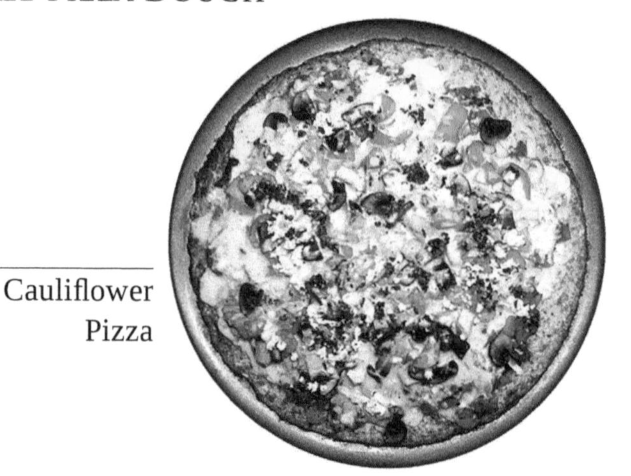

Cauliflower Pizza

Place all dry ingredients in a large mixing bowl. Whisk to mix all ingredients well.

Pour in the water and yeast and mix well with a fork or a spoon.

1 egg white

¼ cup olive oil

2 tbsp low-fat Greek yogurt

Pour these ingredients one at a time, in the mixing bowl, stirring to make sure all ingredients are mixed well together. Place a damp towel and let it rest for about 90 minutes.

Lightly brush a large baking round pizza pan. Scoop the dough in the center of the pan.

Have a small bowl of water next to the pizza pan. Wet your fingers and with your four fingers press to flatten the dough. The dough should be soft and smooth to work with.

Working with your always wet fingertips, open the dough into a round shape.

At this point, the thickness of the round should be about ¼ inch thick. I like this thickness but you can do it a little thinner if you want.

Place the pizza in the middle rack of your preheated oven and bake for 25 minutes.

Remove the pizza dough from the oven.

To assemble the pizza

Pizza sauce recipe – see index.

Spread it on top of the pizza dough, about a ½ inch away from the edges.

1 tbsp grated Romano cheese.

Sprinkle on top of the sauce.

1½ cups shredded low-fat mozzarella

Top the tomato sauce with a thin layer of shredded mozzarella cheese.

Your favorite topping

Use your favorite topping.

½ cup shredded low-fat mozzarella

Sprinkle on top of the toppings.

Return pizza in the oven and bake for another 10 to 15 minutes longer.

Keep checking the pizza in the baking processes. The thickness of the dough, amounts of toppings and different ovens could alter the baking time.

8 slices

GF – VT

Calories in pizza in main ingredients per slice: Rice flour 72. Buckwheat flour 25. Sorghum flour 45. Potato starch 18. Tapioca flour 24. Almond flour 38. Olive oil 60. Total of 282.

Calories in mozzarella cheese per serving: Total of 85.

Nutrients in pizza: The different flours provide a powerful combination of health benefits – see Gluten-free flours section.

NOTE: This recipe makes one large pizza. You could make two smaller pizzas by repeating the process of assembling the pizza and bake them together. If not, place the excess dough in an airtight glass container and refrigerate. It is good for 5 to 6 days. Or freeze in a bag for later use. The frozen dough should be good for a couple of months. However the frozen dough, as is the case of most frozen foods, does not taste the same.

If you are doing a second pizza, bake for 5 to 6 minutes longer.

Cauliflower Pizza Crust

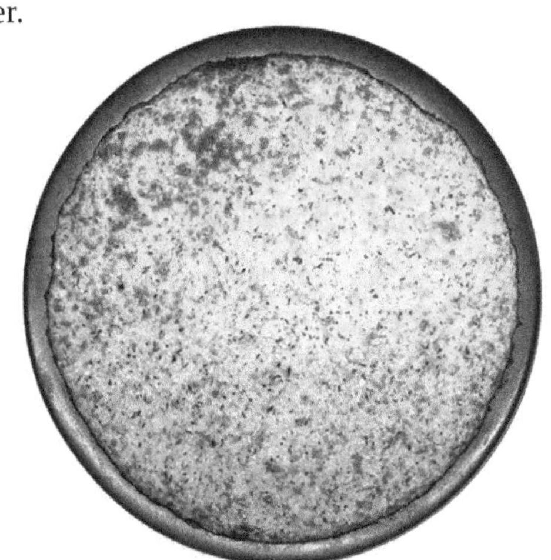

Preheat oven to 400-degrees

Approximately 2 lbs cauliflower – You will need 4 cups cauliflower rice.

Place florets in the food processor, a few at a time, and pulse 2 or 3 times.

4 cups cauliflower rice
2 cloves garlic, minced
2 egg, beaten
1 cup shredded mozzarella
½ cup grated Romano cheese
1 tsp dry thyme
1 tsp dry oregano
1 tsp dry basil
½ tsp black pepper

Place in a mixing bowl along with the cauliflower and mix well by hand.

Lightly brush a large round pizza pan with olive oil. Place cauliflower mixture in the center of the pan and press by hand to open it into about a 12" round crust. With your fingers smooth the edges of the cauliflower crust.

Bake in the preheated oven for about 30 to 32 minutes. Remove from oven.

Tomato sauce – Recipe in the index.

Spread on top of the cauliflower crust.

1 cup shredded mozzarella
Your favorite topping.

Arrange on top of mozzarella.

Return to the oven and bake for 10 to 12 minutes longer.

GF - VT

8 slices

NOTE

Some cauliflower pizza crusts call for steaming the cauliflower before baking and flipping the crust halfway through baking. I found that by steaming the cauliflower, I compromise the character and nutrients, especially vitamin C, of the cauliflower. By flipping the crust, I lose some of the softer texture. It is the general belief that by steaming the cauliflower crust will hold together and without parchment paper will stick on the baking pan. I do not steam, flip or use baking paper with my recipe. To overcome the issues mentioned above, I use a small amount of oil to prevent the sticking part. I also use an extra egg for moistness and bake my crust longer. My technique results in a softer, tastier and healthier crust.

Calories per slice: Crust – Cauliflower 28. Eggs 40. Mozzarella 25. Romano 25. Total of 118

• *Cauliflower contains a high amount of fiber and provides a significant amount of antioxidants. It is high in choline, an essential nutrient for our body, found only in a few foods. Cauliflower, along with broccoli, is one of the best plant-based sources of choline. Cauliflower contains high amounts of vitamin C, which acts as an antioxidant. It is low in calories but high in fiber and water, perfect for low-fat diets. Besides vitamin C, cauliflower contains vitamins K, B6, folate and pantothenic acid. It also includes several minerals, like potassium, magnesium, manganese and phosphorous – overall an impressive nutrition profile.*

Pizza Sauce

1 tbsp olive oil

Heat in a large sauté pan.

½ medium onion, chopped

2 cloves garlic cloves, chopped

Add to the pan. Sauté for 2 to 3 minutes on medium heat

1 tsp red cooking wine

4 Roma tomatoes, chopped

2 cremini mushrooms, chopped

Add to the pan and simmer for 3 to 4 minutes

½ cup vegetable broth

1 tsp dry thyme

1 tbsp dry oregano

1 tbsp fresh basil, chopped

1 tsp black pepper

Add to the pan and simmer for about 8 to 10 minutes. In the last couple of minutes, press the tomatoes in the pan, with the back of a large spoon to a paste consistency.

EL – GF – VT – VG

Calories in the main ingredients: Roma tomatoes 18.

• *Tomatoes are the primary dietary source of the antioxidant lycopene, the most powerful antioxidant which has been measured in foods, and it has been linked to many health benefits. Other vegetables and fruits with lycopene are guavas, watermelon, papaya, grapefruit, sweet red peppers, asparagus, red cabbage, mango, and carrots. The importance of lycopene in tomatoes is because the general population consumed a higher amount of tomatoes than any other foods which contains the antioxidant lycopene. Tomatoes are also a great source of vitamin C, potassium, folate and vitamin K.*

NOTE: The use of mushrooms in the pizza sauce will absorb some of the acidity of the tomatoes. The use of vegetable broth is to balance the acidity.

Garlic Bread

½ cup low-fat butter,

I like to use the Smart Balance® Original Butter.

1 tbsp grated Romano cheese

1 tsp grated Parmesan cheese

1 tbsp olive oil mayonnaise

2 cloves garlic, minced

1 tbsp fresh parsley, minced

Mix well by hand and spread on gluten free bread slices.

Toast the slices in the oven and serve.

Garlic Herb Gluten-free Pasta

3 cloves garlic, roasted and minced

1 tsp dry oregano

1 tsp dry thyme

1 tsp dry basil

1 tsp dry rosemary, minced

1 tsp black pepper

Using the gluten-free pasta recipe, incorporate the above ingredients with the flours, before mixing with the eggs and olive oil.

Pasta

During the decades I spent in the restaurant business, I only used dry pasta when I needed specialty cuts pasta such is fussili, mostaccioli, or pasta shells. Every other pasta such as fettuccine and linguini noodles, pasta sheets for lasagna and manicotti, and the stuffed pasta such as ravioli, tortellini, or agnolotti were freshly made and cooked to order in my restaurant. The freshly made pasta is one of the reasons that our pasta dishes oozed with freshness and flavor. If you pay closer attention to a pasta dish made with dry pasta, most of the flavor is in the sauce. The freshness in the freshly made pasta is incomparable. The truth is that in most restaurants, the dry pasta is cooked and reheated to be served. That is not to say that dry pasta is not good but to point out that freshly made pasta is more superior in the taste.

To make fresh pasta, gluten-free or not, it takes a little bit of practice, but the effort to learn is well worth it. There is a recipe for wheat pasta in the *Recipes to Celebrate Life* section.

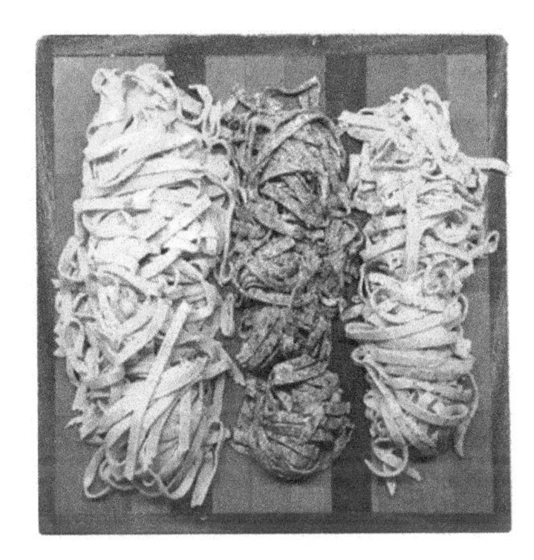

Spinach Gluten-free Pasta

¾ cup frozen organic spinach

Drain well. Place in a food processor and pulse 2 to 3 times. It is important for spinach to be completely dry before mixing with the pasta dough.

Using the pasta recipe, incorporate the spinach along with the wet ingredients when are mixed with the flours.

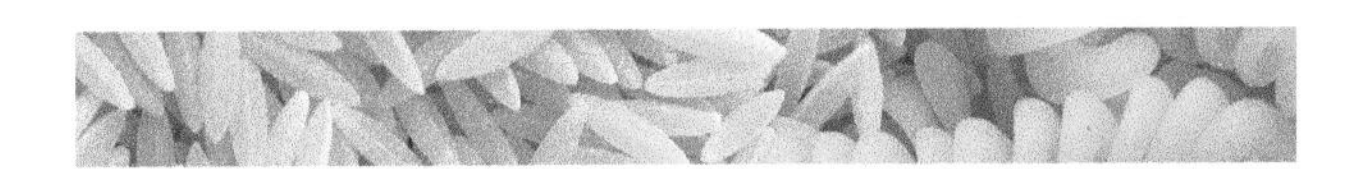

Pasta is bestserved with:

- ***A salad with romaine lettuce or Greek peasant salad.***
- ***With grilled vegetables, especially asparagus, eggplants or artichokes.***
- ***With a spread including sun-dried tomatoes or kalamata olives.***
- ***With a bruschetta that includes either or tomatoes, onions, garlic, grated Parmesan cheese.***
- ***And of course with the traditional garlic bread.***

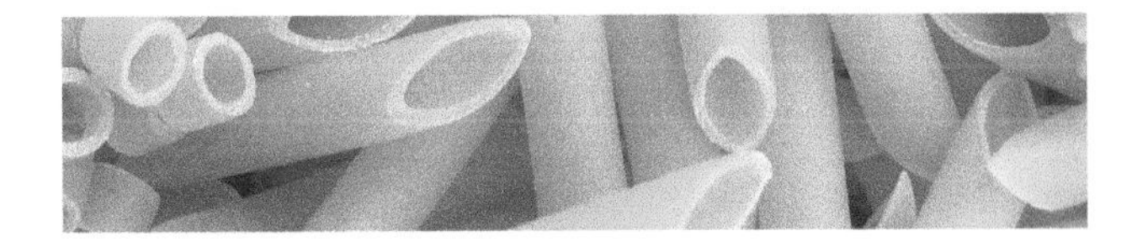

Gluten-free Pasta

1 cup brown rice flour
½ cup white rice flour
½ cup arrowroot flour
2 tbsp flaxseed
½ tsp nutmeg
2 tsp xanthan gum

In a large bowl blend well all the above ingredients.

5 eggs, beaten
1 tbsp olive oil

Add the olive oil into the eggs and slowly pour into the center of the flour mixture, stirring with a wooden spoon into a circular motion to incorporate the wet and dry ingredients.

Dust a working surface with brown rice flour and continue kneading until the dough is smooth.

Divide dough into four parts. Working with one piece at a time, flatten the dough into a rectangle shape.

Dust the piece of the pasta dough with brown flour and using a rolling pin,roll into a wide strip, about 1/8 inch thick. It is important not to make your pasta strip too thin or will break. Gluten-free pasta should be thicker than regular pasta.

Using a hand-crank pasta machine, dust the dough and feed it through the machine to make flat sheets. Your machine should have an attachment of two different pasta cuts.

Use the attachment to make the preferred cut.

If you do not have a pasta machine, roll the dough with a rolling pin, into long strips, into preferred thickness. Dust and fold the width of pasta strip into a flat roll. With a sharp knife, cut the side of the roll into desired pasta size, such as fettuccine or linguini.

Makes 8 servings

Calories in main ingredients: Brown rice 72. White rice flour 36. Total of 108.

Manicotti Spinaci

Sauce
2 tbsp olive oil

Heat in a sauté pan

½ onion chopped
3 cloves of garlic, chopped

Add to the pan and sauté on medium heat for about 2 minutes.

1 tbsp white wine
8 ripe Roma tomatoes, chopped
½ cup vegetable broth
1 tsp dry basil
1 tbsp dry oregano
1 tsp dry thyme
½ tsp black pepper

Add and simmer for 10 to 12 minutes. Set aside.

Preheat oven to 375-degrees.

Manicotti
8 gluten-free pasta sheets.

Pasta sheets should be approximately 4 to 5 inches long. Handmade pasta machine makes pasta sheets 5 to 5½ inches wide.The pasta recipe in this book should make 8 pasta sheets.

Spinach filling
3 cups fresh spinach, chopped
3 cups low-fat mozzarella cheese, shredded
¼ cup Romano cheese, grated
½ cup low-fat feta, crumbled
1 cup low-fat ricotta
1 clove garlic, minced
½ tsp nutmeg
1 tsp. black pepper

Place in a mixing bowl and blend all ingredients well.

Lay the pasta sheets on a working surface.

Divide spinach filling into 8 parts.

Place the filing on the end of each pasta sheet and spread it evenly crosswise.

Roll the pasta sheet tightly over the filling.

Lightly oiled the bottom of a 12"x8" ceramic or glass baking dish.

Place the eight manicotti in and pour the sauce over.

Bake in the preheated oven for about 30 to 35 minutes.

4 servings

GF – VT

Calories in main ingredients per serving: Pasta 27.Roma tomatoes 36. Mozzarella 162. Romano cheese 27. Feta 50. Ricotta 60. Olive oil 60. Total of 422.

Eggplant and Red Pepper Lasagna

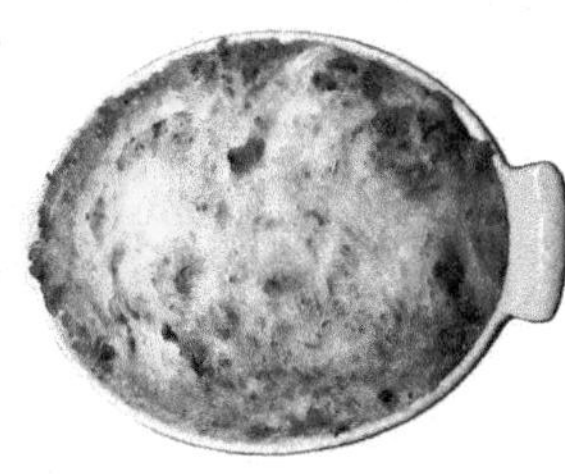

Preheat oven to 350-degrees

¼ cup olive oil

Turn the flat grill to medium heat and pour on the olive oil.

1 eggplant, slice lengthwise, about ¼-inch thick.

You should have six or 7 slices of the eggplant.

1 large red pepper, sliced

Place the vegetables and grill until they are cooked. About 5 to 6 minutes.

Set aside.

2 tbsp olive oil

Heat in a sauté pan on medium heat.

1 small red onion, chopped

2 cloves garlic, chopped

Add to the pan and sauté for 2 to 3 minutes

3 tbsp white cooking wine

8 Roma tomatoes, chopped

1 tbsp capers, chopped

1 tsp dry basil

1 tsp dry oregano

1 tsp dry thyme

1 tbsp fresh Italian parsley, chopped

1 tsp fresh mint, chopped

½ tsp black pepper

Add and simmer for about 7 to 8 minutes until tomatoes break down.

Stir well and remove from heat.

Pasta

6 cups water

Bring to a gentle boil in a stockpot.

2 gluten-free pasta sheets

Pasta sheets should be 10 inches long.

Handmade pasta machine makes pasta sheets 5 to 5 ½ inches wide.

Place in the stockpot and cook for about 4 minutes.

12-inch oval baking dish – approximately 3-inch deep.

Lightly oiled the bottom of the dish.

Place one pasta sheet on the bottom of the baking dish.

Pour half of the sauce over the pasta.

8-oz low-fat ricotta cheese

1 tbsp Parmesan cheese, grated

⅛ tsp cumin

With a spoon scoop out small parts of the ricotta, spreading it on top of the sauce.

Sprinkle Parmesan and cumin on top.

Layer the remaining pasta sheet on top.

Pour the rest of the sauce over pasta.

2 cups low-fat mozzarella cheese, shredded

Cover the sauce with.

Bake in the preheated oven for about 30 to 35 minutes.

GF – VT

4 servings

Calories in main ingredients per serving: Olive oil 119. Roma tomatoes 36. Ricotta 59. Provolone cheese 108. Pasta 27. Total of 322.

Basil Garlic Fettuccine

4 quarts of water

Place in a stockpot and bring to boil.

16-oz gluten-free fresh made fettuccine

Add to the stockpot and cook for about

4 to 5 minutes. The pasta should be al dente.

Drain the liquid and set aside.

3 tbsp olive oil

Heat in a sauté pan.

1 Roma tomato, chopped

6 cremini mushrooms, chopped

1 tsp ground black pepper

Add in, sauté on medium heat for 5 to 7 minutes.

½ cup white cooking wine

½ cup fresh basil, chopped

2 cloves garlic, chopped

¼ cup pine nuts

Add to the pan and continue cooking for 2 to 3 minutes.

The cooked fettuccine

Add and toss the fettuccine with the sauce.

Cook for 1 to 2 minutes.

¼ cup grated Romano cheese

Add to the pasta, stir well, turn off the heat and serve.

2 servings

GF – VT

Calories in main ingredients per serving: Pasta 54. Olive oil 30. Pine nuts 78. Romano cheese 54. Total of 270.

Green Lasagna

Preheat oven to 350-degrees

Sauce

3 tbsp olive oil

Heat in a sauté pan on medium heat

1 green pepper, sliced
1 red pepper, sliced
1 zucchini, sliced
8 cremini mushrooms, sliced
2 cloves garlic, chopped

Sauté for about 4 to 5 minutes.

2 tbsp white cooking wine
8 Roma tomatoes, chopped
1 tsp dry basil
1 tsp dry oregano
½ tsp black pepper

Add and simmer for about 7 to 8 minutes until tomatoes break down.

Stir well and remove from heat.

Pasta

6 cups water

Bring to a boil in a stockpot.

2 gluten-free spinach pasta sheets

Each pasta sheets should be total of 10 inches long.

Handmade pasta machine makes pasta sheets 5 to 5 ½ inches wide.

Place in the stockpot and cook for about 4 minutes.

12-inch oval baking dish – approximately 3-inch deep.

Lightly oiled the bottom of the dish.

Place a pasta sheet on the bottom of the baking dish.

Pour half of the sauce over the pasta.

8-oz low-fat ricotta cheese
1 tbsp Parmesan cheese, grated
⅛ tsp nutmeg

With a spoon scoop out small parts of the ricotta, spreading it on top of the sauce.

Sprinkle Parmesan and nutmeg on top.

Layer the remaining pasta sheet on top.

Pour the rest of the sauce over the pasta.

2 cups low-fat mozzarella cheese, shredded

Cover the sauce with.

Bake in the preheated oven for about 30 to 35 minutes.

GF – VT

Fettuccine with Scallops and Clams

4 quarts of water

Place in a stockpot and bring to boil.

16-oz gluten-free fresh made fettuccine

Add to the stockpot and cook for about 4 to 5 minutes.

Drain the liquid and set aside.

4 tbsps olive oil

Heat oil in a large sauté pan on medium heat .

16-oz bay scallops
10-oz baby clams

Use organic, natural clams in BPA-free can. Drain liquid and wash well.

Add clams and scallops to the pan.

Sauté for 4 to 5 minutes

½ cup white cooking wine
1 cup vegetable broth
l clove garlic, chopped
1 tsp dry thyme
1 tsp white pepper
Juice of ¼ lemon
1 tbsp fresh parsley
1 tbsp fresh basil leaves
1 tsp fresh dill

Add to the pan and simmer for about 4 to 5 minutes.

The cooked fettuccine

Add fettuccine to the sauté pan and continue cooking until fettuccine has absorbed most of the liquid, 3 to 4 minutes.

¼ cup grated Parmesan cheese.

Turn heat off, add grated cheese and blend well.

EL – GF

2 servings

Calories in main ingredients per serving: Pasta 54. Olive oil 60. Clams 119. Scallops 198. Total of 431.

4 servings

Calories in main ingredients per serving: Olive oil 90. Pasta 27. Roma tomatoes 36. Ricotta 59. Mozzarella 108. Total of 320.

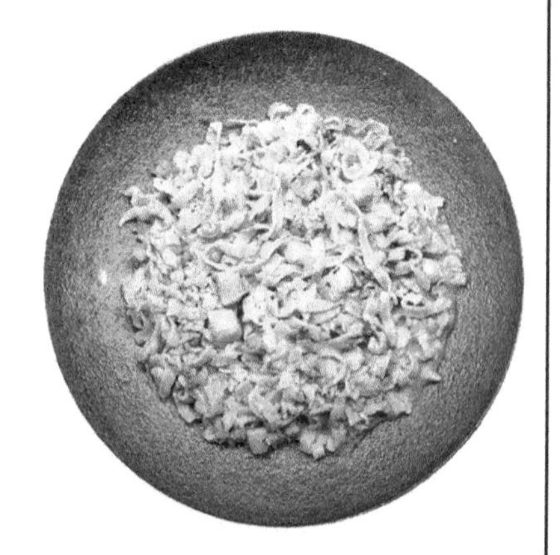

Tomato Pesto Ravioli

Ravioli

1 cup low-fat mozzarella cheese, shredded
⅛ cup Romano cheese, grated
⅛ cup Parmesan cheese
1 tbsp parsley, chopped
1 cup low-fat ricotta cheese
½ tsp nutmeg
1 tsp white pepper
Place in a mixing bowl and blend well by hand.
4 gluten-free pasta sheets, 12 to 14 inches long
Handmade pasta machine makes pasta sheets 5 to 5½ inches wide.
Place the pasta sheets on a working surface.
With a small spoon scoop the ravioli filling and place it on top of the two pasta strips, spacing filling to about 3 inches apart.
1 egg, beaten
Brush the strips lightly around the fillings and cover with the remaining two strips.
With your fingers press the pasta strip gently around each filling.
Using a square ravioli cuter stamp press to make square ravioli.
This recipe makes approximately 20 ravioli.
Fill a medium-size stockpot to about ⅔ full with water and bring to boil.
Place ravioli into the stockpot and cook for about 5 to 6 minutes.
Remove stockpot and drain the water.

Sauce

2 tbsp olive oil
Heat in a sauté pan.
½ onion, chopped
1 cloves garlic, chopped
Sauté on medium heat for about 3 to 4 minutes.
6 cremini mushrooms, chopped
8 Roma tomatoes, chopped
1 tsp dry oregano
1 tsp dry thyme
½ tsp black pepper
1 cup vegetable broth
Add to the pan and continue cooking for another 6 or 7 minutes.

Feta pesto sauce

While sauce is being cooked, prepare the pesto
1 cup of fresh basil
2 cloves of roasted garlic
2 tbsp olive oil
1 tbsp Parmesan cheese
¼ cup walnuts
3-oz feta cheese
Place in a food processor and pulse 1 to 2 times.
Add to the sauté pan, lower the heat, stir well for a minute and turn the heat off.
Add the cooked ravioli into the sauté pan, and gently blend with the sauce.
¼ cup grated Romano cheese
Turn off the heat, add to the pan,toss and serve.

2 servings

GF – VT

Calories in the main ingredients per order: Olive oil 60.
Pasta 54. Roma tomatoes 36.
Mozzarella 170.
Grated cheese 52. Ricotta. 30.
Egg 39. Walnuts 65.
Total of 506.

Artichoke Spinach and Lamb Lasagna

Preheat oven to 350-degrees
3 tbsp olive oil
Heat in a sauté pan on medium heat.
1 small onion, chopped
2 cloves garlic, chopped
Add to the pan and sauté for 2 to 3 minutes.
8-oz ground lamb
Add to the sauté pan and cook for about 4 minutes.
2 tbsp red cooking wine
4 artichoke hearts, chopped
8 Roma tomatoes, chopped
Add and simmer for another 7 to 8 minutes.
1 cup of fresh spinach, chopped
1 tsp dry basil
1 tsp dry oregano
1 tsp dry thyme
1 tsp fresh rosemary, chopped
1 tsp fresh mint, chopped
2 tsp black pepper
Add and simmer for 3 to 4 minutes until tomatoes break down.
Stir well and remove from heat.

Pasta

6 cups water
Bring to a gentle boil in a stockpot.
2 gluten-free pasta sheets
Pasta sheets should be 10 inches long.
Handmade pasta machine makes pasta sheets 5 to 5 ½ inches wide.
Place in the stockpot and cook for about 4 minutes.
12-inch oval baking dish – approximately 3-inch deep.
Lightly oiled the bottom of the dish.

Place one pasta sheet on the bottom of the baking dish.
Pour half of the sauce over the pasta.
⅓ cup low-fat ricotta cheese
⅓ cup low-fat Greek yogurt
Blend in a mixing bowl.
With a spoon, scoop out small parts of the mixture, spreading it on top of the sauce.
1 tbsp Romano cheese, grated
⅛ tsp nutmeg
Sprinkle on top.
Layer the remaining pasta sheet on top.
Pour the rest of the sauce over pasta.
2 cups low-fat mozzarella cheese, shredded
Cover the sauce with.
Bake in the preheated oven for about
30 to 35 minutes.

GF – VT

4 servings

Calories in main ingredients per serving: Olive oil 90. Ground lamb 160. Roma tomatoes 36. Artichoke hearts 76. Pasta 27. Mozzarella cheese 108. Ricotta 32. Greek yogurt 12. Total of 529.

NOTE: Eggplants taste slightly different depending on how they are cooked and what you cook them with. The wide range of potential flavors is one of the reasons that I love to cook with eggplants. The main reason that eggplants change their character is their ability to absorb high amounts of liquids; hence eggplant adopts high quantities of other flavors. But, whatever different flavor penetrate the eggplants, they never lose their luxurious taste. Some people complain about eggplants of being bitter or spongy, but when eggplants are adequately cooked, they achieve tastes that no other fruit or vegetable can. In addition to bringing a unique texture and flavors to recipes, eggplant brings a host of potential health benefits. They are nutrient-dense food. Eggplants are incredibly versatile and can be easily incorporated into your diet. I use them for grilling, salads, soups, or baked. I've heart many tricks to prepare eggplant for cooking; peel the skin, salt the eggplant for several hours, wash and place it between paper towels, and so on. Losing the peel, drenching them with salt or washing them, you lose the essential character of the eggplant – its bitterness, which its the most exciting future. I do none of that – I handle eggplants straight forward. I am careful with the oil used and when I grill them outdoors, I dip them, usually, in a mustard vinaigrette. There are several eggplant recipes in this book, I encourage you to try some of them.

Pasta Fillings

Spinach

½ cups spinach, drained
1 cup mozzarella cheese,
¼ cup Romano cheese, grated
¼ cup feta
1 cup ricotta
1 clove garlic, chopped
½ tsp. nutmeg
1 tsp. black pepper
Mix all ingredients well.
Makes 30 to 35 stuffed pasta.

Cheese

1½ cup mozzarella cheese, shredded
¼ cup Parmesan cheese, grated
1 tbsp fresh parsley, chopped
1 cup ricotta cheese
½ tsp. nutmeg
1 tsp white pepper
Mix all ingredients well.

Makes 20 to 25 stuffed pasta.

You can use the fillings to make square or round ravioli, tortellini, half-moon agnolotti or other stuffed pasta. My suggestion for best tasting stuffed pasta is to stuff the pasta with a rich tasting filling and use a mild tasting sauce.

Anchovies are trending, especially in cosmopolitan US cities influenced by Southern European foods and culture. Innovative chefs find ways to incorporate the unique taste of anchovies in various dishes. Anchovies for me is a take it or leave it food. Growing up, anchovies were an occasional food for our family, however, its taste is so distinctive, it stays with you for a long time. When I moved to America, on the mention of anchovies, I saw people grimace their faces into a sour expression as if anchovies were the most disgusting thing on earth. Coming from a place where anchovies are a delicacy I was perplexed with this reaction. Consequently, people were unaware that their beloved Ceasar salad's dressing is made with anchovies or when they eat in an Italian restaurant some the favorite foods, like the puttanesca sauce, have anchovies in them. Additionally, some of the ready-made sauces like Worcestershire sauce have anchovies.

I must admit that sometimes I yearn for the taste of anchovies. While in the restaurant business, there were a couple of times after the restaurant closed, I baked a mini pizza with anchovies and kalamata olives and loved every bite if it.

The recipe below, with gluten-free pasta and tomato-anchovy sauce is a testament of the unique taste anchovies add to a recipe.

Fettuccine with Anchovy and Caper Tomato Sauce

Pasta

4 quarts of water

Place in a stockpot and bring to boil.

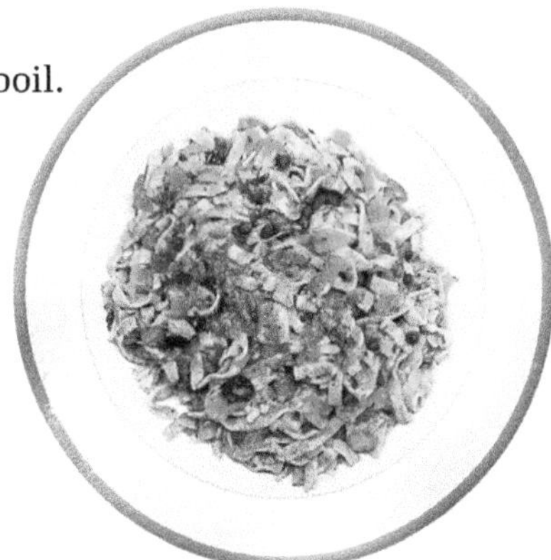

16-oz gluten-free fresh made fettuccine

Add to the stockpot and cook for about 4 to 5 minutes.
Drain the liquid and set aside.

Sauce

2 tbsp olive oil

Heat in a large sauté pan.

½ onion, chopped
4 cloves garlic, chopped

Add to the pan and sauté on medium heat for 2 to 3 minutes.

¼ cup red cooking wine
6 Roma tomatoes, chopped
8 anchovy fillets, chopped
2 tbsp capers
¼ cup pitted Kalamata olives, chopped
1 cup vegetable broth

Add to the pan and continue cooking on medium heat for another 5 minutes.

1 tbsp fresh Italian parsley, chopped
1 tbsp fresh basil, chopped
1 tsp dry oregano
1 tsp dry thyme
½ tsp black pepper
¼ tsp ground cloves

Add to the pan and cook for another 8 to 9 minutes.

The cooked Fettuccine

Add to the pan and blend with the sauce.
Continue cooking for another 2 to 3 minutes.

¼ cup grated Romano cheese

Turn the heat off, add to the pan and toss with the pasta.

2 servings

GF

Calories in main ingredients per serving: Pasta 54. Olive oil 119. Roma tomatoes 36. Anchovies 13. Kalamata olives 22. Romano cheese 55. Total of 299.

Breakfast

*"This idiosyncratic chef is a kitchen magician,
a candidate for culinary sainthood."*
New Times

*"The Raspberry-Stuffed Toast, composed of small round baguette slices,
stuffed with raspberries and cream cheese, dipped in egg batter and fried, then
topped with an orange almond sauce."*
The Best of Phoenix – Phoenix Magazine

THE COMPLICATED WORLD OF BAKING METHODS

As I mentioned in an earlier section, cooking and baking must be handled with a different approach. The two fundamental principles of baking are, the proportion of liquid to flour and the method used to merge the dry and wet ingredients. If this step is not done correctly, it will result in a disastrous outcome that cannot be corrected, unlike in cooking when you can "fix" the texture and taste by adding more spices or thickeners along the way. If you are looking for information in various books or online for baking at home, most likely you will be confused and sometimes discouraged to do what otherwise it should be a fun experience. There are the methods of Rubbing-in which is similar to Cutting-in. There is the Melting method, the Whisking method which is similar to the Whipping method. And there is the Roll-in method, the Creaming method, the All-in method, which is like the Quick method, also called the Muffin method, and so on. Ultimately all these methods are various techniques to, mainly, produce different textures in cakes and rarely used in home cooking. If you are new to baking or you are trying to further educate yourself about the amazing world of baking, in trying to define the various baking methods people come up with, your head will be spinning for days. If you follow a recipe, it should explain how to mix and bake your ingredients. The two common methods, especially with gluten-free baking, are the creaming and quick methods. The quick method is beneficial in gluten-free baking because you are working with "naked" flours, stripped of the protection gluten provides for safe baking.

Simply put the creaming method is one that blends fats, like butter, with sugar until creamy and then beaten eggs are slowly added to the mixture. This is the traditional method and the basis for cookie and cake making. A soft cake or chewy cookie is the product of the creaming method. The creaming method incorporates air into the dough while mixing. The air, with the help of baking soda or baking powder, is what helps the cake or cookies rise.

The quick method, also called the muffin method, is one of the simpler of all other methods. It is a technique where the dry ingredients, such as flour and the liquid ingredients, like beaten eggs and milk, are mixed in different bowls and then quickly combined. Once the two are combined and stirred together very briefly the finished batter is ready to be baked. The advantages of the correctly done quick method in gluten-free baking will produce a light and airy product since the gentle blending protects your defenseless gluten-free flours. The batter will be somewhat lumpy and much thinner than it would be when using the creaming method. The quick baking method is mainly used for muffins, pancakes, quick breads, and waffles. Since muffins are defined by their "peak-top," they must be baked in higher temperatures. The high heat cooks the edges of the muffin quickly and forces the batter to rise. If you over-mix the batter in the quick method, then you will, most likely, end up with rubbery muffins and quick breads, dense pancakes or doughy waffles.

Quick method: Place the flour and other dry ingredients in a large bowl and mix them with a wire whisk until thoroughly blended. Combine beaten eggs with the rest of the wet ingredients in a separate bowl, pour the mixture slowly in the center of the dry ingredients and stir with a wooden spoon until all ingredients are just combined. This step should take a few seconds. For muffins and quick breads, a thick and lumpy muffin batter is good. The lumps will go away when they bake, for pancakes and waffles stir a bit longer to a little smoother mixture. Note: If you use too much liquid or fruit in the bread or muffins, they will be wet in the center and if you use too many dry ingredients, your bread or muffins will be dense – these facts are correct especially when working with gluten-free flours.

Smoothie Formula

My triple crown spices are cinnamon, turmeric and ginger. For a powerful health punch, chia seeds and flaxseed. And to go the extra mile, protein power with nutrients. The above items along with almond milk are the basics in my smoothies. You could create your smoothie by adding some of the following items.

- Lemon
- Apples
- Oranges
- Bananas
- Pineapple
- Mango
- Carrots
- Celery
- Parsley
- Kale
- Mint
- Spinach
- Yogurt

Choose a combination of these items and add ice and water to adjust the consistency of your smoothie.

- *Cinnamon a healing spice that contains large amounts of highly potent polyphenol antioxidants. It is so powerful that cinnamon can be used as a natural food preservative. Cinnamon also includes a small amount of vitamin E, niacin, vitamin B6, magnesium, potassium, zinc, and copper.*
- *Ginger is a natural source of vitamin C, magnesium, potassium, copper, and manganese.*
- *Turmeric contains thymol, a potent antioxidant and it is an excellent source of vitamin C, vitamin A, fiber, riboflavin, iron, copper, and manganese. It has good amounts of calcium and manganese, vitamin B6, folate, phosphorus, potassium, and zinc.*
- *Chia seeds contain healthy omega-3 fatty acids, carbohydrates, protein, fiber, antioxidants, and calcium.*
- *Flaxseed Is a rich source of healthy fat, antioxidants, and fiber. The seeds contain protein, lignans, and the essential fatty acid omega-3.*

Pancakes

Most of my pancake recipes need no syrup; some of the ingredients used are natural sweeteners. Please taste the pancakes before adding additional sweeteners. When using syrup, I recommend the use of maple syrup.

Pumpkin Sweet Potato Pancakes

STEP 1

1 medium size sweet potato

Boil the potato covered with water for about 12 to 15 minutes, until potato is slightly underdone. Cool and peel the potato. Pulse it in the food processor 2 to 3 times. Set aside.

½ cup quick oats

Grind in a food processor into a flour consistency. Set aside.

STEP 2

1 cup brown rice flour
The oat flour
1 tsp cinnamon
1 tsp nutmeg
1 tsp arrowroot

Place ingredients in a large mixing bowl and stir with a wooden spoon to blend well.

1 egg, beaten
1¼ cups unsweetened almond milk
1 tbsp olive oil

Pour in the center of the flour mixture and stir until all ingredients are just combined.

2 tbsp low-fat Greek yogurt
1 cup pumpkin puree
The mashed sweet potato

Add to the mixing bowl and stir to incorporate in the batter.

Oiled a flat top grill with 4 tablespoons of olive oil, pour mixture on the grill using a ladle and cook well on one side, about 3 to 4 minutes. Flip the pancakes and cook for another 3 to 4 minutes.

Makes 6 pancakes

GF – VT

Calories of main ingredients per pancake: Eggs 13. Olive oil 20. Pumpkin puree 14. Sweet potato 19. Brown rice flour 95. Oat flour 24. Total at 185.

Carrot Cake Pancakes

2 cups gluten free pancake mix
½ tsp cinnamon
¼ tsp nutmeg

Place ingredients in a large mixing bowl and stir with a wooden spoon to blend well.

1½ cup unsweetened coconut milk
2 eggs, beaten
4 tbsp olive oil

Pour in the center of the flour mixture and stir until all ingredients are just combined.

2 large carrots

Run the carrots in a food processor's shredding plate. they should have

1 cup shredded carrots.
½ cup fresh pineapple, chopped
¼ cup raisins
¼ cup walnuts, chopped

Add to the mixing bowl along with the carrots and stir to incorporate in the batter.

Oiled a flat top grill with 4 tablespoons of olive oil, pour mixture on the grill using a ladle and cook well on one side, about 3 to 4 minutes.

Flip the pancakes and cook for another 3 to 4 minutes.

Makes 6 large pancakes

GF – VT

Calories of main ingredients per pancake: Coconut milk 22. Egg 26. Raisins 21. Walnuts 22. Pancake mix 24. Total 89.

Buckwheat Cherry and Pear Pancakes

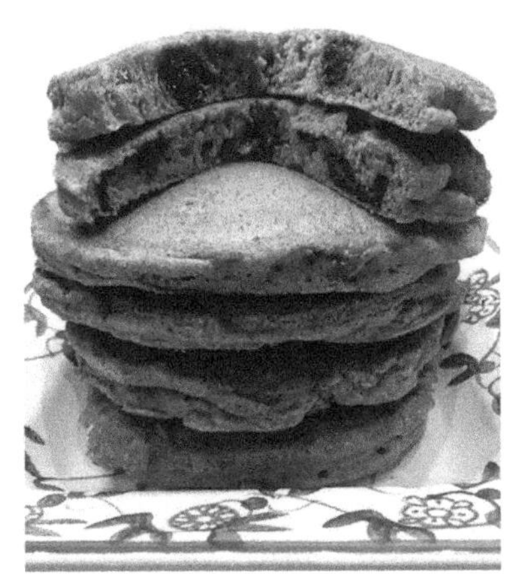

1½ cup gluten-free pancake mix
1 cup buckwheat flour
1 tbsp arrowroot
1 tsp cardamom

Place ingredients in a large mixing bowl and stir with a wooden spoon to blend well.

1 cup unsweetened coconut milk
½ cup unsweetened almond milk
2 egg, beaten
4 tbsp olive oil

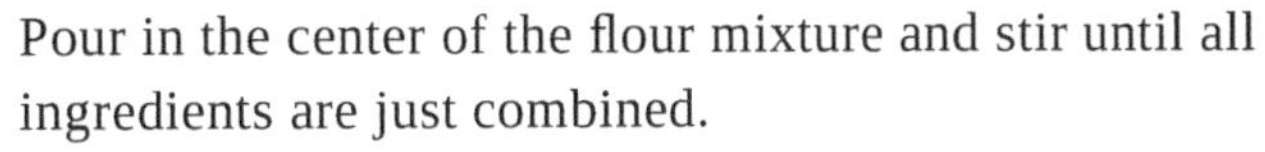

Pour in the center of the flour mixture and stir until all ingredients are just combined.

1 ripe pear peeled and chopped.
1 cup dark cherries, chopped. Use frozen or fresh when in season.
⅛ tsp vanilla extract

Add to the mixing bowl and stir to incorporate in the batter.

Oiled a flat top grill with 4 tablespoons of olive oil, pour mixture on the grill using a ladle and cook well on one side, about 3 to 4 minutes.

Flip the pancakes and cook for another 3 to 4 minutes.

Makes 6 large pancakes

GF – VT

Calories of main ingredients per pancake: Eggs 26. Olive oil 40. Pear 17. Cherries 15. Pancake flour 36. Buckwheat 67. Soy milk 16. Total at 217.

Tips for cooking PANCAKES

- **Use the quick mixing method – do not over-mix.**
- **Do not make ahead of time.**
- **Only flip once.**
- **Do not use much oil.**
- **Make sure oil is hot before pouring the batter.**
- **It is best to use a flat-top grill. If not available use a thick sauté pan.**

Pumpkin Oat and Raisin Pancakes

1 cup gluten-free pancake mix
1 tsp arrowroot
1 tsp cinnamon
½ tsp cloves
1 tbsp flaxseed

Place ingredients in a large mixing bowl.

1 cup quick oats

Place oats in a food processor and grind them to a flour consistency. Add to the mixing bowl and stir with a wooden spoon to blend well.

1½ cups almond milk
4 tbsp olive oil

Pour in the center of the flour mixture and stir until all ingredients are just combined.

1 cup pumpkin puree
½ cup raisins

Add to the mixing bowl and stir to incorporate in the batter. Oiled a flat top grill with 4 tablespoons of olive oil, pour mixture on the grill using a ladle and cook well on one side, about 3 to 4 minutes. Flip the pancakes and cook for another 3 to 4 minutes.

Makes 6 large pancakes

GF– EL – VT – VG

Calories of main ingredients per pancake: Pumpkin puree 14. Olive oil 60. Quick oats 26. Pancake flour 24. Raisins 21. Total at 145.

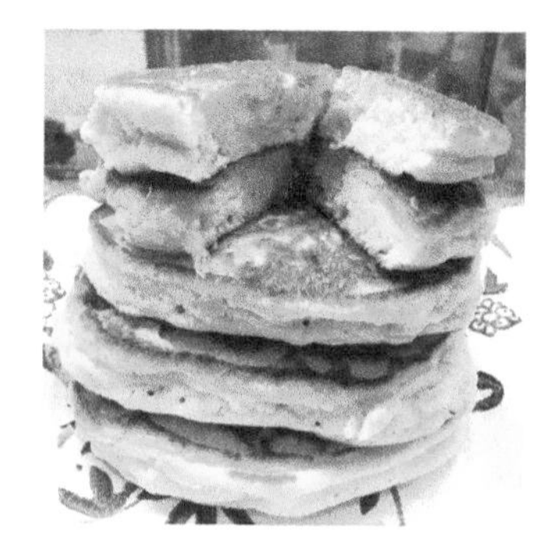

Mango Banana Pancakes

½ cup coconut flour
1½ cup gluten-free pancake mix
1 tbsp arrowroot
½ tsp cardamom

Place ingredients in a large mixing bowl and stir with a wooden spoon to blend well.

1 cup unsweetened coconut milk
½ cup low-fat milk
2 eggs, beaten
4 tbsp olive oil

Pour in the center of the flour mixture and stir until all ingredients are just combined.

1 large banana, mashed
1 mango, peeled and chopped – about 1 cup.

Add to the mixing bowl and stir to incorporate in the batter. Oiled a flat top grill with 4 tablespoons of olive oil, pour mixture on the grill using a ladle and cook well on one side, about 3 to 4 minutes. Flip the pancakes and cook for another 3 to 4 minutes.

Makes 6 large pancakes

GF – VT – Omit egg for EL, VG

Calories of main ingredients per pancake: Coconut milk 8. Olive oil 20. Banana 21. Mango 34. Egg 26. Coconut flour 54. Pancake flour 36. Low-fat milk 17. Total at 216.

Potato Feta Pancakes

STEP 1

1 large potato, peel and shredded
½ large red onion, chopped

Grilled on a flat grill with 1 tbsp olive oil unlit soft. About 4 to 5 minutes.

Set aside and let them cool.

STEP 2

1½ gluten-free pancake mix

Place ingredients in a large mixing bowl.

1 egg
1 ½ low-fat milk
4 tbsp olive oil

Pour in the center of the flour mixture and stir until all ingredients are just combined.

The grilled potato
The grilled red onion
½ cup crumbled feta cheese
1 tsp black pepper

Add to the mixing bowl and stir to incorporate in the batter. Oiled a flat top grill with 4 tablespoons of olive oil, pour mixture on the grill using a ladle and cook well on one side, about 3 to 4 minutes. Flip the pancakes and cook for another 3 to 4 minutes.

Makes 6 large pancakes

GF – VT

Calories of main ingredients per pancake: Potato 28. Egg 13. Pancake flour 36. Olive oil 60. Feta 33. Soy milk 25. Total at 195.

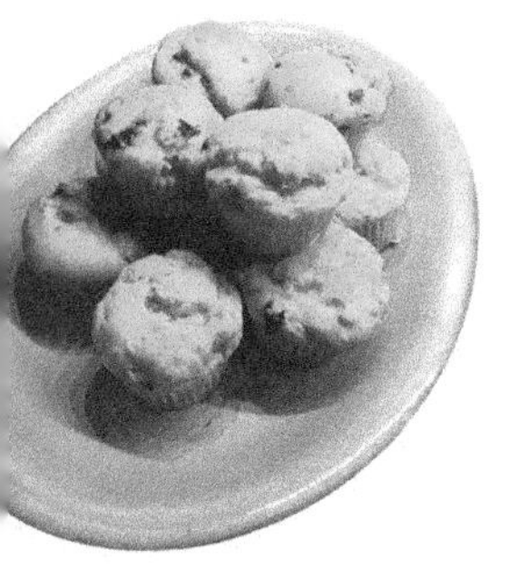

MUFFINS

For muffins use the quick mixing method, also known as the muffin mixing method. The muffin recipes in this book are made with two different batters:

One is simple with muffin mix flour, the other with a combination of flours. If you are like me that does not make muffins often, the muffin mix is more practical. Muffin flours are much improved and with a little "doctoring-up" it makes a good muffin.

PUMPKIN, WHITE CHOCOLATE MUFFINS

Preheat oven to 400-degrees

3 cups gluten-free muffin mix
¼ tsp nutmeg

Place ingredients in a large mixing bowl and stir with a wooden spoon to blend well.

½ cup low-fat milk
½ cup unsweetened almond milk
½ cup olive oil
2 eggs, beaten

Pour in the center of the flour mixture and stir until all ingredients are just combined.

½ cup pumpkin puree
1 cup white chocolate chips

Add to the mixing bowl and stir to incorporate in the batter. Using an ice cream scoop, pour the batter into paper lined 12-muffin pan cups. Fill the cups to about ¼ inch from the top. Bake in the preheated oven for about 22 to 25 minutes. Let muffins cool before removing from the cups.

Makes 12 muffins

GF – VT

Calories of the main ingredients per muffin: Muffin mix 128. Olive oil 5. Eggs 13. White chocolate chips 38. Pumpkin puree 7. Milk 8. Total of 199.

BANANA, APPLES AND OATS MUFFINS

Preheat oven to 400-degrees

3 cups gluten-free muffin mix
¼ tsp cinnamon

Place ingredients in a large mixing bowl and stir with a wooden spoon to blend well.

½ cup low-fat milk
½ cup unsweetened almond milk
½ cup olive oil
2 eggs, beaten

Pour in the center of the flour mixture and stir until all ingredients are just combined.

½ apple, peeled and chopped
1 banana, chopped
½ cup quick oats
1 tbsp unsweetened applesauce

Add to the mixing bowl and stir to incorporate in the batter. Using an ice cream scoop, pour the batter into paper lined 12-muffin pan cups. Fill the cups to about ¼ inch from the top. Bake in the preheated oven for about 22 to 25 minutes. Let muffins cool before removing from the cups.

Makes 12 muffins

GF – VT

Calories of the main ingredients per muffin: Muffin mix 128. Olive oil 5. Eggs 13. Banana 9. Oats 7. Applesauce 5. Milk 8. Total of 173.

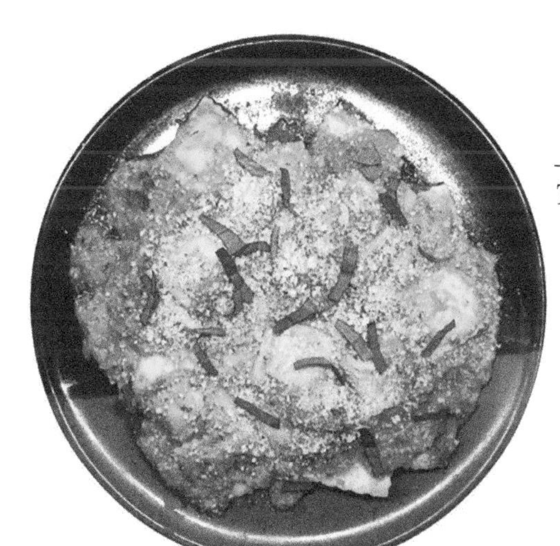

Tomato Pesto Ravioli

Blueberry, Mango and Walnut Muffins

Preheat oven to 400-degrees

3 cups gluten-free muffin mix
¼ tsp nutmeg
1 tsp flaxseed

Place ingredients in a large mixing bowl and stir with a wooden spoon to blend well.

½ low-fat milk
½ cup unsweetened coconut milk
½ cup olive oil
2 eggs, beaten

Add slowly to the bowl, mixing with a wooden spoon until dough is smooth.

½ mango, peeled and chopped
1 cup fresh blueberries
2 tbsp low-fat Greek yogurt
½ cup walnuts, chopped

Add to the mixing bowl and stir to incorporate in the batter.

Using an ice cream scoop, pour the batter into paper lined 12-muffin pan cups.

Fill the cups to about ¼ inch from the top.

Bake in the preheated oven for about 22 to 25 minutes.

Let muffins cool before removing from the cups.

Makes 12 muffins

GF – VT

Calories of the main ingredients per muffin: Muffin mix 128. Olive oil 5. Eggs 13. Mango 17. Walnuts 7. Blueberries 7. Milk 8. Total of 185.

Muffin Recipe

½ cup rice flour
1 cup brown rice flour.
1/8 cup arrowroot flour
½ cup sorghum flour
1 cup gluten-free muffin mix
1/8 cup tapioca flour
1 tsp baking power
¼ tsp cinnamon

Place ingredients in a large mixing bowl and stir with a wooden spoon to blend well.

1 cup unsweetened almond milk
2 eggs, beaten
½ cup olive oil
1 tsp vanilla extract

Pour in the center of the flour mixture and stir until all ingredients are just combined.

Add 1½ to 2 cups of fillings.

Add to the mixing bowl and stir to incorporate in the batter.

Bake in a preheated 400-degree oven for about 22 to 25 minutes.

Makes 12 muffins

Calories of the main ingredients per muffin: White rice flour 24. Brown rice flour 48. Muffin mix 43. Arrowroot 13. Sorghum 18. Olive oil 5. Eggs 13. Total of 164.

Peach, Strawberry and Dates Muffins

Preheat oven to 400-degrees

4 dried soft dates, pitted

Place in the food processor with 1 tsp of water and pulse to a paste.

3 cups gluten-free muffin mix
¼ tsp cinnamon

Place ingredients in a large mixing bowl and stir with a wooden spoon to blend well.

½ low-fat milk
½ cup unsweetened coconut milk
½ cup olive oil
2 eggs, beaten

Pour in the center of the flour mixture and stir until all ingredients are just combined.

1 small peach, peeled and chopped or use ½ cup frozen peaches, chopped
1 cup fresh strawberries, chopped
2 tbsp low-fat Greek yogurt
¼ cup walnuts, chopped
The date paste

Add to the mixing bowl and stir to incorporate in the batter. Using an ice cream scoop, pour the batter into paper lined 12-muffin pan cups. Fill the cups to about ¼ inch from the top.

Bake in the preheated oven for about 22 to 25 minutes.

Let muffins cool before removing from the cups.

Makes 12 muffins

EL – GF – VT

Calories of the main ingredients per muffin: Muffin mix 128. Olive oil 5. Eggs 13. Peach 6. Strawberries 4. Walnuts 11. Dates 19. Total of 186.

Chocolate, Raspberry Muffins

Preheat oven to 400-degrees

3 cups gluten-free muffin mix

Place ingredients in a large mixing bowl and stir with a wooden spoon to blend well.

½ cup unsweetened coconut milk

½ cup low-fat milk

½ cup olive oil

2 eggs, beaten

¼ tsp vanilla extract

Pour in the center of the flour mixture and stir until all ingredients are just combined.

1 cup fresh raspberries

1 cup mini chocolate chips

Add to the mixing bowl and stir to incorporate in the batter.

Using an ice cream scoop, pour the batter into paper lined 12-muffin pan cups. Fill the cups to about ¼ inch from the top.

Bake in the preheated oven for about 22 to 25 minutes.

Let muffins cool before removing from the cups.

Makes 12 muffins

GF – VT

Calories of the main ingredients per muffin: Muffin mix 128. Olive oil 5. Eggs 13. Milk 8. Chocolate chips 69. Total of 223.

Cherry Almond and Blueberry Muffins

Preheat oven to 400-degrees

3 cups gluten-free muffin mix

2 tsp flaxseed

Place ingredients in a large mixing bowl and stir with a wooden spoon to blend well.

½ unsweetened almond milk

½ cup low-fat milk

½ cup olive oil

2 eggs, beaten

¼ tsp vanilla extract

Pour in the center of the flour mixture and stir until all ingredients are just combined.

1 cup fresh blueberries

1 cup frozen dark cherries, defrosted and cut in halves

½ cup sliced almonds

Add to the mixing bowl and stir to incorporate in the batter.

Using an ice cream scoop, pour the batter into paper lined 12-muffin pan cups.

Fill the cups to about ¼ inch from the top.

Bake in the preheated oven for about 22 to 25 minutes.

Let muffins cool before removing from the cups.

Makes 12 muffins

GF – VT

Calories of the main ingredients per muffin: Muffin mix 128. Olive oil 5. Eggs 13. Milk 8. Blueberries 7. Cherries 6. Almonds 22. Total of 189.

The muffin recipe on page 142 is my recipe using various gluten-free flours.

Lemon Filling

¼ cup coconut sugar

3 tbsps arrowroot

¾ cup almond milk

Whisk in a saucepan.

1 egg yolk

1 tbsp finely chopped lemon zest

Add and mix with the whisk.

Place saucepan over medium heat and cook until mixture thickens, 3 to 4 minutes.

Remove from the heat.

¼ cup juice of a lemon

1 tbsp low-fat organic butter

Add to the pan and stir well.

NOTE: Use this filling for muffins or quick breads.

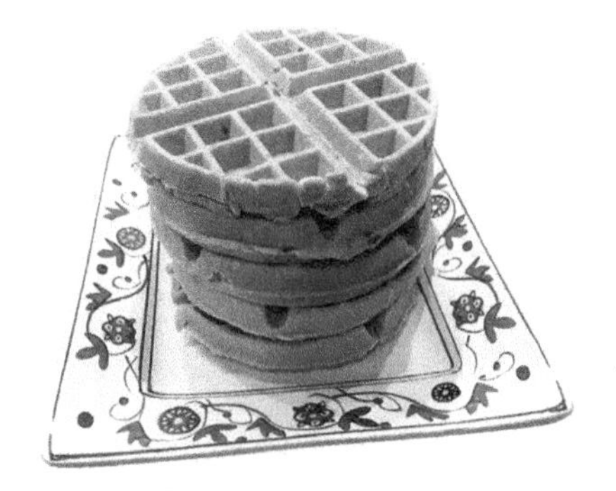

Waffles

Forget all the waffles you've had before. No syrup is needed, just serve with fruits as a topping.

Waffle Recipe

½ cup almond flour
½ cup brown rice flour
¼ cup potato starch
¼ cup sorghum flour
½ cup tapioca flour
1 tbsp arrowroot

Place in a large mixing bowl.

3 eggs

Separated in two small mixing bowls.

1 cup unsweetened soy milk
2 tbsp olive oil
1 tbsp baking powder
1 tsp cinnamon
1 tsp pure vanilla extracted

Add to the bowl with the egg yolk and mix well.

Mix all above ingredients, except the egg whites, with the flours.

Pour slowly in the mixing bowl and blend well with a fork.

With a fork, whip the egg whites until stiff and add them into the rest of the mixture.

Mix well.

2 tbsp sugar-free applesauce
1 banana, mashed
¼ cup of raisins

Add to the waffle mixture and mix gently.

Let the mixture rest for a few minutes.

It is best to use a flip waffle maker with a temperature control.

Heat up the waffle iron to between 375 to 400-degrees.

Lightly spray the waffle iron with oil.

When the iron is heated, use a soup ladle to pour the waffle batter into the iron, close and flip the waffle iron.

When the green light indicated that the waffle is done, flip it back, open and remove. If you don't have a flip waffle iron – heat up the waffle plate, lightly spray with oil, pour in batter. It cooks in 5 to 6 minutes.

The amount of batter pour into the waffle iron is determined on the size of the plate.

This recipe makes 5 to 6 large round waffles.

EL – GF – VT

Calories of the main ingredients per waffle: Almond milk 50. Brown rice flour 48. Potato starch 24. Sorghum flour 20. Tapioca flour 31. Eggs 32. Soy milk 22. Olive oil 40. Banana 17. Raisins 20. Total of 304.

NOTE: I use applesauce, bananas and raisins for add-ons in this recipe. However, you can substitute with any other ingredients.

Eggs

Eggs are a good source of high-quality protein, omega-3, riboflavin, vitamin B12, selenium and contain other essential nutrients. Both white and brown standard eggs contain the same type and amount of nutrients. Eggs are low in saturated fat, but high in cholesterol. The egg whites are fat and cholesterol free. The egg white accounts for most of the egg's liquid weight and contains more than half the total protein, chloride, potassium, sulfur, riboflavin, and niacin of the egg. The egg yolk contains most of the iron, copper, manganese, phosphorus, iodine, and calcium and the vitamins A, D, and E. The egg is one of the few natural foods that contain vitamin D. Eggs are an important and versatile ingredient for cooking, as their particular chemical makeup is literally the glue of many important baking reactions. Bottom line: Whole eggs are among the most nutritious foods on the planet, containing a little bit of almost every nutrient you need. They are also cheap, easy to prepare and pair well with almost any food.

NOTE: There are different cooking techniques to prepare a frittata or an omelet. For the frittata, the two common ways are to bake or on a stove-top. Since as far as I remember, I used the stove-top to oven method for the frittata. For the omelet, I get best results when it is cooked on a flat grill and cover it after folding. Making a fluffy frittata or an omelet is rather simple. For best results, I add 1 tablespoon of milk to every 4 to 6 eggs. Beat the eggs well with a wire whisk, and most important do not overcook your eggs. A good frittata should not be over-baked. If the color of its top is deep golden-brown, the interior is over-baked. The best frittatas have a texture that is light and fluffy with a tan color. Here is what I do; I cook the frittata on the stove-top, keeping the heat at medium-low, just until the edges have set, which takes a few minutes. The low temperature will allow the eggs to set with the rest of the ingredients. Then I transfer it to a preheated oven to finish it.

Following are some samples of my favorites, however you could use any fillings you like.

It is essential to cook any vegetables before pouring the eggs into the pan. This is especially important when using vegetables with high water content, like mushrooms or zucchini.

Frittatas are good for breakfast lunch or dinner.

Mediterranean Frittata

Preheat oven to 350-degrees

4 tbsp olive oil

1 medium size potato, peeled and sliced

Heat oil in a sauté pan, add potatoes and sauté on medium heat for about 4 to 5 minutes.

4 artichoke hearts, sliced

2 hearts of palm, half sliced

Add to the sauté pan and cook for 1 to 2 minutes longer.

8 extra large eggs

1 tbsp low-fat milk

Beat well in a mixing bowl with a wire whip.

¼ cup feta cheese, crumbled

Add eggs and feta to the sauté pan and cook for 2 to 3 minutes longer.

Lightly brush with olive oil the bottom and sides of a round shallow baking dish, transfer mixture into a baking dish.

½ cup shredded mozzarella cheese

Sprinkle on top of the egg mixture and bake in the preheated oven for 6 to 8 minutes.

Let it set for a few minutes, sliced and serve.

Cooking time varies according to the number of ingredients used.

GF – VG

6 servings

Calories in the main ingredients per serving: Olive oil 40. Potato 18. Artichoke hearts 17. Hearts of palm 15. Eggs 104. Feta cheese 16. Mozzarella cheese 29. Total of 239.

Avocado Crabmeat Omelet

Prepare the vegetables before cooking the eggs.

1 small avocado, chopped

1 green onion, chopped

4-oz crabmeat

2 slices of Swiss cheese

Set aside.

3 tbsp olive oil

Heat in a medium size sauté pan or use a flat grill if available.

Making an omelet on a flat grill it is much easier to fold it.

6 eggs

1 tbsp low-fat

Beat the eggs and cream well with a wire beater.

Add to the pan and let cook on medium heat for about 2 minutes. The bottom should be firm and set, but the top should look moist.

Place the avocado, green onions and crabmeat in the center of the eggs. Turn your heat to low. Fold the one end of the omelet with a spatula over the filling and fold again to place the seam down.

2 slices of swiss cheese

Place on top of the omelet, cover the pan and let cook for 2 to 3 minutes.

GF – VT

3 servings

Calories in the main ingredients per serving: Avocado 78. Crabmeat 37. Swiss cheese 46. Olive oil 79. Eggs 156. Total of 393.

Frittata Muffins

In this recipes the frittatas are baked in muffin trays.
Preheat oven to 350-degrees
8 large eggs, beaten in a large mixing bowl
1 tbsp low-fat milk
Beat well in a mixing bowl with a wire whip.
6 mushrooms, sliced
½ cup sun dried tomatoes, chopped
1 avocado, chopped
½ cup feta cheese, crumbled
¼ cup low-fat ricotta cheese
1 tsp black pepper
Add to the bowl with the eggs and mix well.
Lightly brush with olive oil the cups of a 12 muffin cup tray. With a soup ladle pour mixture into the muffing cups, leaving a little room on the top of the cup, (about ¼ inch.)
Bake in the preheated oven for about 15 to 18 minutes.
Let frittatas set for about 10 minutes before removing from the cups.

GF – VT

12 muffin cups

Calories in the main ingredients per egg muffin: Eggs 52. Sun dried tomatoes 10. Avocado 27. Feta cheese 16. Ricotta cheese 7. Total off 112.

Country Eggs

3 tbsp olive oil
Heat in a sauté pan.
2 Roma tomatoes, chopped
Add to the sauté pan and cook in low heat for 2 to 3 minutes.
6 large eggs, beat well in a mixing bowl
¼ cup feta cheese, crumbled
Add to the pan and scrambled the eggs until lightly cooked.

2 servings

GF – VT

Calories in the main ingredients per serving. Olive oil 60. Roma tomatoes 18. Eggs 234. Feta cheese 50. Total of 362.

Sweet Potato Hash

4 tbsp olive oil
Heat in a large sauté pan.
1 large sweet potato, peeled and large cut
Add to the pan and sauté on medium heat for about 8 minutes.
1 onion, chopped
1 green bell pepper, chopped
2 cloves garlic, chopped
1 tbsp balsamic vinegar
Add to the pan and continue cooking for another 3 to 4 minutes.
6 mushrooms, sliced
1 tsp black pepper
1 tsp fresh rosemary, chopped
1 tbsp balsamic vinegar
1 tsp dry thyme
Add to the pan and cook for 3 to 4 minutes longer.

4 servings

EL – GF – VT – VG

Calories in the main ingredients per serving. Olive oil 60. Sweet potato 29. Total of 89.

Grilled Potatoes with Vegetables

4 tbsp olive oil
Heat in a flat grill.
2 medium potatoes, sliced
Add to the grill and cook on medium heat for about 6 minutes.
1 small onion, sliced
8 mushrooms, sliced
1 red pepper, sliced
Add to the grill and cook for another 5 to 6 minutes.
1 tsp black pepper

EL – GR – VT – VG

4 servings

Calories in the main ingredients per serving. Olive oil 120. Potatoes 82. Total of 202.

Quick Breads

A toasted quick bread slice is enjoyable for breakfast or a snack, especially the banana walnut mango bread. The cinnamon raisin bread makes a flavorful French toast. The lemon date bread is a delicious light summer dessert.

NOTE: If you bake you quick bread at too hot temperature will cause the outer portion of your bread to cook too quickly and be undercook in the middle. If you use too much liquid or fruit the bread will be wet in the center if you use too much dry ingredients your bread will be dense – these facts are correct especially when working will gluten-free flours.

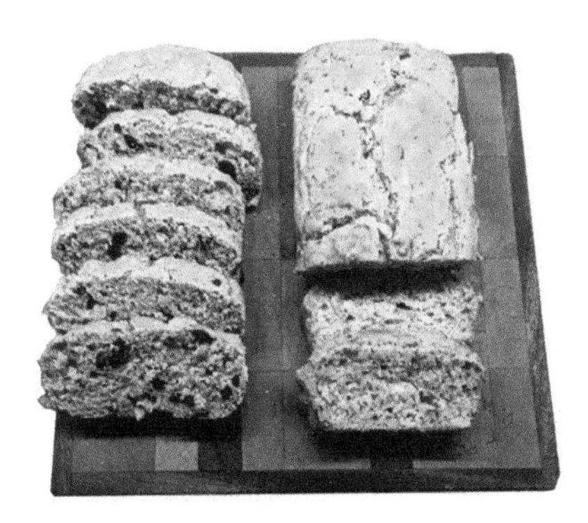

Cinnamon Raisin Bread

Preheat oven to 350-degrees

½ cup rolled oats
½ cup brown rice flour
½ cup almond flour
1 cups gluten-free muffin mix
1 tbsp arrowroot
1 tbsp flaxseed
2 tsp baking powder
1 cup raisins
1 tbsp coconut sugar
1 tsp cinnamon

Place in a mixing bowl and blend well.

2 large eggs, beaten
1 cup unsweetened almond milk
2 tbsp olive oil
½ tsp pure vanilla extract

Mix in a separate bowl. Pour slowly into the dry ingredients and thoroughly mix.

½ cup walnuts, chopped

Add to the batter and mix.

Lightly grease with olive oil an 8"x4"x2½" glass or ceramic bread baking pan.

Pour in the mixture and bake in the preheated oven for for 40 to 45 minutes.

Remove from oven and let cool before removing the bread.

Serves 12

GF – VT

Calories of the main ingredients per serving: Oats 10. Brown rice flour 24. Almond flour 25. Muffin mix 43. Raisins 42. Olive oil 20. Total of 164.

Banana Walnut Mango Bread

Preheat oven to 350-degrees.

½ cup brown rice flour
½ cup coconut flour
1 cup muffin mix flour
¼ cup arrowroot
1 tbsp flaxseed
2 tsp baking powder
¼ tsp nutmeg

Place in a mixing bowl and blend well.

2 eggs, beaten
2 tbsp olive oil
1 unsweetened cup coconut milk

Mix in a separate bowl. Pour slowly into the dry ingredients and thoroughly mix.

½ cup walnuts, chopped
1 ripe banana, mashed
½ mango, peeled and chopped

Add to the bowl and mix well.

Lightly grease with olive oil an 8"x4"x2½" glass or ceramic bread baking pan.

Pour in the mixture and bake in the preheated oven for for 40 to 45 minutes.

Remove from oven and let cool before removing the bread.

Calories of the main ingredients per serving: Brown rice flour 24. Coconut flour 39. Muffin mix 43. Bananas 17. Olive oil 20. Walnuts 22. Total of 165.

Date Lemon Bread

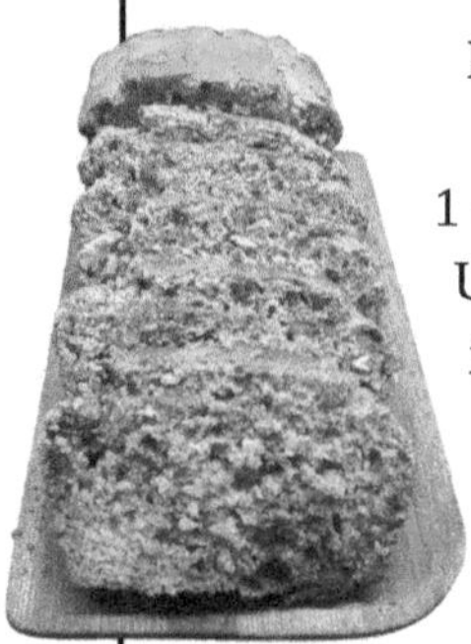

Preheat oven to 350-degrees

1 cup dried dates, Using soft dates is important to limit the water usage to pulse the dates. Too much liquid will make your bread mushy.

2 tsp water

Place in the food processor and pulse 2 or 3 times. Set aside.

½ cup brown rice flour
½ cup almond flour
1 cup muffin mix flour
¼ cup tapioca flour
2 tbsp arrowroot
1 tbsp flaxseed
2 tsp baking powder
¼ tsp ground ginger
½ tsp cinnamon

Place in a mixing bowl and blend well.

2 eggs, beaten
1 tbsp juice from a lemon
1 tbsp lemon peel, chopped
1 cup unsweetened almond milk
2 tbsp olive oil

Mix in a separate bowl. Pour slowly into the dry ingredients and thoroughly mix.

½ cup pecans, chopped
The date paste

Add to the batter and mix. Lightly grease with olive oil an 8"x4"x2½" glass or ceramic bread baking pan. Pour in the mixture and bake in the preheated oven for 40 to 45 minutes.

Remove from oven and let cool before removing the bread.

Serves 12

GF – VT

Calories of the main ingredients per serving: Dates 52. Brown rice flour 24. Almond flour 25. Muffin mix 43. Raisins 42. Olive oil 20. Pecans 30. Total of 236.

Basic Gluten Free Quick Bread Recipe.

Preheat oven to 350-degrees

½ cup brown rice flour
½ cup almond flour
1 cup muffin mix flour
¼ cup tapioca flour
2 tbsp arrowroot
1 tbsp flaxseed
1 tsp baking powder

Place in a mixing bowl and blend well.

2 eggs, beaten
1 cup unsweetened almond milk
2 tbsp olive oil

Mix in a separate bowl. Pour slowly into the dry ingredients and mix thoroughly.

Add 1½ cups add-ons and spices.

Lightly grease with olive oil an 8"x4"x 2½" glass or ceramic bread baking pan.

Pour in the mixture and bake in the preheated oven for 40 to 45 minutes.

Remove from oven and let cool before removing the bread from the pan.

Home cooking is making a comeback

There was a time when families gathered around the dinner table to share a meal. A time when the dining table was most likely the only time of the day when a family could reconnect. And then, things changed. Our busy lifestyle was undoubtedly one of the factors which lead us to find alternatives to easier and quicker meals for the family. And so began the emergence of fast food and casual restaurants. The home dining table was replaced with drive in food pick-ups and other quick options for meals. This is the main reason that has caused obesity to reach an all time high. However, research shows that recently there is a new trend towards dining at home. Today there are more convenient ways to cooking at home, it has become easier to find ideas about new recipes and to learn about the food quality. Sometimes you do not need research to understand a trend; the evolution of the home kitchen is the best indication of the importance of home cooking. The forgotten area of the home, with the dark brown cabinets of long ago, evolved into being the heart of the house. Open kitchens connected to the dining rooms have become the new living rooms. It is where people gather and cross paths. In the past, cooking was a thing to do, a chore, but today, the kitchen has become a place of creative art. I believe that people today are placing much more emphasis on what they eat and how they live, and the realization that food brings family and friends together is finally sinking into the social consciousness. There is no question eating at home is a better approach for your health, economically and socially. When a plate of food reaches the restaurant table, you do not know how your food was prepared and what quality ingredients were used. There is nothing wrong to occasionally enjoy indulgent food in a favorite restaurant. However, eating at home allows you to control your portion sizes and you know exactly what is on your plate. The toxicity in cooking is exceptionally high with the oils that most restaurants use for frying foods, especially the deep-fried ones. It is not likely that the restaurant will use healthy oils - such as pure coconut oil, extra virgin olive oil or pure avocado oil. The use of cheap iodized salt in excess is common in the restaurant kitchen also. Hidden added sugars, and compounds to enhance flavor are usually included in many restaurant sauces. In addition to the health risks when eating out too often, it is far more expensive. It is not that the restaurant purposely charges a high price; it is because restaurants must raise their prices to keep up with rising labor, rent and overall overhead costs. Besides the social benefits of eating at home, countless studies over the years have asserted that families who sit down and enjoy meals together at a table tend to be healthier. Eating at home can feel like a daunting task, especially if you are new to cooking or you have limited time to prepare a meal. My advice is to start small and work up to more involved dinners. In this book, many recipes take less than thirty minutes to prepare. The secret is to have an organize kitchen and have all the ingredients needed at hand. I've heard people say that eating out is a treat. While that can be true, I beg to differ. I believe that eating a home-cooked flavorful, healthy meal is the ultimate treat. The notion that all meals must be prepared by laboring in the kitchen for hours is also a myth. My new book can be a guide to introduce new flavors and healthier alternatives to your family. Learning new ways to blend various herbs and spices, the use of natural, healthier ingredients and the knowledge of food chemistry will limit your time in the kitchen.

A study published in June 2018, by the NPD Group, a leading global information company, states that last year over 80 percent of meals were prepared and eaten at home. The study also shows that eat at home meals will grow over the next five years. In addition, in-home meal preparation is also aided by the modern conveniences of grocery delivery. Today, the meals prepared at home, are a much higher percentage than a decade ago, according to research from NPD Group Inc.

I've heard plenty of criticism that the younger generations are eating out too much and are developing unhealthy eating habits. Despite the criticism that millennials are always going out to eat, it is encouraging to know that they are the driving force for the shifting environment to healthier eating. According to a study released on September 22, 2016, by OTA, the Organic Trade Association, parents in the 18 to 34-year-old age range are now the biggest group of organic buyers in America. Millennial parents account for 52 percent of organic buyers, Generation X parents made up 35 percent of parents choosing organic, and Baby Boomers 14 percent. Organic sales in the U.S. in 2015 posted new records, up to a robust 11 percent from the previous year, according to OTA's 2016 Organic Industry Survey.

In 2018, U.S. organic food sales saw exceptional growth. According to Nielsen Homescan household projected data, organic food sales during the 52 weeks ending November 28, 2018, rose nearly 9% over the previous period. Millennials and Hispanics made significant contributions to the sales spike, spending more during this period than the last, respectively.

In another indication that home cooking is making a comeback is the increased cookbook sales. Publisher's Weekly reports that sales of print cookbooks rose 21 percent in 2018 compared with 2017, according to data collected by NPD Bookscan.

There are many reasons why several reports showing that healthier foods are steadily on the rise. A meal at home is fresher, more nutritious and higher quality while eating in a friendlier environment with social activities. It is after all the home cooking and dining that helped to push organic sales to unprecedented levels. The U.S. organic market in 2018 broke through the $50 billion marks for the first time, with sales hitting a record $52.5 billion, up 6.3 percent from the previous year, according to the 2019 Organic Industry Survey released by the Organic Trade Association.

The changes in eating mentality and behavior shouldn't come as a surprise. The new generations are better informed and better educated about nutrition. The future of healthier foods is looking bright. As I mentioned in an earlier post, knowledge is power and today we have plenty of knowledge.

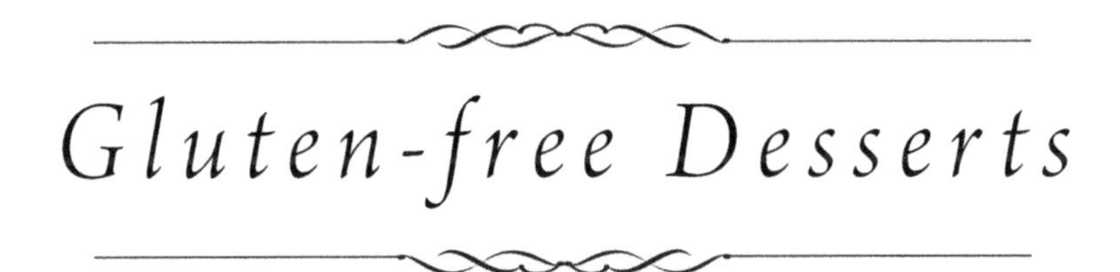

Gluten-free Desserts

"A larger-than-life force of nature known as Nick Ligidakis, he is a restaurateur legend in the Valley."
New Times

"When it comes to cheesecakes at Nick's, nothing succeeds like success. These are some of the most decadent cheesecakes in the planet."
Best of Phoenix

Sweeteners

Even though refine sugar and artificial sweeteners are under increased scrutiny because of their unhealthy impact and side effects, their general consumption is on the rise. It is a puzzling fact since there is research to back the claims of the damage they do to our health. Some sweeteners must be used when it comes to desserts, some breakfast items and drinks – there is no way around it. However, for those who follow a healthy diet or must avoid unhealthy sweeteners for medical reasons the most frequent question is what kind of sweetener to use while avoiding refined sugar, some artificial sweeteners or fructose fruit syrup. The answer is that there are plenty of healthy alternatives. Sugar is overly processed and high quantities of it will do much damage to your health. Natural sweeteners are sugar sources that are somewhat in a pure state. The less refined products maintain their vitamins, minerals and antioxidants, and some fiber. Plus, some of these natural sweeteners like banana puree, date paste and natural fruit jams provide fruit-health benefits. Following a healthy lifestyle does it mean that we have to give up the sweetness entirely. You can substitute unhealthy refined sugars, artificial sweeteners and fructose fruit syrup with various natural sweeteners. I like to introduce my preferences for natural sweeteners as a healthier alternative.

Fruit Sweeteners

On the top of my list are the natural fruit sweeteners. The prominent fruits to be used as sweeteners are dates and bananas. Dates are loaded with potassium, copper, iron, manganese, magnesium and vitamin B6. They are easily digested and help to metabolize proteins, fats and carbohydrates. To use dates as sweetener, you must make a date paste; soak dates in hot water until soft, for about an hour. Add the soaked dates to your food processor, along with a little water and blend until smooth. Add a bit more water if needed to create a thick paste. Date paste can be used in many recipes. Use it in cookie, muffin, pie, or cake recipes to reduce sugar and boost the nutrients. Usually, a half cup of date paste will substitute 1 cup of sugar. The drawback with dates is that they are high in calories. One dry date contains about 65 calories. Bananas are sweet with a subtle flavor, making them an excellent natural sweetener. To make a banana puree, place them in your food processor with a bit of water and blend to the consistency of applesauce. To give the banana puree an extra flavor, substitute the water with lime juice. Bananas can be used as an equal amount to sugar. For 1 cup of sugar, replace it with 1 cup of banana puree. One cup of bananas contains about 200 calories. Berries, apples, pears and grapes are great sweetener either as fruit or pure fruit jam which has no sugar or pectin added, or a fruit jam made by yourself. Fruit jams can be used as an equal amount; 1 cup of sugar replace it with 1 cup of fruit jam. Using fruit sweeteners as an alternative to sugar will change the consistency of your recipe. You either have to use less liquid or more thickener to bring your recipe to desired consistency. It takes a bit of practice, but it is well worth the effort to not only produce a heather food for your family but to create new tastes. The fruit sweeteners will boost the flavor of your recipes.

Honey

Diluted honey, thinned out with other elements, has always been around. However, since health-conscious people are looking for a healthier alternative and honey was the first choice on the list, its popularity lately has sky-rocketed. With the increased demand in the last few years, some honey producers invented many adulterate and sophisticated methods; therefore, the impurity of honey became more complicated. Pure honey is packed with enzymes, antioxidants, iron, zinc, potassium, calcium, phosphorous, and vitamins B6, niacin and riboflavin. Once the honey is refined, it loses most of the health benefits. A pure label on the honey jar does not guarantee at all that it is not diluted with water and further sweetened with other syrups. It is relatively safe to buy local raw honey directly from a trusted beekeeper. Local honey comes from the bees that live in your neighborhood and is well known to be a great immune booster against allergies. It is believed that the darker the honey, the richer the flavor and the greater the health benefits. Unfortunately, you can not cook with honey in high temperatures. Some people believe that heating honey in high temperatures turns into toxic and kills people. That is simply a myth. The main reason you do not use raw honey while baking in high heat is that it changes its make-up and destroys the enzymes, minerals and vitamins. It is essential to look for raw, organic, unfiltered honey, and treat it like sugar when it comes to measurements. One tablespoon of raw homey contains about 65 calories. Raw honey is a superfood.

Coconut Sugar

My attraction to coconut sugar as a natural sweetener is about its low glycemic index and rich mineral content. Coconut sugar is made from the sweet nectar of flower buds of the coconut palm. It is packed with polyphenols and phytonutrients. Coconut sugar contains iron, zinc, calcium, potassium, antioxidants, and phosphorous, Coconut sugar is versatile and now available in many markets. I like coconut sugar because of its appealing taste; it comes with hints of date and caramel flavors, which gives an added flavor into your recipe. Another reason I like coconut sugar is that it is not as sweet as regular sugar. One of the reasons my desserts had an influential flavor is because the sugar was not the overbearing factor in the taste. I've used limited amounts of sugar or other flavors, like potent flavor fruits, vanilla or cinnamon to balance the sugary aftertaste. The measurement of coconut sugar in recipes is just like traditional sugar. It is a bit coarser than regular sugar and if you like a more delicate texture, pulse it in your food processor for a couple of times. Coconut sugar is hands down my first choice to use as a dry, granulated form. It is more expensive than another natural sweetens but well worth the price. One tablespoon of coconut sugar contains 45 calories.

Xylitol

Xylitol is a sugar alcohol with implanted sweetness. Xylitol contains neither alcohol nor sugar; it is a powder, typically extracted from birch wood; hence the word xylitol, from the Greek roots Xylo- which means "wood" and "–itol" signifying sugar alcohols. Researchers first discovered its oral health benefits decades ago. It was first used in Finland and it has been used as a sweetener in European countries. Xylitol has a pleasant sweetness ideal as a sugar substitute and quickly becoming an excellent choice for a sweetener. Whereas some sweeteners may cause health risks, studies show that xylitol has real health benefits. It doesn't spike blood sugar and eliminates the bacteria in your mouth. If you're looking for a healthier alternative to regular sugar, xylitol is one of the best choices. Xylitol is a white crystalline substance that looks and tastes like sugar. It can be used the same way you would use sugar teaspoon for teaspoon. Xylitol has 30 calories per tablespoon.

Stevia

Stevia is a leafy herb and has been used for centuries by native South Americans. The leaves of the herb are sweeter than sugar – some research talks about being 200 times as sweet as sugar. The overbearing sweetness is what I don't like about stevia. If you have to use a cup for cup in your recipe to substitute regular sugar, then your final baking product will be unbearably sweet. If you could manage to cut down the sweetness whiteout compromising the texture, stevia is an excellent alternative to sugar. Stevia is an ideal natural sweetener; has zero calories, zero carbohydrates and none known side effects. Stevia is part of the sunflower family; therefore, along with the sweetness, there is an earthy, nutty flavor. Because the gluten-free flours, mainly coconut flour, are "naked" absorb much moistness and adapt quickly to other flavors, they will break down some of the stevia's sweetness. Stevia is excellent for a drink sweetener where you can regulate the taste.

Real Maple Syrup

The pure maple syrup adds a pleasant flavor to foods and is excellent as an alternative to regular pancake syrup for pancakes and waffles. It can be used for baking as well. Maple syrup contains a small amount of minerals, such as manganese and zinc. Regular Pancake syrup on the supermarket shelves is one of the most unhealthy foods for your body. Using pure maple syrup as a sweetener for pancakes and waffles, you avoid high fructose corn syrup, caramel color, salt, sodium hexametaphosphate, and preservatives such as sodium benzoate and sorbic acid, ingredients included in most regular pancake syrups. One tablespoon of maple syrup has 52 calories.

Agave

Agave syrup, depending on processing, it can contain anywhere up to 95 percent fructose while heavily processed agave nectar brings little to the table in terms of nutrition. Agave syrup is extremely high in fructose and high in sugar, carbs and calories, has been associated with several negative health effects. Agave syrup comes from the sweet substance of the blue agave plant that grows primarily in Mexico. It is the same plant that produces tequila. While processing methods can vary, most involve enzymes and chemicals. Agave, being much higher in fructose and sugar than plain sugar, is a sweetener which makes regular sugar look healthy in comparison. Therefore it is likely not suitable for your healthy diet. It contains 60 calories per tablespoon.

Agave does not make my healthy list.

Biscotti is an old-time Southern European treat, unknown to the American general public until the coffee shops became a trend in America. Biscotti is a natural partner to coffee. Its texture should be crisp and dipping it in coffee softens and enriches its flavor. Biscotti keeps well for a long time in an airtight container. But I doubt they stay on your counter for more than a few days because they are addictive. Baking times vary due to their size and the oven used. When baking the dough rolls, make sure they are baked enough to be sliced easily. When you "dry" the biscotti in the second phase of baking, the color should be light brown when done. You can turn them midway through baking the second phase of baking if you like them equally brown on both sides. If they seem a bit soft when done, do not be a concern. Biscottis are harden once cooled. They taste better the second day and much better the third day.

Instructions on how to bake the biscotti

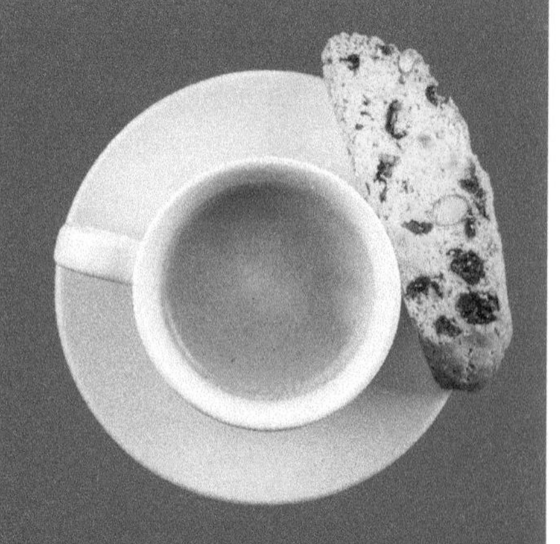

- Remove dough and divide it into two parts. Lightly knead each portion and roll into a cylinder, about 16 inches long.
- It is best (and easier) to use a 12x17 baking pan. Lightly brush the baking pan with olive oil and place the rolls on the baking pan, about 3 inches apart from each other. Press gently to flatten the top of each roll and form a half oval top shape.
- Bake in your preheated oven for about 20 to 25 minutes. Remove from oven, let cook for a few minutes. Once cool enough to handle the dough, carefully remove, one piece at a time, place on a cutting surface and with a sharp knife, gently slice the dough into about ¾ inch slices.
- Place the biscotti slices flat on the baking pan, return to the oven and bake for another 15 to 20 minutes until the biscottis turn light brown. Remove from oven and let cool before removing from the baking pan.

Makes 40 to 45 biscotti

GF – VT

Calories for the main ingredients per biscotti: Butter 8. Coconut oil 10. Coconut sugar 16. Eggs 7. Gluten-free flour 17. White rice flour 18. Brown rice flour 12. Almond flour 13. .Anise vs. Fennel

When it comes to cooking and baking, anise is not to be confused with fennel. Some believe that those two are interchangeable in recipes. This is incorrect. While the aroma is similar, the taste is not. The fronds of fennel have leaves resembling dill, the bulb is citrusy, and the seed is extremely licorice; all parts of fennel can be used for cooking. From the anise plant, you can only use their seed for flavoring. The anise seed has a very distinct flavor that is at once spicy and sweet with a mild licorice accent. Fennel is a plant that its parts carry several different flavors and anise is a seed with a more intense flavor, especially the licorice one.

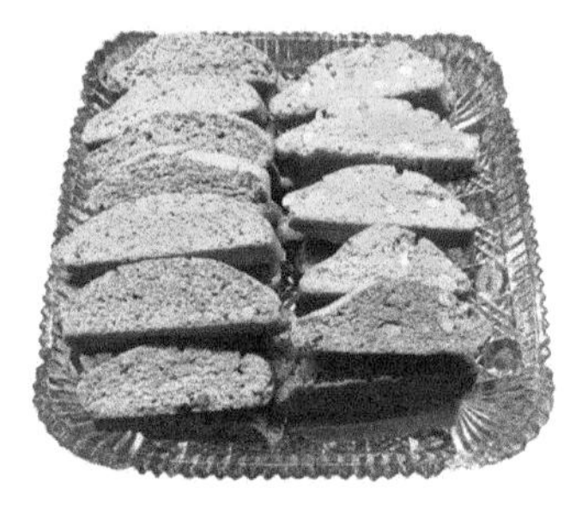

Anise Biscotti

Preheat oven to 375-degrees

½ cup butter, low-fat, organic
¼ cup olive oil
1 cup coconut sugar

Blend well with your mixer on slow speed.

4 eggs

Add to the mixing bowl and continue mixing on slow speed. Once eggs are blended with butter and oil, turn off the mixer.

2 cups gluten-free flour
1½ cups white rice flour
1 cup brown rice flour
1 cup almond flour
¼ cup tapioca
¼ cup arrowroot
2 tsp baking powder
1 tsp baking soda
1 tsp nutmeg

Add to the mixing bowl and blend on slow speed.

⅛ tsp anise extract
1 tsp ground anise seeds

Add and continue mixing until all ingredients are blended well.

Almond Biscotti

Preheat oven to 375-degrees

½ cup butter, low-fat, organic
¼ cup organic extra virgin coconut oil
1 cup coconut sugar

Blend well with your mixer on slow speed.

4 eggs

Add to the mixing bowl and continue mixing on slow speed. Once eggs are blended with butter and oil, turn off the mixer.

2 cups gluten-free flour
1½ cups white rice flour
1 cup brown rice flour
1 cup almond flour

¼ cup tapioca
¼ cup arrowroot
2 tsp baking powder
1 tsp soda
1 tsp nutmeg
Add to the mixing bowl and blend on slow speed.
⅛ tsp vanilla extract
1 cup slivered almonds
Add and continue mixing until all ingredients are blended well.

Basic Biscotti Dough

Use this recipe for more biscotti variations.
Add flavors or other add-ons.
½ cup butter, low-fat, organic
¼ cup organic extra virgin coconut oil
1 cup coconut sugar
Blend well with your mixer on slow speed.
4 eggs
Add to the mixing bowl and continue mixing on slow speed. Once eggs are blended with butter and oil, turn off the mixer.
2 cups gluten-free flour
1½ cups white rice flour
1 cup brown rice flour
1 cup almond flour
¼ cup tapioca
¼ cup arrowroot
2 tsp baking powder
1 tsp baking soda
1 tsp nutmeg

Almond Butter Cookies

Preheat over to 375-degrees
¾ cup butter, low-fat, organic
1 cup coconut sugar
½ cup xylitol sugar
Place in the mixer's bowl and cream together on low speed.
2 eggs
¼ cup almond butter
Add and blend well.
1¼ cups brown rice flour
¾ cup gluten-free flour
¼ cup tapioca flour
1 tbsp arrowroot
½ tsp baking soda
¼ cup almond meal
Add to the mixer and blend.
Brush lightly with oil a baking sheet.
Use a medium ice cream scoop and form dough balls.
Space the dough balls a couple of inches apart. Bake for 10 to 12 minutes.

Makes 20 medium size cookies

Calories per cookie: Butter 27. Coconut sugar 36. Xylitol sugar 10. Brown rice flour 33. Gluten-free flour 20. Almond meal 7. Almond butter 19. Total of 152.

Oatmeal Cookies

Preheat over to 375 degrees
1 cup butter, low-fat, organic
1 cup coconut sugar
½ cup xylitol sugar
Place in the mixer's bowl and cream together on low speed.
2 eggs
⅛ tsp pure vanilla extract
Add and blend on slow speed.
½ cup oat flour
1¼ cups brown rice flour
¼ cup tapioca flour
1 tbsp arrowroot
1 cup quick oats
1 tsp baking soda
½ tsp cinnamon
½ tsp nutmeg
Add and blend on slow speed.
1 cup raisins
Add to the mixer and blend.
Brush lightly with oil a baking sheet.
Use a medium ice cream scoop and form dough balls.
Space the dough balls a couple of inches apart. Bake for 10 to 12 minutes.

Makes 20 medium size cookies

Calories per cookie: Butter 36. Coconut sugar 36. Xylitol sugar 10. Brown rice flour 33. Oat flour 10. Quick oats 8. Raisins 25. Total of 158.Food extracts are solutions containing the flavor compound of a particular food as the primary ingredient. There should be no sugar in pure extracts, just a very concentrated flavor with some alcohol. It is best to use only pure organic extracts. Because of the concentrated flavor, it does not take much to add a specific flavor into your recipe. There are many extract flavors in the market today but I only, periodically, use a few. There is no reason to use fruit flavor extracts when you can get the flavor from the fruit itself. The most used flavor is vanilla. Sometimes I will use almond, anise, hazelnut, pistachio, or caramel extracts. Again, as long they are pure and organic, they are perfectly safe for your health.

Coconut Date Cookies

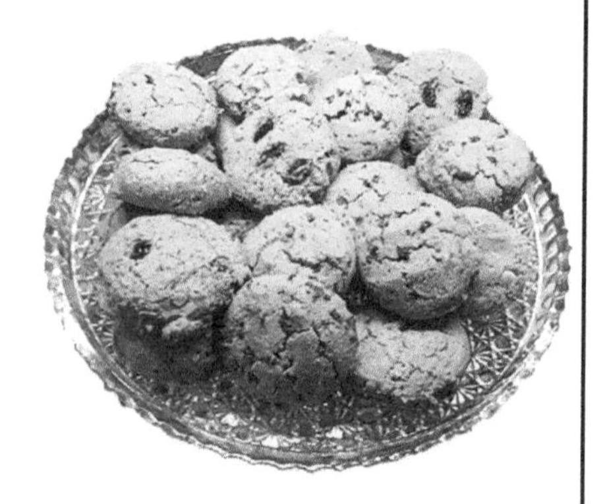

Preheat over to 375 degrees
1 cup butter, low-fat, organic
1 cup coconut sugar
½ cup xylitol sugar
Place in the mixer's bowl and cream together on low speed.
2 eggs
⅛ tsp pure vanilla extract
Add to the mixer and blend well
1¼ cups brown rice flour
¾ cup coconut flour
¼ cup tapioca flour
1 tbsp arrowroot
½ tsp baking soda
¼ cup shredded coconut, unsweetened
¾ cup pitted dates, chopped
⅛ tsp nutmeg
Add and blend on slow speed.
½ cup white chocolate chips
Add to the mixer and blend.
Brush lightly with oil a baking sheet.
Use a medium ice cream scoop and form dough balls.
Space the dough balls a couple of inches apart. Bake for 10 to 12 minutes.

Makes 20 medium size cookies

Calories per cookie: Butter 36. Coconut sugar 36. Xylitol sugar 10. Brown rice flour 33. Coconut flour 17. Coconut 4. Dates 20. White chocolate chips 22. Total of 178.

Chocolate Chip Cookies

Preheat over to 375 degrees
1 cup butter, low-fat, organic
1 cup coconut sugar
½ cup xylitol sugar
Place in the mixer's bowl and cream together on low speed.
2 eggs
⅛ tsp pure vanilla extract
Add to the mixer and blend well.
1¼ cup brown rice flour
¾ cup white rice flour
¼ cup tapioca flour
1 tbsp arrowroot
½ tsp baking soda
Add and blend on slow speed.
½ cup mini semisweet chocolate chips
Add to the mixer and blend.
Brush lightly with oil a baking sheet.
Use a medium ice cream scoop and form dough balls.
Space the dough balls a couple of inches apart. Bake for 10 to 12 minutes.

Makes 20 medium size cookies

Calories per cookie: Calories per cookie: Butter 36. Coconut sugar 36. Xylitol sugar 10. Brown rice flour 33. White rice flour 22. Chocolate chips 20. Total of 157.

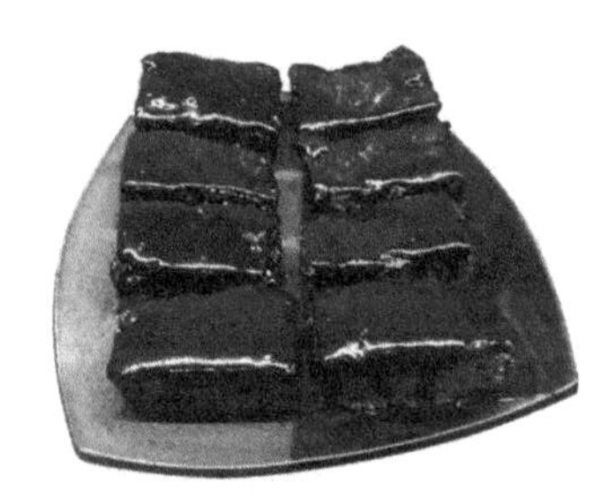

Fig Date Raspberry Brownies

Preheat over to 350 degrees
½ cup butter, low-fat, organic
¼ cup coconut sugar
Place in the mixer's bowl and cream together on low speed.
3 eggs
Add and blend on slow speed.
1 banana, mashed
1 cup dried figs, California
1 cup pitted dates, chopped
Pulse above ingredients 2 to 3 times in the food processor.
Add to the mixer.
½ cup gluten-free flour
½ cup coconut flour
1 tbsp arrowroot
1 tbsp flaxseed
½ tsp baking powder
Add to the mixer and blend on low speed
½ cup fresh raspberries
½ cup pecans, chopped
½ cup white chocolate, melted
Add to the mixer and mix gently.
Pour mixture in an 8"x8" inch class baking pan and cook in the preheated oven for 55 to 60 minutes.

Topping
1 cup semisweet chocolate chips
In a boiling pot gently heat 3 to 4 cups water.
Place chocolate in a mixing bowl and place the bowl over the water. Stir occasionally.

¼ cup almond milk, heated
Add to the chocolate and stir well and remove from the heat. When brownies are done, remove from oven and pour the chocolate mixture on top. Refrigerate for at least 1 hour before serving.

Makes 20 small brownies

Calories of the main ingredients per brownie: Butter 18. Coconut sugar 9. Eggs 11. Figs 25. Dates 25. Gluten-free flour 14. Coconut flour 12. Pecans 17. White chocolate 22. Chocolate chips 40. Total of 193.

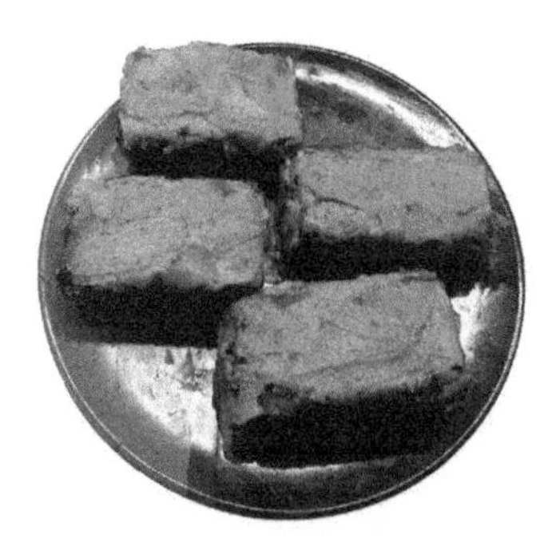

Caramel Brownies

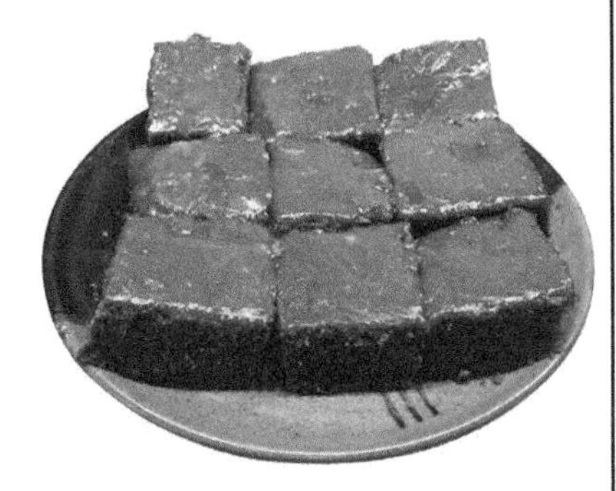

Caramel sauce
¾ cups unsweetened coconut milk
½ cup coconut sugar
1 tbsp low-fat butter
⅛ tsp vanilla extract
1 tsp honey
Combine ingredients in a saucepan
and simmer for about 30 minutes,
until liquid thickens.
Preheat over to 350-degrees

Brownies
½ cup butter, low-fat, organic
¼ cup coconut sugar
Place in the mixer's bowl and cream
together on low speed.
3 eggs
Add and blend on slow speed.
½ cup coconut flour
¼ cup brown rice flour
Add to the mixer and blend on low speed
1 cup semisweet chocolate, melted
2 tbsp caramel sauce. Save the rest of the sauce.
½ cup pecans, chopped
Add to the mixer and mix gently.
Pour mixture in an 8"x8" inch class baking pan and cook in the preheated oven for 55 to 60 minutes.

Topping
½ cup white chocolate chips
Place the saucepan with the caramel sauce on low heat. Add to the white chocolate and stir until melted. When brownies are done, remove from oven and pour the chocolate mixture on top. Refrigerate for at least 1 hour before serving.
Makes 20 small brownies
Calories of the main ingredients per brownie: Butter 36. Coconut sugar 27. Eggs 11. Coconut flour 12. Pecans 17. Brown rice flour 7. Chocolate 40. White chocolate 22. Total of 172.

Peanut Butter Brownies

Preheat over to 350-degrees
½ cup butter, low-fat, organic
½ cup coconut sugar
Place in the mixer's bowl and cream together on low speed.
2 eggs
Add and blend on slow speed.
1 banana, mashed
¾ cup low-fat peanut butter
Add to the mixer.
1 cup brown rice flour
½ cup almond flour
1tbsp cocoa powder
1 tbsp flaxseed
1 tsp baking powder
Add to the mixer and blend on low speed
¼ cup almond milk
½ cup pitted dates, chopped
Add to the mixer and mix gently. Pour mixture in an 8"x8" class baking pan and cook in the preheated oven for 55 to 60 minutes.

Topping
1 cup semisweet chocolate chips
In a boiling pot gently heat 3 to 4 cups water.
Place chocolate in a mixing bowl and place the bowl over the water. Stir occasionally.
¼ cup low-fat peanut butter
½ cup almond milk

When chocolate is melted, add to the above ingredients, stir well and remove from the heat.
When brownies are done, remove from oven
and pour the chocolate mixture on top.
Refrigerate for at least 1 hour before serving.
Makes 20 small brownies
Calories of the main ingredients per brownie: Butter 18. Coconut sugar 18. Low-fat peanut butter 50. Brown rice flour 28. Dates 13. Chocolate 40. Total of 177.

My method for chocolate truffles is easy and versatile. The cake recipe is the basis for making a variety of truffles.

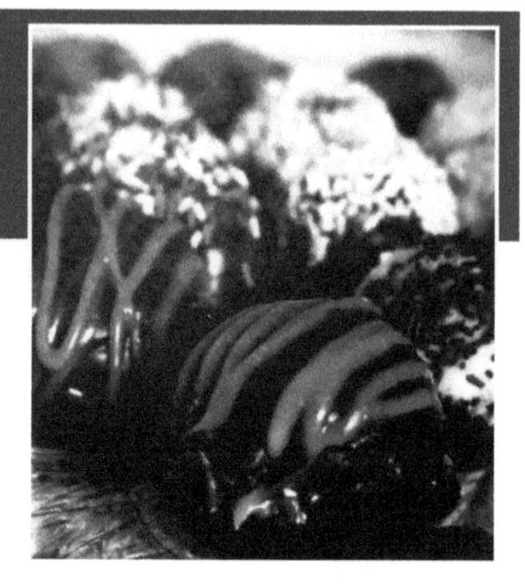

Chocolate Truffles

Preheat oven to 350-degrees
1¾ cup gluten-free baking flour,
1 cup coconut sugar
½ cup xylitol sugar
1½ tsp baking powder
1½ tsp baking soda
1 cup cocoa powder
Blend well in a mixer.
3 eggs, beaten
1¼ almond milk
½ cup pure coconut oil
Add to the mixer and blend well on slow speed.
Lightly oil a 10-inch springform pan.
Pour mixture in the pan and bake in the preheated oven for 40 to 45 minutes.
Let the cake cool before removing from the pan.

NOTE: Use a baking flour which contains various blends of flours, including sweet rice flour, xanthan gum and tapioca.

Truffle mixture

16 oz semisweet chocolate
Melt in a double boiler
The baked cake
Break up the cake in large pieces and place it in the bowl of your mixer.
8 oz low-fat, soft, unsalted butter.
Add to the mixer and blend on slow speed.
¼ cup heavy cream
The melted chocolate
Add to the mixer and blend until mixture is smooth.
Refrigerate for about 2 hours.
You can use part of the mixture and refrigerate the rest for later use.

The entire dough makes, 40 to 45 truffles.

To make 12 truffles, use 2 cups of the truffle mixture and add the flavors listed in Truffle Variations on the following page.

Icing the Truffles

8 oz semisweet chocolate
¼ cup heavy cream.
Melt in a double boiler.
2 cups truffle mixture
Scoop out the mixture with a medium size ice cream scoop.
Roll the truffle ball between your hands to smooth them out.
Place the icing on a flat baking tray and roll the truffles in the icing.
Refrigerate the tray for about 1 hour or so until the chocolate icing is firm.
Roll the truffles between the palms ofyour hand and place them on a tray.

Truffle decoration

The primary decoration for truffles is either cocoa powder or chocolate sprinkles.
Roll the truffles in either or the cocoa or the sprinkles and serve.

TRUFFLE VARIATIONS

Raspberry

½ cup frozen raspberries, drained well

Add to 2 cups of truffle mixture and blend.

Prepare icing and follow the steps of coating and decorating.

Suggested decorating; cocoa powder.

Caramel

3 tbsp of caramel sauce

See the caramel brownies recipe on how to make your caramel sauce.

Add to 2 cups of truffle mixture and blend.

Prepare icing and follow the steps of coating and decorating.

Suggested decorating; Ground hazelnuts.

Rum

1 tbsp dark rum

Add to 2 cups of truffle mixture and blend.

Prepare icing and follow the steps of coating and decorating.

Suggested decorating; White chocolate sprinkles.

Orange cappuccino

1 tbsp orange zest, finely chopped

1 tsp ground espresso coffee

Add to 2 cups of truffle mixture and blend.

Prepare icing and follow the steps of coating and decorating.

Suggested decorating; Chocolate vermicelli.

Other truffle flavors

Cherry, use frozen cherries

Mint, use mint extract

Peanut, use 1 tbsp peanut butter or create your own

Other truffle decorations

Chopped nuts

Chocolate shavings

Toasted coconutor use your imagination.

Pie Crust

Makes crust for 2 pies

5 cups flour

2 tsp xylitol sugar

1 cup low-fat butter, chilled

1 cup butter substitute, chilled.

I use Smart Balance© Original

2 egg yolks

1 cup cold water

2 tbsp milk

1 tsp white vinegar

To make crust in the food processor

Place flour and sugar and pulse 2 times.

Add butter and spread and pulse 3 to 4 times.

Add egg yolks and pulse 2 to 3 times.

Add water, milk and vinegar and pulse 2 to 3 times.

Done.

Divide dough in two parts. Pour some extra flour on a working surface. Knead and flatten the dough and roll out with a rolling pin.

To make crust in a mixer

Place flour, sugar, butter and spread in the mixing bowl and blend on slow speed.

Add eggs, mix well.

Add water, milk and vinegar, and gently blend into a smooth dough.

For gluten-free crust

Substitute flour with gluten-free baking flour.

Use a baking flour which contains various blends of flours, including sweet rice flour, xanthan gum and tapioca.

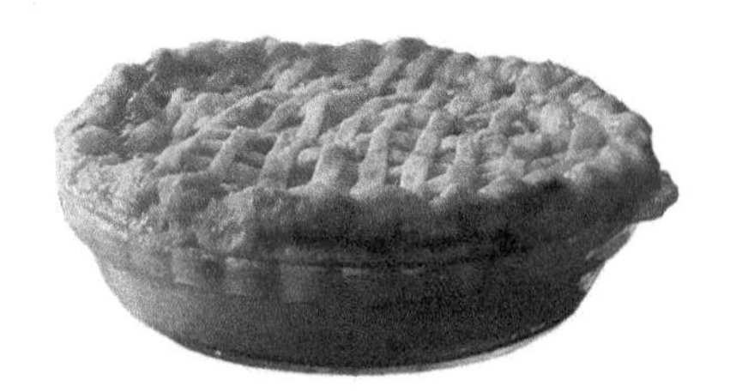

HOW TO USE THE PIE CRUST

To make a fluted edge pie crust

Roll the dough into a 12-inch round. Place it into a lightly oiled pie plate. Press gently into the pie plate. Trim ragged edges with a knife or
kitchen shears. Fold the overhanging dough under to create a thick rim.

Pinch sections of the dough with one hand while pushing against it with the index finger of the opposite hand to flute the edges of the crust.

To make a lattice edge pie crust

Divide the pie crust recipe into two parts.

Roll the one dough into the desired size. Place it into a lightly oiled pie plate.

Press gently into the plate. Roll the remaining dough into a 12 to 14-inch round. Using a pizza cutter, cut the dough into one-inch strips, or to the desired thickness.

Place one strip across the center of the pie top. Place another strip across the top to form a cross. Using a weaving pattern; placing a strip across horizontally and another vertically, about one inch apart, complete the lattice pattern. Cut the edges of the strips in about one inch beyond the edges of the pie plate. Fold the bottom crust into the strips and flute the edges.

Class pie plates are the best to use for pie baking.

Do not oil the pie plate.

When using a glass pie plate, bake in a slightly
lower temperature and bake a bit longer. Glass
holds heat better and produces a browner bottom crust.

CHERRY BERRY PIE

Preheat oven to 350-degrees.

For this pie, you need to make a lattice edge pie crust, using a 10-inch round and a deep glass pie plate.

12 oz fresh cranberries
¼ cup water
Juice of half orange

Place water and orange juice in a large saucepan. When warm, add the cranberries and cook for 5 to 6 minutes.

2 cups pitted dark cherries
2 cups pitted red cherries

Add to the pan and continue cooking for another 5 to 6 minutes.

Turn off the heat.

1 cup coconut sugar
1 tsp cinnamon
1 tsp ground cloves
2 tbsp arrowroot
juice of ½ lemon

Add to the saucepan and blend well.

Pour into the prepared pie crust and complete the lattice design crust.

Bake in the preheated oven for 50 to 55 minutes

8 servings

Calories in pie filling per serving: Cranberries 20. Cherries 45. Coconut sugar 90. Total of 155.

NOTE: I use a combination of dark and red cherries. You can use one or the other. If not in season youcan use frozen cherries.

APPLE CHERRY PIE

Preheat oven to 350-degrees.

For this pie, you need to make a lattice edge pie crust, using a 10-inch round, deep glass pie plate.

6 red apples, peeled and sliced
½ cup coconut sugar
2 tbsp arrowroot
1 tsp cinnamon
juice of ½ lemon

Place ingredients into a mixing bowl and blend well with a wooden spoon. Pour mixture into the pie crust.

3 cups dark cherries, cut in halves
1 tbsp orange peel

2 tbsp low-fat butter, softened
½ tbsp coconut sugar
1 tsp nutmeg
Mix well in a bowl and pour on top of the apple filling and complete the lattice design crust.
Bake in the preheated oven for 60 to 65 minutes.
8 servings
Calories in pie filling per serving: Apples 62. Coconut sugar 90. Dark cherries 34. Low-fat Butter 13. Total of 201.

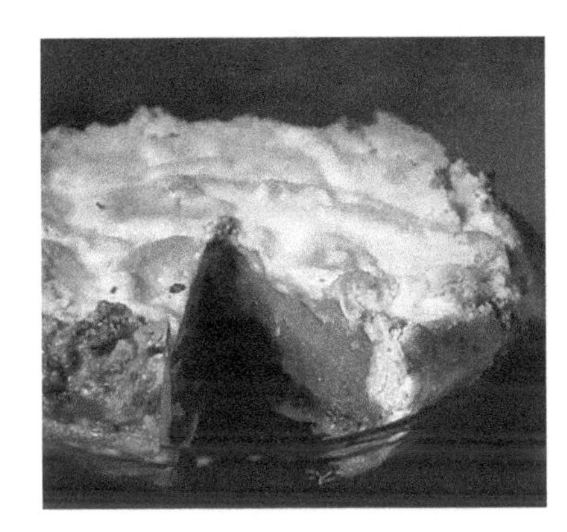

Walnut Pear Pie

Preheat oven to 350-degrees
Prepare a fluted edge pie crust, using a 10-inch round and deep glass pie plate.

Filling

8 pears, peeled and sliced
2 tbsp arrowroot
½ cup xylitol sugar
1 tsp nutmeg
¼ cup low-fat butter, melted
1 tbsp juice from a lemon
1 tsp white wine vinegar
Place all ingredients in a mixing bowl, blend well and pour into the pie crust.

Topping

2 tbsp low-fat butter
1 tsp coconut sugar
Blend gently with a mixer.
1 egg
1 tbsp low-fat Greek yogurt
½ cup walnuts, grated
1 tbsp almond milk
Add and mix well.
8 oz white chocolate, melted
Blend with the rest of the ingredients.
Spread topping over the Pie filling.
Bake in the preheated oven for 70 to 75 minutes

8 servings

Calories in pie filling per serving: Pears 96.
Sugar 30. Walnuts 33. White Chocolate 55.
Total of 214

Caramel Pecan Pie

Caramel sauce
¾ cups unsweetened coconut milk
½ cup coconut sugar
1 tbsp low-fat butter
⅛ tsp vanilla extract
1 tsp honey
Combine ingredients in a saucepan and simmer for about 30 minutes, until liquid thickens. Set aside
Preheat oven to 350-degrees.
Prepare a fluted edge pie crust, using a 10-inch round, deep glass pie plate.
Filling
¼ cup low-fat butter
½ cup coconut sugar
In a mixer, mix gently in low speed.
3 eggs
¾ cup pure maple syrup
1 tsp bourbon vanilla extract
½ tsp cinnamon
½ tsp nutmeg
2 tbsp coconut flour
Add to the mixer and blend well.
1 cup pecan pieces
The caramel sauce
Add and mix thoroughly.
Pour into the prepared pie crust and bake for 65 to 70 minutes.
8 servings
Calories in pie filling per serving: Coconut sugar 90. Low-fat butter 15. Eggs 30. Maple syrup 75. Pecans 94.Total of 306.

Gluten-free Cheesecake Crust

1 cup almond meal
1 cup gluten-free graham crackers
1 cup oats
½ cup coconut sugar
½ cup butter low-fat, melted

Blend well in a mixing bowl.
To place the homemade graham crackers in the food processor and pulse to crumbs. 8 or 9 crackers should make 1 cup crumbs.
I included the graham cracker recipe because I like the graham cracker crust.
If you do not want to use graham crackers substitute with 1½ cups almond meal and 1½ cups oats.

Calories with graham crackers per serving: Graham crackers 49. Almond meal 42. Oats 22. Coconut sugar 26. Low-fat butter 51. Total of 190.
Calories without graham crackers: Almond meal 32. Oats 25. coconut sugar 20. Low-fat butter 39. Total of 116.

How to prepare the crust
Use a 10-inch springform pan. Lightly oiled the pan and press the crust against the bottom and sides of the pan. The crust on the side of the pan will help to keep your cheesecake smooth and creamy.

How to melt chocolate
Place the chocolate in a mixing bowl. Set the bowl over a stockpot with barely simmering a small amount of water. I like to use a mixing bowl larger than the size of the stockpot, so the bottom of the mixing bowl does not touch the water. Occasionally stir the chocolate. Do not overheat.

Carrot Cake

Preheat oven to 350 degrees
½ cup low-fat butter, melted
½ cup pure coconut oil
1 cup coconut sugar

In a mixer, mix gently in low speed.

3 eggs

Add to the mixer and blend.

1½ cups gluten-free flour
½ cup brown rice flour
½ cup almond flour
1 tbsp arrowroot
1 tsp baking soda
1 tsp baking powder
1 tsp cinnamon
½ tsp vanilla extract

Add to the mixer and blend on slow speed.

1 cup fresh pineapple

Place in a food processor and pulse 1 or 2 times.
Add to the mixer, including the liquid.

2½ cups carrots, shredded
¼ cup raisins
¾ cup walnuts, chopped

Add and thoroughly blend.
Lightly oiled a 10-inch springform pan for a round cake or 13"x9" glass or ceramic pan for a rectangular cake.
Bake in the preheated oven for 45 to 50 minutes.
Remove from oven and let it cool.

Frosting
16 oz low-fat cream cheese
½ cup xylitol sugar

Cream well in a mixer.

1/8 cup low-fat Greek yogurt
½ tsp vanilla extracted
½ cup grated walnuts
½ cup unsweetened shredded coconut
1 tsp honey

Add to the mixer and blend.
Remove cake from the pan and spread the icing over the entire cake.

14 servings

Gluten-free Graham Crackers

Preheat oven 350-degrees

¾ cup almond meal
1 cup brown rice flour
½ cup arrowroot
½ cup coconut sugar
1 tsp baking powder
¼ tsp vanilla extract

Mix in a mixing bowl and place in the food processor.

1/3 cup low-fat butter, cold

Add the cold butter in the food processor and pulse 2 times. The mixture should be coarse. Remove and return mixture to the mixing bowl.

⅓ cup almond milk
2 tbsp honey

Add to the bowl and stir with a wooden spoon to thoroughly mix. Dust lightly with brown rice flour a large piece of parchment paper (about 12"x18") Place dough on top and press to flatten. Dust the top of the dough with brown rice flour lightly and cover it with another piece of parchment paper. With a rolling pin open the dough to a rectangle, about ¼-inch thick. Remove top paper and transfer dough, with the bottom paper into a 12"x18" baking pan. Score dough into small rectangles and stamp top with a fork. Bake in the preheated oven for 18 to 20 minutes, until crackers are lightly brown. Remove, cool completely and break crackers along score lines.

Makes 24 crackers

Calories per cracker: Almond meal 18. Brown rice flour 24. Coconut sugar 15. Low-fat butter 24. Honey 5. Total of 86.

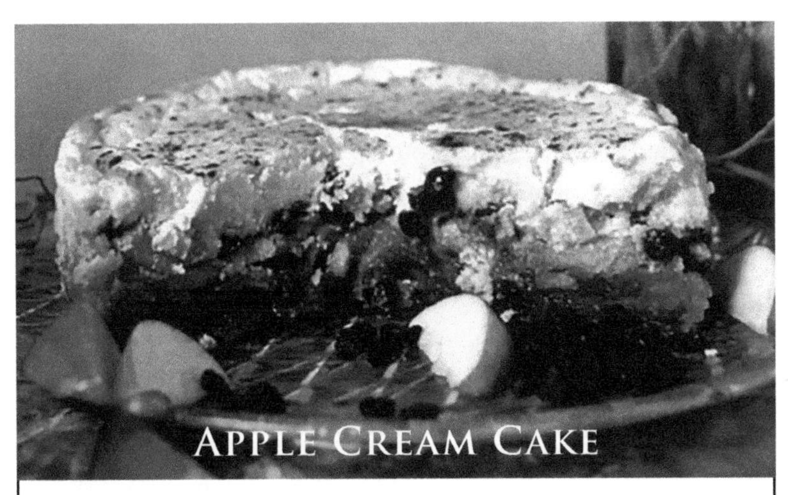

Apple Cream Cake

Preheat oven to 350-degrees

½ cup almond meal
1 cup oats
½ cup coconut sugar
⅛ cup butter low-fat, melted

Blend well in a mixing bowl.
Press crust on the bottom of a 10-inch springform pan.

Apple filling

4 apples, peeled and thinly sliced
½ cup coconut sugar
¼ cup arrowroot
½ cup raisins
½ tsp cinnamon

Mix well in a mixing bowl and pour into the springform pan.

Cream filling

1 lb low-fat cream cheese
¼ cup xylitol sugar

Cream together in a medium speed of your mixer.

3 eggs

Add and mix thoroughly.

½ cup sour cream
¼ cup Greek yogurt
1 tbsp juice of a lemon
½ tsp vanilla extract
2 tbsp heavy cream
¼ cup brown rice flour

Add to the mixer and blend well. Pour over the apple filling.
Bake for 1 hour. Turn oven off and let cake sit in the oven for 35 to 40 minutes.
Refrigerate for 8 to 10 hours before serving.

Makes a 10-inch round cake

16 servings

Strawberry Cheesecake

Preheat oven to 350-degrees
Prepare a cheesecake crust, covering bottom and sides of a 10-inch springform pan.

Filling

1 lb cream cheese
1 cup xylitol sugar
Cream together in a medium speed of your mixer.
4 eggs
Add and mix thoroughly.
2 cups real Greek yogurt
1 tbsp juice of a lemon
1 tbsp arrowroot
1 tsp vanilla
8 oz white chocolate, melted
Add to the mixer and blend well.
6 strawberries cut in large pieces
Mix to incorporate the strawberries. Pour mixture into prepared crust and bake for 1 hour.
While the cheesecake is being baked, prepare the topping.

Topping

7 to 8 strawberries, chopped
¼ cup xylitol sugar
¼ cup water
1 tbsp arrowroot
In a saucepan, combine all ingredients.
Bring to a boil. Cook and stir 2 to 3 minutes.
20 to 22 large strawberries, cut in halves
Place strawberries and strawberry glaze in a large mixing bowl and gently mix.
Refrigerate the topping.
After baking the cheesecake for 1 hour, turn the oven off and let sit for 45 minutes longer.
Refrigerate 12 to 14 hours.
Remove the springform pan and place the strawberries, cut-side down, on top of the cheesecake.
18 servings

Calories in a cheesecake batter per serving: Cream cheese 89. Xylitol sugar 20. Eggs 18. Greek yogurt 9. These calories do not include the add-ons in the various cheesecakes.

Tips about creamier and smoother cheesecake:
The crust on the side of the springform pan.
Cream well the cream cheese with the sugar.
Bake in low temperature, ideally in 350-degrees.
Finish baking your cheesecake with the oven off.

In my original cheesecakes, I used sour cream. However, for a healthier choice, I substitute sour cream with real Greek yogurt. It is essential to use real Greek yogurt. In my opinion, the FAGE brand is the closest to the authentic Greek yogurt I had growing up in Greece. Let's face it when you make desserts; there will be extra calories. But we can substitute ingredients without compromising with the quality of the recipe. Using Greek yogurt is healthier and cuts down the calories of the sour cream to about one-third.

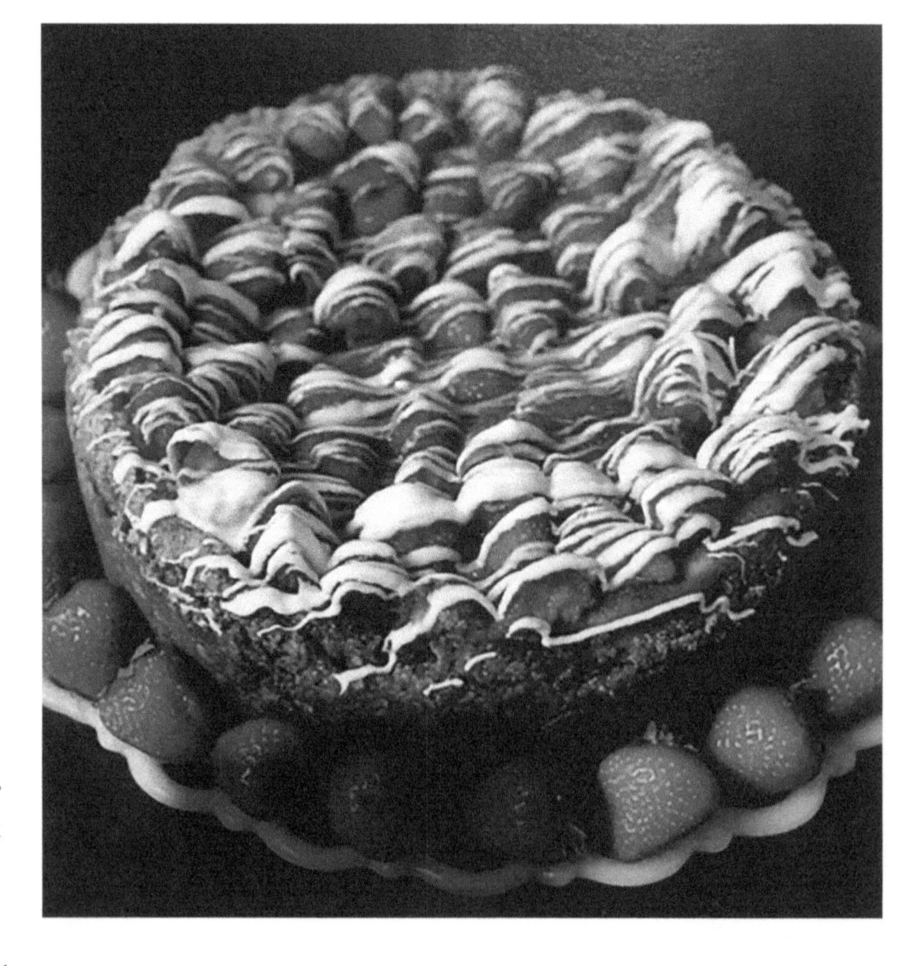

Pumpkin White Chocolate Cheesecake

Preheat oven to 350-degrees

Prepare a cheesecake crust, covering the bottom and sides of a 10-inch springform pan.

Filling

1 lb cream cheese

1 cup xylitol sugar

Cream together in a medium speed of your mixer.

4 eggs

Add and mix thoroughly.

1 tbsp juice of a lemon

1 tsp vanilla

1 cup pumpkin puree

1 lb white chocolate, melted

½ cup real Greek yogurt

½ cup heavy cream

Mix well, pour the mixture into prepared crust and bake for 1 hour.

While the cheesecake is being baked, prepare the topping.

Topping

¾ cup white chocolate

Melt over a double boiler.

¾ cup real Greek yogurt

½ cup xylitol sugar

½ cup pumpkin puree

When chocolate is melted, add the rest of the ingredients, stir to blend well, remove from heat and set aside.

After baking the cheesecake for 1 hour, pour topping over the top, return to oven, turn the oven off and let sit for 45 minutes longer. Refrigerate 12 to 14 hours before removing from the pan.

18 servings

Chocolate cake

Preheat oven to 350-degrees

1¾ cup gluten-free baking flour

1 cup coconut sugar

½ cup xylitol sugar

1½ tsp baking powder

1½ tsp baking soda

1 cup cocoa powder

Blend well in a mixer.

3 eggs, beaten

1¼ almond milk

½ cup pure coconut oil

Add to the mixer and blend well on slow speed.

Lightly oiled a 10-inch springform pan.

Pour mixture in the pan and bake in the preheated oven for 40 to 45 minutes.

Let the cake cool before removing from the pan.

It is easier to remove the cake from a springform pan.

14 servings

Calories per serving: Flour 50. Coconut sugar 52. Xylitol sugar 26. Cocoa powder 14. Coconut oil 67. Eggs 16. Total of 225.

NOTE: Use a baking flour which contains various blends of flours, including sweet rice flour, xanthan gum and tapioca.

NOTE: This recipe can be used to make a barcake.

Use an 8"x4"x2½" glass or ceramic baking dish.

Or use a 7½"x6" rectangular baking dish for birthday cakes.

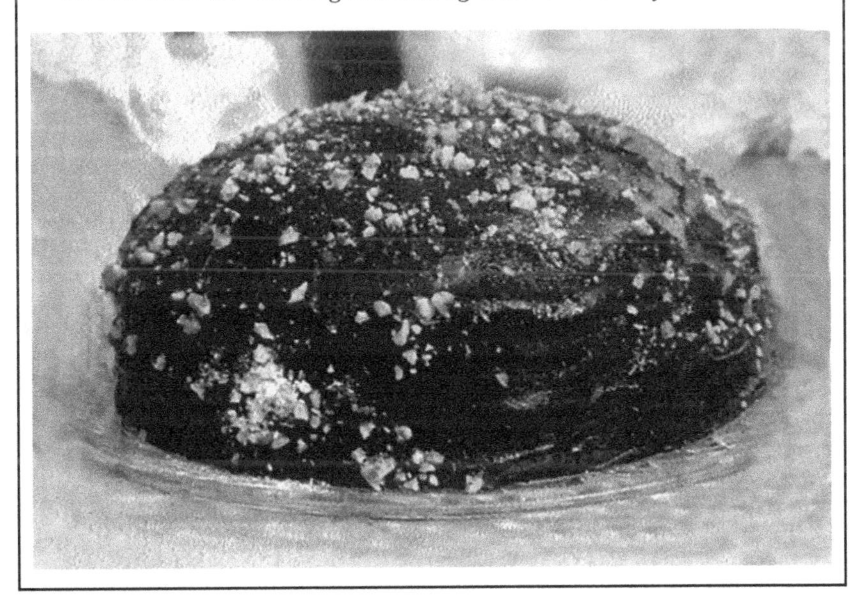

Raspberry Banana Cake

8 oz frozen raspberries

Defrost, save 3 tbsp of the liquid and drain the rest.

2 bananas, thinly sliced

Raspberry simple syrup

3/4 cup water

¼ cup coconut sugar

3 tbsp raspberry liquid

Bring to a boil in a small pan reduce heat and simmer for 3 to 4 minutes. Set aside.

6 oz semisweet chocolate

Melt in a double boil over low heat. When chocolate is melted, turn off the heat.

8 oz white chocolate

Melt in a separate double boil low heat. Turn off the heat.

Chocolate shavings

4 large pieces of parchment paper.

Place 4 tbsp of semisweet chocolate on the one piece of the paper. Cover it with another piece of paper and with a rolling pin roll out the chocolate into paper-thin. Place it into your freezer.

Repeat the process with the white chocolate; paper - 3 tbsp chocolate – paper – roll out to paper-thin. Place it into your freezer.

Assembling the cake

4 cups whipping cream

1 tsp pure vanilla extract

Beat on high speed with the wire whip of your mixer until the cream reaches stiff peaks.

Remove from the mixer and divide the cream into three separate bowls. Refrigerate one of the bowls with the cream for a later use.

Chocolate cake

Using a round cake, barcake or birthday cake format takes the same steps to build the cake.

Slice it in three horizontal slices. Place one slice on a serving platter. With a spoon, sprinkle some of the raspberry simple syrup to moisten the cake. Slowly pour the melted white chocolate into one of the bowls with the cream, constantly blending with a spatula. Spread half of the mixture on the cake and place the sliced bananas over the cream.

Top the bananas with the second piece of cake and pour some of the raspberry syrup over to soak the cake. Slowly pour the melted semisweet chocolate in the other bowl with the cream, constantly blending with a spatula. Spread the entire mixture on the cake and place the raspberries over the cream.

Top the raspberries with the third piece of cake and pour some raspberry simple syrup to moisten the cake.

Use the remaining white chocolate mixture from the first bowl to ice the top and sides of the cake.

Decorating the cake

You need a pastry bag with a closed star tip

Remove the third bowl of the cream from the refrigerator and fill the pastry bag with. Pipe a simple design around the cake edges; Hold your pastry bag at an angle, squeeze, pull the bag towards you moving your hands and into a circular motion go around the cake edges. It is relatively simple, but it takes a bit of practice.

The chocolate shavings

Remove the parchment papers from the freezer, remove the top paper and break the thin chocolate into pieces.

Use the dark shaving for the sides of the cake and the white ones for the top.

If you do not want to use a pastry bag, decorate your cake with just the chocolate shavings.

16 servings

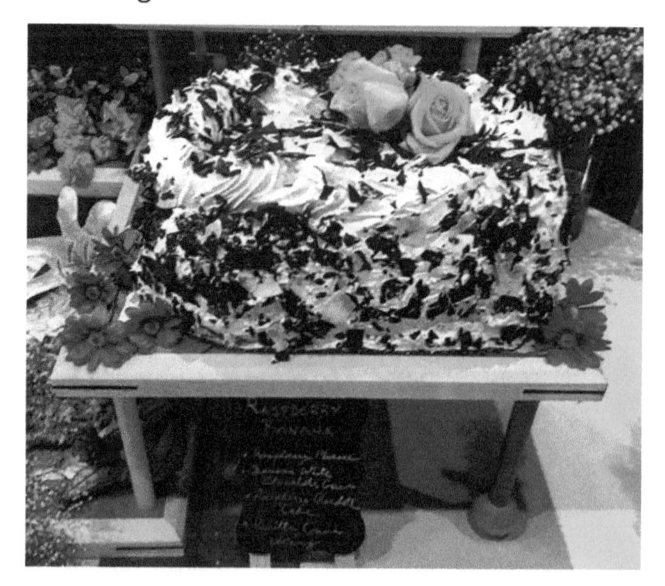

Why all baking authorities insist on baking cakes at 350-degrees? In just about every cookbook, the 350-degree is the standard temperature to bake cakes. What is it about that number? Is it going to be a national disaster if the oven's dial is a few numbers off?

To understand the over temperature obsession, we must realize what is going on during the baking time of a cake – when a gooey batter transforms into an irresistible delight. On every step during the complex process of transformation, there is a chemical reaction and that reaction is based on the oven temperature. In lower temperatures, these chemical reactions occur slowly. The rise of the batter begins at the outer crust and gradually reacts towards the center of the dough. In higher temperatures, the process moves on at a fast pace; therefore, there is an uneven distribution of temperature to all parts of the dough. Consequently, a cake baked around 300 to 325 degrees is much lighter, but the crust of the cake will be relatively soft. A cake baked between 375 to 400 degrees will have crusty edges and dried texture. Baking your cake in 350 degrees is the ideal temperature to bake a cake that is light in texture and with a firm crust. However, a few degrees, more or less, will not make much difference. The point is that every oven is deferent. You must pay attention to the accuracy of your oven to predict the outcome of your cake. If you do not get the results you like, adjust the temperature of your oven. The 350-degree oven is the benchmark to start baking cakes, but you are in control to adjust the temperature dial up or down a bit.

Peanut Butter Cheesecake

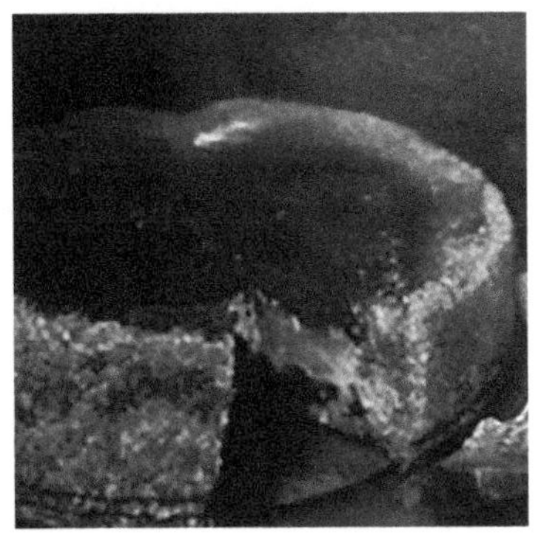

Preheat oven to 350-degrees

Prepare a cheesecake crust, covering bottom and sides of a 10-inch springform pan.

Filling

1 lb cream cheese
1½ cups xylitol sugar

Cream together in a medium speed of your mixer.

1 cup creamy low-fat peanut butter

Add to the mixer and blend well.

5 eggs

Add and mix thoroughly.

1 cup real low-fat Greek yogurt
1 tbsp juice of a lemon

Add to the mixer and blend well.

1 cup semisweet chocolate chips

Mix to incorporate the chocolate chips. Pour mixture into prepared crust and bake for 1 hour.

While the cheesecake is being baked, prepare the topping.

Topping

¾ cup semisweet chocolate chips

Melt over a double boiler

1 cup real Greek yogurt
½ cup xylitol sugar

When chocolate is melted, add the rest of the ingredients, stir to blend well, remove from heat and set aside.

After baking the cheesecake for 1 hour, pour topping over the top, return to oven, turn the oven off and let sit for 45 minutes longer.

Refrigerate 12 to 14 hours before removing from the pan.

18 servings

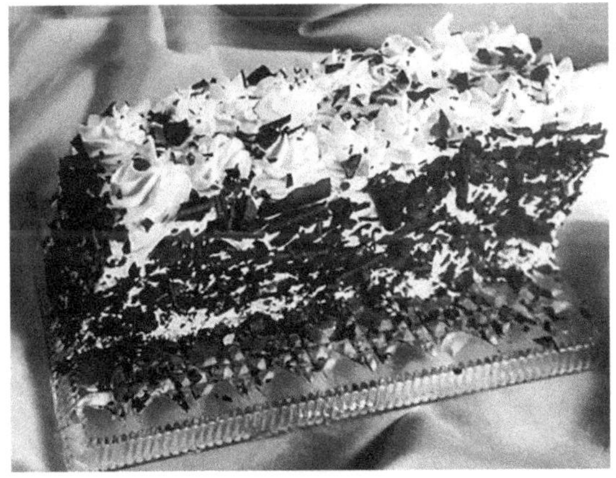

Bar Cake

This cake is based on one of my first recipes

Sweet Chocolate Death

Toasted almonds

2 cups of sliced almonds

Place on a baking pan and toast in a 350-degree oven, 6 to 8 minutes or until light brown.

Chocolate icing

12 oz semisweet chocolate

Melt in a double boiled over low heat.

1½ cups heavy cream

Place in a small pot and gently heat the cream. Add to the melted chocolate stir to a smooth mixture.

Simple syrup

1 cup water

¼ cup coconut sugar

Bring to a boil in a small pan, reduce heat and simmer for 3 to 4 minutes. Set aside.

Chocolate cake

Slice it in three horizontal slices. Place one slice on a serving platter. With a spoon, sprinkle some of the simple syrup to moisten the cake. Pour about one-third of the icing on top of the cake and spread it evenly with a pastry spatula. Set the rest of the icing on the side. Place the second cake slice on top of the cake slice with the icing. With a spoon, sprinkle some of the simple syrup to moisten the cake.

Quick chocolate mousse

4 oz semisweet chocolate

Melt in a double boiled over low heat. Remove from the heat

1½ cups whipping cream

Beat on high speed with the wire whip of your mixer until the cream reaches stiff peaks. Remove from the mixer and fold in the melted chocolate, stirring with a plastic spatula.

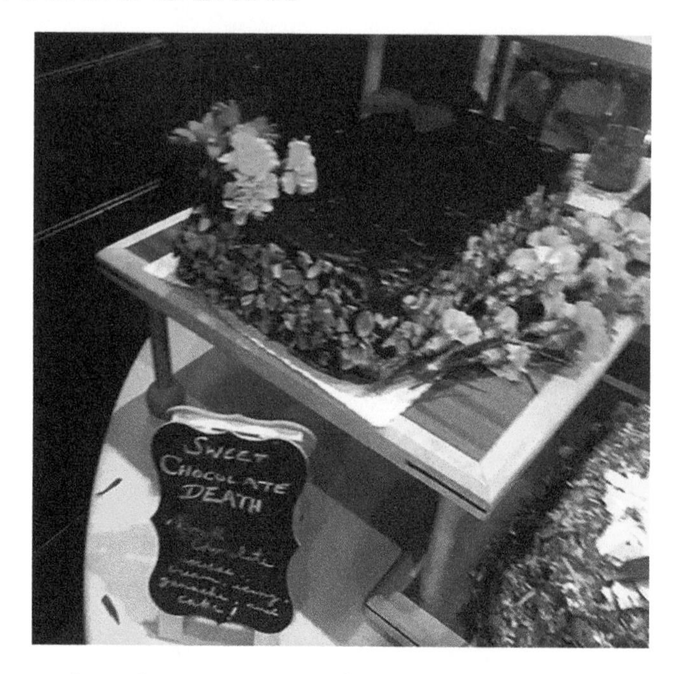

Spread mousse on top of the second cake slice and spread it evenly with your pastry spatula.

Top it with the third cake slice. Press the top slice with the palm of your hands. With your pastry spatula smooth any excess icing or mousse on the sides of the cake.

Remaining icing

Gently reheat the remaining icing on the double boiler. Pour the icing on to the center of the cake and let it run over the cake. There will be some icing running over on the sides of the cake. With your pastry spatula, spread the excess icing around the cake.

Toasted almonds

Cover the sides of the cake with.

16 servings

"The best diet is the one that allows for the occasional indulgence"

Foods to Celebrate Life's Special Moments

"I watched magic being made"

In 1989, Nick Ligidakis was on his way to becoming a Valley culinary legend. We interview Romeo Taus, one of the renown chefs in the Valley who study under Ligidakis.

"I liked his food, I liked his energy, I liked his concept...Remember, this was when Wolfgang Puck was starting to put goat cheese on pizza, and Nick had that flair...I was his towel boy in his cooking classes. I would listen to him talk about food and I would just salivate... Nick was the original farm-to-fork chef in Phoenix. He was a true artist, he never cared about making money. He just cared about making the best food. It showed in the greatness of his food...When he cooked, I watched magic being made."

New Times – The Best in the Valley

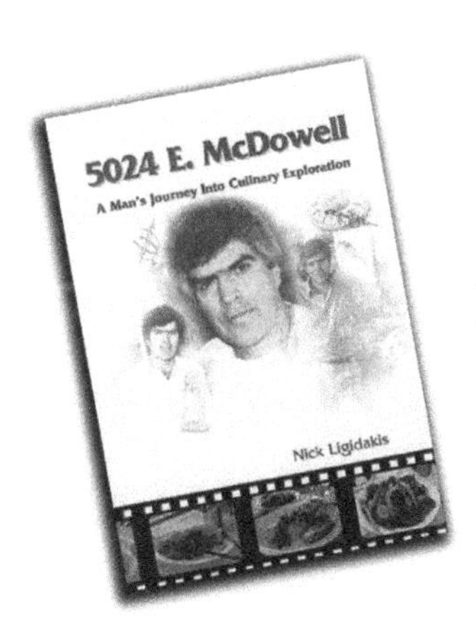

Recipes from my cookbook

5024 E. McDowell

Over 400 original recipes

My family loves the Raspberry Stuffed Toast. It is the most requested dish for brunch.

Raspberry Stuffed Toast

16 slices of French banquette, about ½ inch thick

Lay on a working surface.

8 oz cream cheese
½ cup raspberries, fresh or frozen
¼ cup sugar-free raspberry jam

Place in a bowl and mix well. With a spoon place the mixture on top of the 8 slices. Top the mixture with the other 8 slices to resemble a sandwich.

Gently press the bread slices together.

Turn your flat grill on (or use a sauté pan)

3 eggs
2 tbsp heavy cream
½ tsp nutmeg
½ tsp cinnamon

Place in a mixing bowl and beat with a fork.

¼ cup olive oil

Pour on the grill, heat for a minute.

Dip the 8 pieces of the stuffed bread, one at a time, into the egg batter and place on top of the grill.

Cook well on both sides, about 3 to 4 minutes on each side.

Place the raspberry stuffed toast on a serving platter.

¼ cup sugar-free orange jam
2 tbsp sliced almonds
3 tbsp heavy cream

Place in a sauté pan and cook on medium heat, stirring, for 2 to 3 minutes.Pour sauce over the stuffed toast and serve.

3 to 4 servings

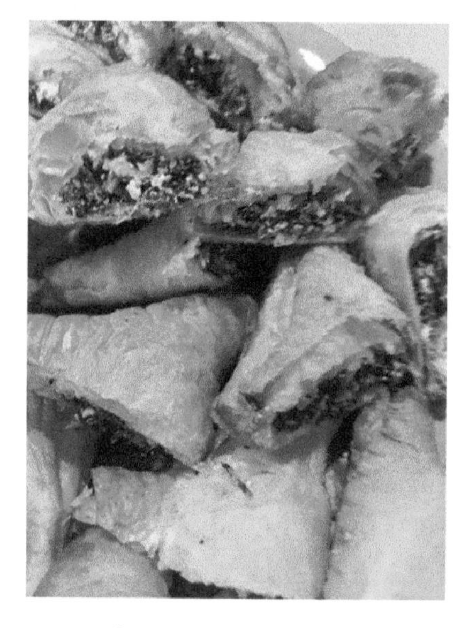

Spinach Puffs

Preheat oven to 375-degrees.

2 cups frozen chopped spinach, drain well
1 cup feta cheese, crumbled
¼ cup pine nuts
½ onion, finely chopped
2 green onions, finely chopped
1 tsp fresh dill, chopped
1 tsp fresh mint, chopped
½ tsp black pepper
½ tsp cinnamon
1 egg
1 tbsp olive oil
1 tbsp milk
2 tbsp grated Parmesan cheese

Mix all ingredients well in a mixing bowl.

16 pieces of puff pastry dough, approximately 4"x4" inches

Lay the puff pastry on a working surface, wet the edges lightly with watter and place 2 to 2½ tbsp filling on the center of the dough. Fold the dough into a triangle and press gently with a fork to seal the edges.

Lightly brush with olive oil 2 large baking pans.

Bake for about 18 to 20 minutes, until pastry is golden brown.

Serve with Horseradish sauce.

Horseradish Sauce
1 cup sour cream
½ cup olive oil mayonnaise
2 cloves garlic, finely chopped
1 tsp black pepper
1 tsp prepared horseradish
½ tsp Worcestershire sauce
1 tsp Dijon mustard

Mix well with a fork and serve with the spinach puffs.

NOTE: You can make the squares smaller or bigger if you like. Follow the same process and place less or more filling in the center of the dough.

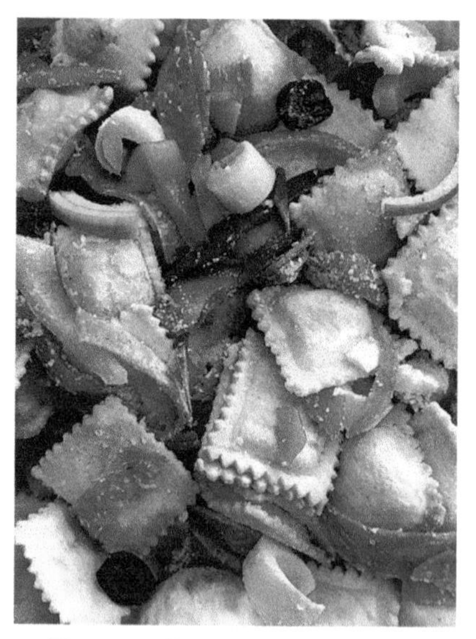

Fried Ravioli Salad

1 lb cheese ravioli
½ cup olive oil

Heat olive in a large sauté pan. Add ravioli a few at a time and lightly brown on both sides. Place in a large salad bowl.

2 tbsp grated Romano cheese
2 tbsp grated Parmesan cheese

Add to the bowl and toss with the ravioli. Let it cool.

1 red bell pepper, sliced
½ green bell pepper, sliced
½ red onion, chopped
3 hearts of palm, sliced
1 cup artichoke hearts, quartered
8 pea pods, remove strings, sliced
½ cup sliced black olives
¼ lb Italian salami, cut into strips
Add to the bowl.
¼ cup mustard vinaigrette dressing
Add to the bowl, toss and serve.

4 servings

Mustard Vinaigrette Dressing

1 cup olive oil
¼ cup red wine vinegar
1 clove garlic, chopped
¼ of a small onion, minced
1tsp dry basil
1 tsp black pepper
1 tsp dry dill weed
1 tbsp dry oregano
1 tbsp dry thyme
½ tsp dry rosemary
⅛ cup Dijon mustard
Place in a mixing bowl and mix with a wire whisk.
Refrigerate in a glass jar.

It makes about 16 oz dressing.

There is never a family gathering without this recipe.

Asparagus Chicken

Preheat oven to 375-degrees
2 - 8 oz chicken breasts
Place chicken on a cutting board. Gently pound chicken with a meat mallet to flatten.
4 pieces of sliced ham
Place 2 pieces on the center of each chicken breast.
4 slices of provolone cheese
Place 2 pieces on top of each ham slices.
6 asparagus spears, cut off the tough bottom parts
Place 3 asparagus on each top of provolone cheese.
Roll chicken breasts tightly, making sure the ham, provolone and asparagus are entirely enclosed with the chicken.
½ cup flour
1 cup breadcrumbs
1 egg
Place ingredients on 3 separate bowls. Beat the egg.
¼ cup olive oil
Heat in a large sauté pan on medium heat.
Roll the stuffed chicken breasts on the flour, then on the egg and coat them with the breadcrumbs. Add to the pan, seam down, and sauté for about 5 to 6 minutes. Turn and sauté for another 5 to 6 minutes.
Remove chicken and place on a baking dish. Bake for 15 to 18 minutes.
In the meantime, prepare the sauce.
1 tbsp olive oil
Heat in a small sauté pan.
2 tbsp sliced almonds
6 mushrooms, sliced
Add to the pan and sauté on medium heat for 4 to 5 minutes.
1 tbsp white wine
½ tsp black pepper
1 cup heavy cream
Add to the pan, turn heat to low and simmer for 3 to 4 minutes.

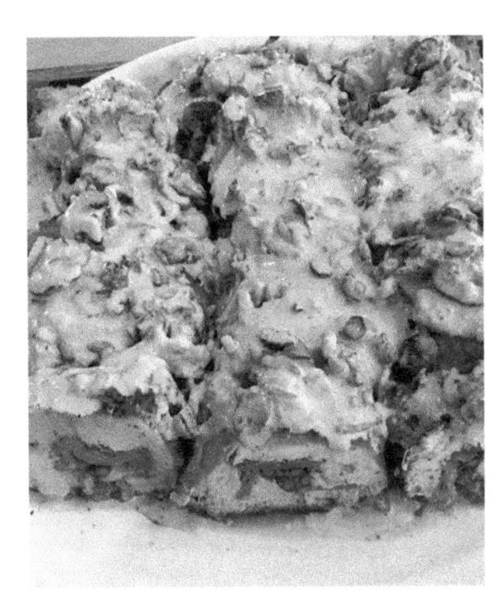

2 tbsp grated Romano cheese.
Add to the pan and stir until sauce is thickened, 1 to 2 minutes.
Remove chicken from the oven, place on a cutting board and sliced into about 1 inch thick rolls.
Place sliced chicken on a serving platter, top with the sauce and serve.

2 servings

Chicken Palm

4 tbsp olive oil
  Heat in a sauté pan.
2 - 8 oz chicken breasts
  Sauté on medium heat, until lightly brown on one side, about 6 to 7 minutes.
¼ cup white cooking wine
  Turn chicken and add the wine.
1 cup artichoke hearts, sliced
3 hearts of palm, sliced
½ cup pecan pieces
  Add to the pan and cook for 5 to 6 minutes, until chicken is cooked.
½ cup heavy cream
1 tsp black pepper
1 tbsp Dijon mustard
  Add to the pan, lower the heat and cook for about 3 to 4 minutes.
  Remove chicken breasts and place them on a serving plater.
¼ cup Swiss cheese
  Add to the pan, stir until cheese is melted. Remove from heat and pour over chicken.
2 servings
  It is best to serve over cooked fettuccine.

Chicken Plaka

4 tbsp olive oil
  Heat in a sauté pan.
2 - 8 oz chicken breasts
  Sauté on medium heat, until lightly brown on one side, about 6 to 7 minutes.
  Turn chicken.
½ onion, chopped
2 cloves garlic, chopped
  Add to the pan.
Juice of ½ lemon
  Squeeze over chicken. Cook for about 3 to 4 minutes.
6 mushrooms, sliced
½ cup artichoke hearts, chopped
1 tsp black pepper
  Add and cook for about 3 to 4 minutes longer.
2 tbsp white cooking wine
½ cup heavy cream
  Add, lower the heat and cook for 3 to 4 minutes, until the cream is thickened.
  Place chicken on a serving plater and pour the sauce over.
2 servings
  It is best to serve over cooked fettuccine.

Peppery Steak

4 tbsp olive oil
  Heat in a sauté pan.
14 to 16 oz New York steak, sliced
  Add to the pan and sauté on medium heat for about 4 to 5 minutes.
2 tbsp red cooking wine
  Add to the pan and sauté for about 2 minutes.
½ onion, sliced
½ red onion, sliced
½ red bell pepper, sliced
½ green bell pepper, sliced
2 cloves garlic, chopped
  Add to the pan and cook for about 5 to 6 minutes.
6 mushrooms, sliced
1 tbsp sliced black olives
1 tbsp sliced green olives
1 tsp black pepper
  Add to the pan and cook for another 2 to 3 minutes.
1 tsp soy sauce
1 tbsp Worcestershire sauce
2 tbsp steak sauce
  Add to the pan and cook for another 2 to 3 minutes, stirring occasionally.
  Remove from heat and serve.
2 servings
It is best served with rice pilaf.

Greco Roman Steak

4 tbsp olive oil
  Heat in a sauté pan.
14 to 16 oz rib-eye steak, sliced
  Add to the pan and sauté on medium heat for about 4 to 5 minutes.
2 tbsp red cooking wine
1 clove garlic, chopped
½ cup sun-dried tomatoes, sliced
¼ cup capers
  Add to the pan and cook for another 2 to 3 minutes.
1 tbsp fresh basil
1 tbsp dry oregano
1 tbsp dry thyme
½ cup feta cheese, crumbled
  Add to the pan, lower heat, simmer for 2 to 3 minutes, stirring occasionally.
  Remove from heat and serve.
2 servings

Roasted Leg of Lamb with Oven Potatoes and Farro Risotto

  Marinate the lamb overnight.
1 leg of lamb with the bone in, approximately 10 to 12 lbs
  Place in a roasting pan.
1 cup olive oil
  Rub the lamb with it.
Juice of 2 lemons
  Pour over the lamb.
4 cloves of garlic, finely chopped
  Rub over the lamb.

2 tbsp dry oregano
2 tbsp dry thyme
2 tbsp dry basil
1 tbsp black pepper
1 tbsp rosemary
Mix in a bowl and sprinkle over the lamb.
Refrigerate overnight.
Start cooking the leg of lamb 3 to 3½ hours before dinner.
Preheat oven to 375-degrees.
10 medium size potatoes, peeled and cut into 3 pieces each.
Remove lamb from the refrigerator. Place potatoes around the lamb. Add 2 cups of water to the pan.
1 lb butter
2 cups white cooking wine
Place in a pan and heat gently until the butter is melted.
Pour over lamb and potatoes.
Bake for 40 to 45 minutes, basting lamb and potatoes with the juice from the pan.
Turn heat to 325-degrees and cook, occasionally basting, for approximately 3 hours longer, until lamb is cooked. Serve lamb and potatoes on a large plater.
Serve with Farro Risotto
12 to 14 servings

Farro Risotto

4 cups water
4 cups vegetable broth
Bring liquids into a gentle boil on medium heat.
2 cups farro
Add farro. Total cooking time is about45 to 50 minutes.
When you start cooking the farro, prepare the vegetables.
2 tbsp olive oil
Heat in a sauté pan.
1 onion, chopped
3 cloves garlic, chopped
2 shallots, chopped
1 red bell pepper, chopped
Add to the pan and sauté for about 5 to 6 minutes
¼ cup white cooking wine
2 portobello mushroom, cut in pieces
6 artichoke hearts, chopped
1 tbsp capers
1 tsp fresh rosemary, chopped
1 tbsp Italian parsley, chopped
1 tsp black pepper
Add to the pan and sauté for another 4 to 5 minutes. Remove from heat.
In about 40 minutes into the cooking process of farro, add the vegetables to the pot. Stir well. Continue cooking for another 10 minutes. By this time the liquid should be absorbed and farro should be soft.
Remove and serve

A family favorite, especially for the young ones.

Mostaccioli Primo

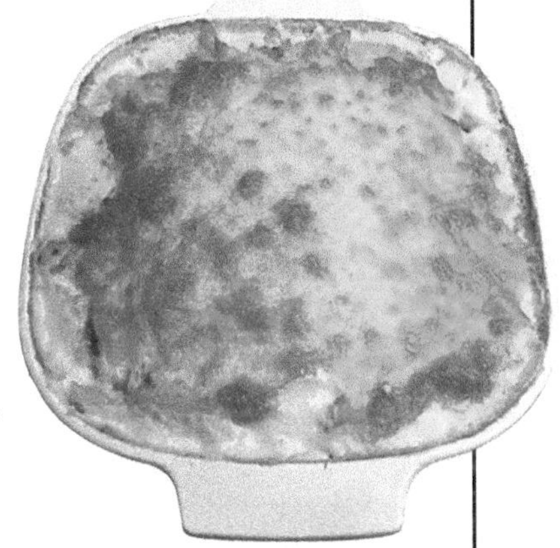

Heat oven to 350-degrees
8 cups water
In a boiling pot, bring to a gentle boil on medium heat.
8 oz mostaccioli pasta
Add to the pot an boil for about 8 to 10 minutes, until mostaccioli is al dente.
Remove and drain the excess water.
3 tbsp olive oil
Heat in a large sauté pan.
½ onion, chopped
½ cup artichoke hearts, chopped
Add to the pan and sauté for 4 to 5 minutes.
¼ cup white cooking wine
2 cups heavy cream
½ cup ricotta cheese
2 tbsp grated Parmesan cheese
Add to the pan and simmer, stirring for 2 minutes.
Add the cooked mostaccioli to the pan, turn off the heat, stir well and place mixture in a large glass or ceramic baking dish.
6 oz shredded mozzarella cheese
Spread on top of mostaccioli.
Bake in the preheated oven for about 20 minutes to 22 minutes, until mozzarella is lightly browned.
2 servings

Fresh pasta recipe

2 cups durum wheat flour
2 cups semolina flour
Blend in your mixer slow speed
6 eggs
6 tbsp olive oil
4 tbsp water
Add to the mixer and gently mix well
Dust a working surface with semolina and continue knead the dough until smooth.
Divide dough into six parts.
Working with one piece at a time, flatten the dough into a rectangle shape.
Dust the dough piece with flour and using a rolling pin,roll into a wide strip, about 1/8 inch thick.
Using a hand-crank pasta machine, dust the dough and feed it through the machine to make flat sheets.
Run the sheets through your preferred cut of the pasta machine.
Prepare as much pasta needed and refrigerate the rest in storage bags.
This recipe makes, approximately,
18 servings

Linguini Pesce

6 cups water
In a boiling pot, bring to a gentle boil on medium heat.
8 oz fresh linguini pasta
Add to the pot an boil about 5 to 6 minutes, until linguini is al dente.
Remove and drain the excess water.
4 tbsp olive oil
Heat in a large sauté pan.
6 mushrooms, sliced
6 asparagus, discard hard bottom part and cut to pieces
2 cloves garlic, chopped
Add to the pan and sauté on medium heat for about 3 to 4 minutes.
8 oz medium-sized shrimp, peeled and washed.
½ cup crabmeat
Add to the pan, cook for 3 to 4 minutes.
2 tbsp white cooking wine
1 tsp black pepper
1 tsp fresh basil, chopped
½ tsp fresh rosemary, chopped
Add and cook for another 3 to 4 minutes.
Cooked linguini
1 cup heavy cream
Add to the pan, lower the heat and continue cooking for 2 to 3 minutes.
3 tbsp grated Parmesan cheese
Add to the pan, stir well and let cook for 1 to 2 minutes.
2 servings

Fusilli Primavera

10 cups water
In a boiling pot, bring to a gentle boil on medium heat.
4 oz white fusilli pasta
4 oz green fusilli pasta
Add to the pot an boil for about 8 to 9 minutes, until pasta is al dente.
Remove and drain the excess water.
4 tbsp olive oil
Heat in a sauce pan.
½ onion, chopped
½ red onion chopped
2 cloves garlic, chopped
½ red bell pepper
½ green bell pepper
½ cup broccoli florets, cut into pieces
1 small zucchini, sliced
Add to the pan and sauté on medium heat for 6 to 7 minutes.
¼ cup white cooking wine
4 mushrooms, sliced
2 artichoke hearts, chopped
1 tbsp sliced black olives
1 tbsp sliced green olives
1 tsp black pepper
Add to the pan and continue cooking for another 5 to 6 minutes.
Cooked fusilli pasta
½ cup heavy cream
Add to the pan, stir well and cook for 2 to 3 minutes.
2 tbsp grated Romano cheese
Add, stir well to blend cheese and pasta and remove from heat.
2 servings

I use this sauce for gyro on flat pita. You can use this sauce for salad dressings, vegetable deep or with grilled pita bread.

Yogurt Dressing

1 cucumber, peeled and cut in pieces
2 green onions, chopped
Place in a food possessor and pulse 2 or 3 times.
Drain excess liquid.
1 cup olive oil mayonnaise
1 tbsp grated Parmesan cheese
½ cup sour cream
2 cups real Greek yogurt
Juice of 1 lemon
1 tsp Dijon mustard
1 tsp black pepper
Place all ingredients in the bowl and mix well.
Refrigerate in a jar.
Lemon acts as a natural preservative and will keep sauce fresh for about 60 days in your refrigerator.

This simple dressing is one of the best recipes I've created. Use it as a salad dressing, vegetable dip, to make potato salad, on eggs, or eat it by the spoonful.

Feta Dressing

3 cups feta cheese, crumbled
2 tbsp red wine vinegar
3 tbsp olive
2 cups olive oil mayonnaise
2 cloves garlic, chopped
1 tsp dry thyme
1 tsp dry basil
1 tbsp dry oregano
1 tsp black pepper
In a mixing bowl, mix all ingredients well with a spatula.
Refrigerate in jars.
Good for 2 months.
Vinegar and garlic act as natural preservatives.

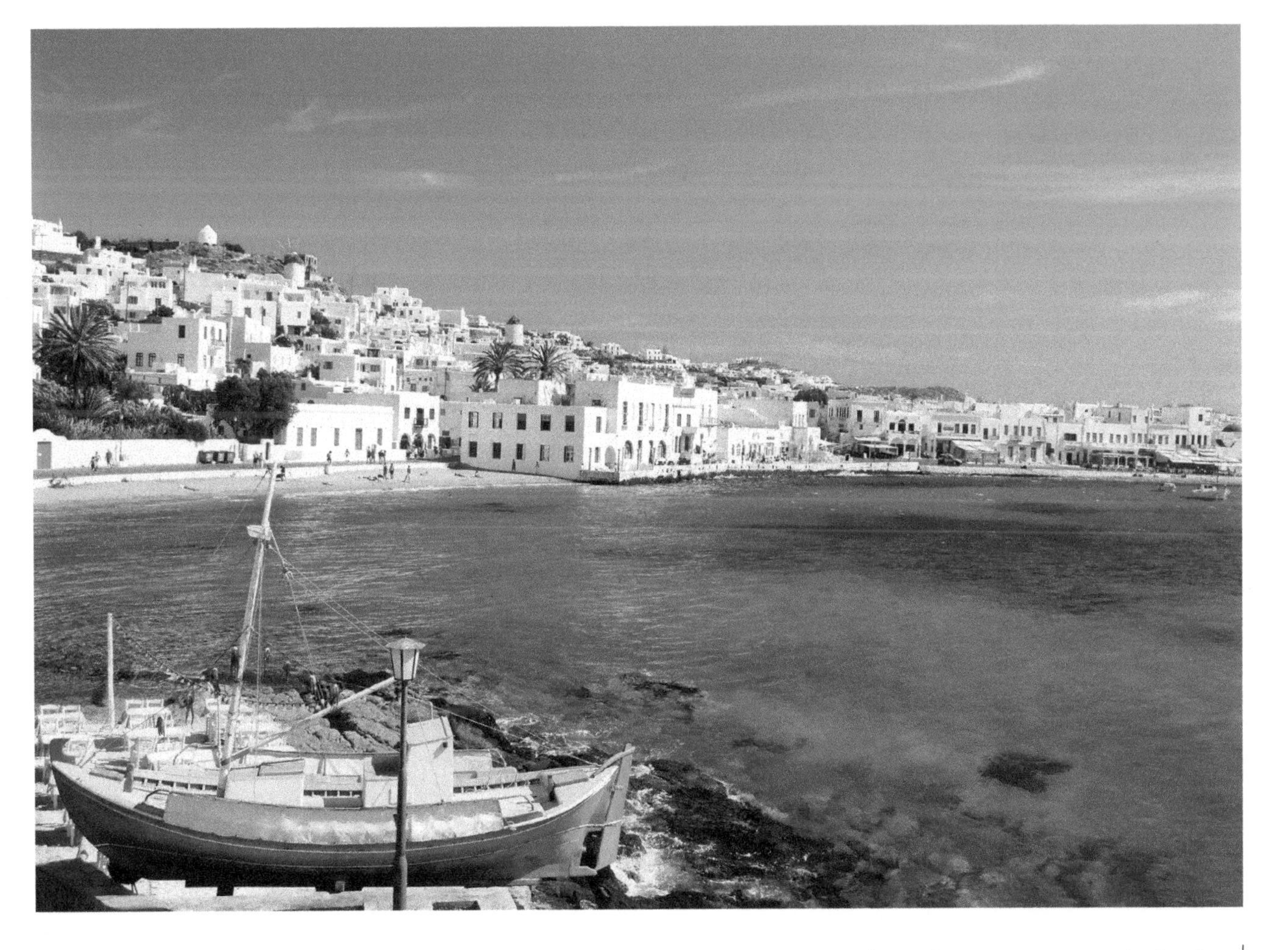

Gyros Recipe

2 lbs. lean ground beef
2 lbs. ground lamb
1 small onions, grated Juice of
Juice of 1 lemons
3 cloves garlic, chopped
2 eggs
¼ cup cornmeal
1 tbsp dried basil
1 tbsp black pepper
1 tbsp dried oregano
1 tbsp fresh parsley, chopped
1 tbsp fresh mint leaves
2 tbsp dried thyme
1 tbsp cumin
2 tbsp ground mustard

Place all ingredients in the bowl of your mixer and mix well. Place the gyros meat in large plastic bags and flattened it to about 2 inches thick blocks.
Freeze until the mixture is slightly frozen. To make gyros sandwiches, slice part of the block into thin slices and grill on a flat grill or sauté in a sauté pan.
Wrap it in pita bread with tomatoes, onions, lettuce and yogurt sauce.

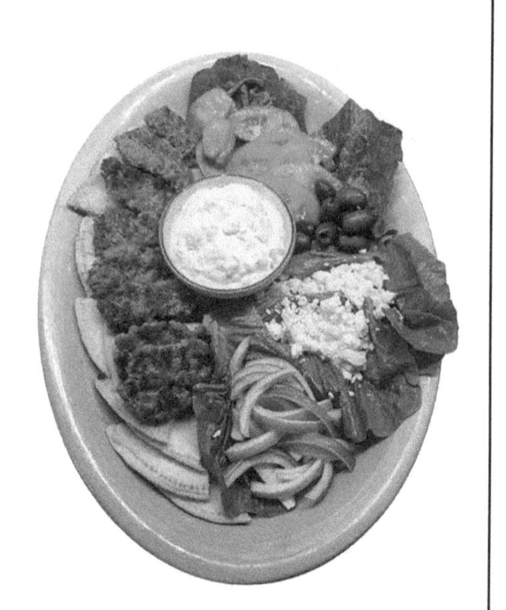

Best flat pita sandwich ever. An addictive taste that will stay with you forever.

Feta Gyros Pita

¾ cup of feta dressing.
Set aside.
3 tbsp olive oil
Heat on a flat grill or a sauté pan
12 gyro meat slices,
See gyros recipe.
1 cup artichoke hearts, quartered
Add to the grill and cook until gyros is cooked, 4 to 5 minutes.
Place in the mixing bowl with the dressing and mix well with a fork.
2 flat pita bread
Place on the grill and grill for about 1 minute on each side.
2 pieces of aluminum foil or parchment paper.
Lay the foil/paper on a working surface.
Centered the pita on the foil and fold foil around the pita bread.

White Gyros

1 lb ground turkey
1 lb ground chicken
1 tsp orange zest
Juice of ½ lemons
1 tbsp dry oregano
1 tbsp dry basil
1 tsp fresh rosemary, minced
1 tsp ground mustard
1 tsp cumin
½ tsp white pepper
½ tsp cinnamon
½ tsp nutmeg
Place in a mixing bowl of your mixer.
Gently mix to incorporate the ingredients.
½ small onion onions, large cut
3 mushrooms
1 artichoke heart
2 cloves garlic
1 stalk of celery, large cut
Pulse the above ingredients in a food processor 2 to 3 times.
Transfer to the mixing bowl and mix well with the rest of the ingredients on slow speed.
It is best if refrigerate a couple of hours before using.
Cook on a flat grill or a sauté pan.
Slice and serve in pita bread with tomatoes, avocado and feta dressing or make turkey burgers and serve with yogurt sauce.
Freeze extra meat.

Artichoke Chicken Pita

3 tbsp olive oil
Heat on a flat grill.
8 oz chicken breast, cut into pieces
¼ onion, sliced
Place on the grill and cook for about 5 to 6 minutes.
1 cup artichoke hearts, sliced
Add to the grill and cook for another 4 to 5 minutes.
½ cup yogurt dressing

Place in a mixing bowl.
Remove chicken mixture from the grill and toss with the sauce.

2 flat pita bread
Place pitas on the grill and grill for about 1 to 2 minutes on each side.

2 pieces of aluminum foil or parchment paper.
Lay the foil/paper on a working surface.
Centered the pita on the foil and fold foil around the pita bread.

2 servings

Spartan Pita

3 tbsp olive oil
Heat on a flat grill or sauté pan.

¼ onion, thinly sliced
¼ red onion, thinly sliced
½ green bell pepper, thinly sliced
Add to the grill and cook for about 2 to 3 minutes

½ cup artichoke hearts, sliced
1 small zucchini, thinly sliced
6 mushrooms, sliced
2 heats of pal sliced
¼ cup of sliced green olives
Add to the grill and cook for another 4 to 5 minutes.

2 tbsp Italian dressing
Add to the grill and toss with the vegetables.
Remove and place in a mixing bowl.

2 flat pita bread
4 slices of Provolone cheese
Place pitas on the grill and cook for about 1 to 2 minutes on each side.
Place 2 slices of provolone cheese on each pita.

2 pieces of aluminum foil or parchment paper.
2 pieces of aluminum foil or parchment paper.
Lay the foil/paper on a working surface.
Centered the pita on the foil and fold foil around the pita bread.

2 servings

On my post about Herbs and Spices, page 24, I wrote, "In every one of my recipes, I try to combine as many as the four flavors without one overpowering the others. The day that I can combine the four tastes in harmony, I will have invented the perfect taste." This recipes comes nearly to a perfection of tastes.

Goat Shrimp

12 jumbo shrimp
Peeled, leave tail on and butterflied.
Lay shrimp on a working surface

½ cup sun-dried tomatoes, chopped
½ cup feta cheese, crumbled
Mix in a bowl. Place mixture on the open shrimp.

24 thin strips of bacon
Using two strips for every shrimp, enclose filling in the shrimp and wrap bacon around the shrimp.
Make sure, top and sides of the shrimp are wrapped well.

1 tsp black pepper
1 tsp dry basil
1 tsp oregano
1 clove garlic, chopped
Mix in a small bowl.

½ lemon
½ cup olive oil
Pour olive oil in a large sauté pan
Heat it to medium high and add Shrimp, 4 or 5 at a time.
Cook well on one side, turn, squeeze some lemon on top and sprinkle with the spices.
Repeat with the rest of the shrimp, adding a bit more oil if needed.

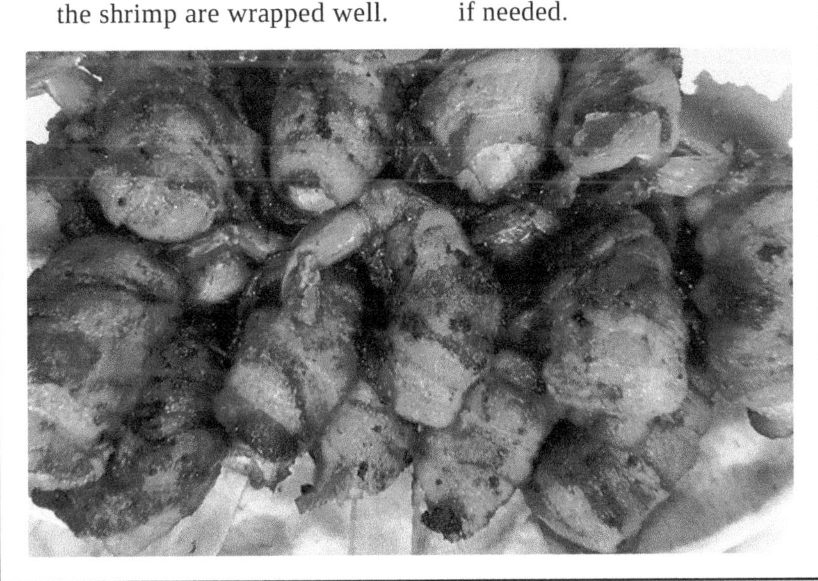

Desserts

*"Each one of us bent our heads in prayers of thanks
to the Grecian God of desserts."*
Java Magazine

*"In his legendary restaurant, Nick makes a dessert named Sinful Act.
It is a diabolical, multi-layer chocolate creation."*
Best of Phoenix

*"Some of us find reading Nick's dessert menu
better than erotic poetry."*
Arizona Republic

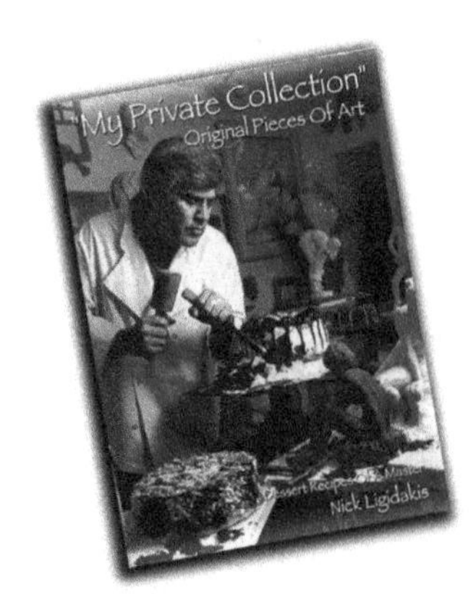

Recipes from my dessert book
My Private Collection
Over 300 original recipes

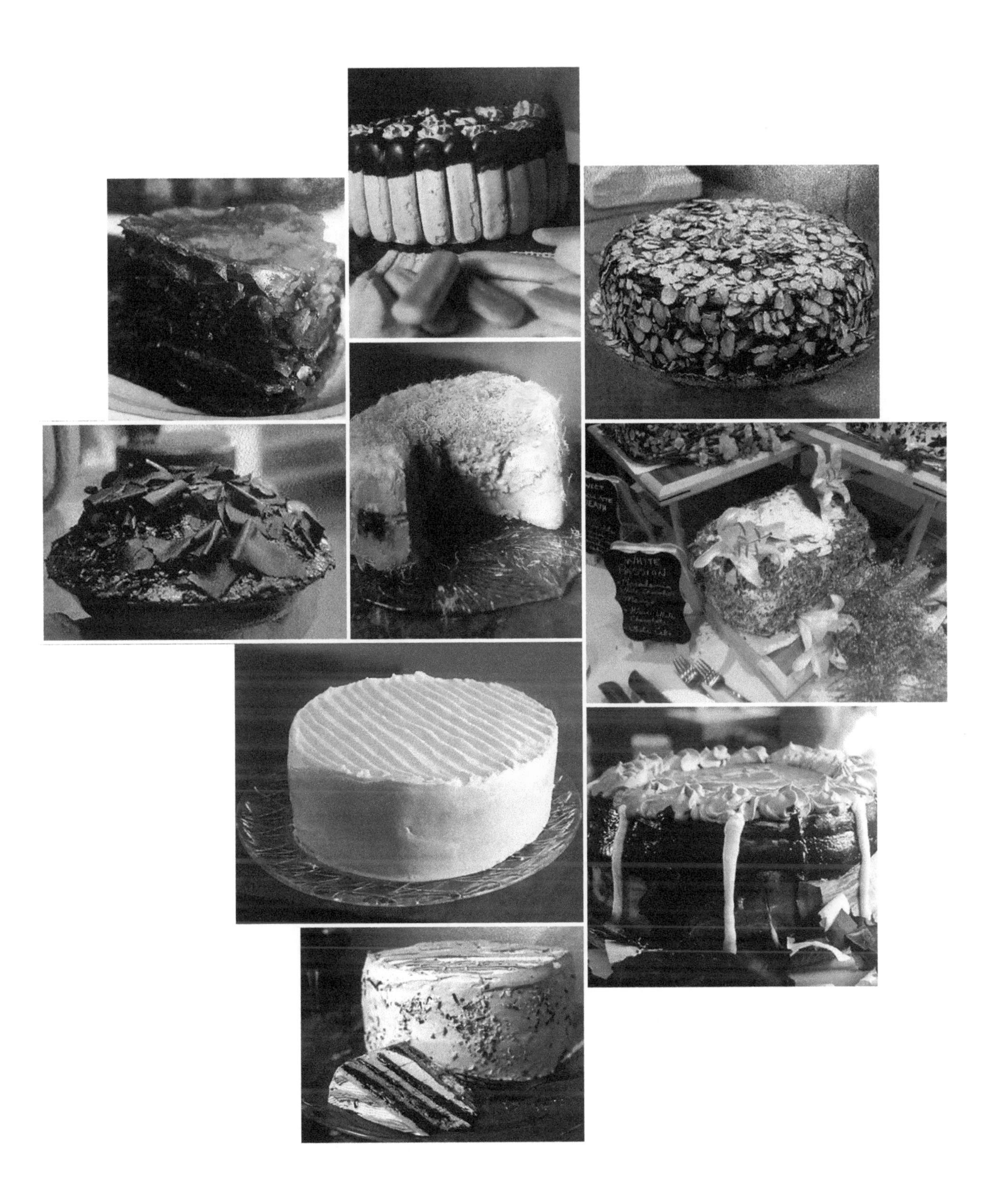

Cheesecake Crust

2 cups graham cracker crumbs
1 cup oats
½ cup coconut sugar
¾ cup butter low-fat, melted
Blend well in a mixing bowl.
Prepare the crust for baking.
Use a 10-inch springform pan. Lightly oiled the pan and pressed the crust against the bottom and sides of the pan. The crust on the side of the pan will help to keep your cheesecake smooth and creamy.

¾ cup sour cream
½ cup granulated sugar
½ cup frozen raspberries, well drained
When chocolate is melted, add the rest of the ingredients, stir to blend well, remove from heat and set aside.
After baking the cheesecake for 1 hour, pour topping over the top, return to oven, turn the oven off and let sit for 45 minutes longer. Refrigerate 12 to 14 hours before removing from the pan.

18 servings

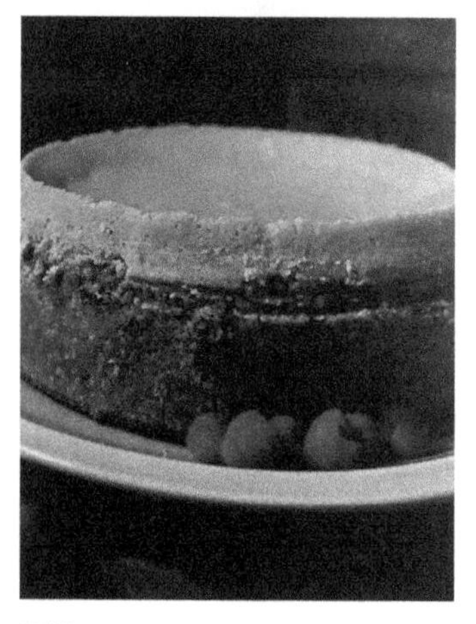

Red Berry Cheesecake

Preheat oven to 350-degrees
Prepare a cheesecake crust, covering the bottom and sides of a 10-inch springform pan.
16 oz white chocolate
Melt in a double boiler.

Filling
1 lb cream cheese
1 cup xylitol sugar
Cream together on a medium speed of your mixer.
4 eggs
Add and mix thoroughly.
1 tbsp juice of a lemon
1 tsp vanilla
16 oz white chocolate, melted
1 cup sour cream
½ cup heavy cream
½ cup frozen raspberries, well drained
½ cup fresh boysenberries
Add to the mixer. Mix well, pour the mixture into prepared crust and bake for 1 hour.
While the cheesecake is being baked, prepare the topping.

Topping
¾ cup white chocolate
Melt over a double boiler.

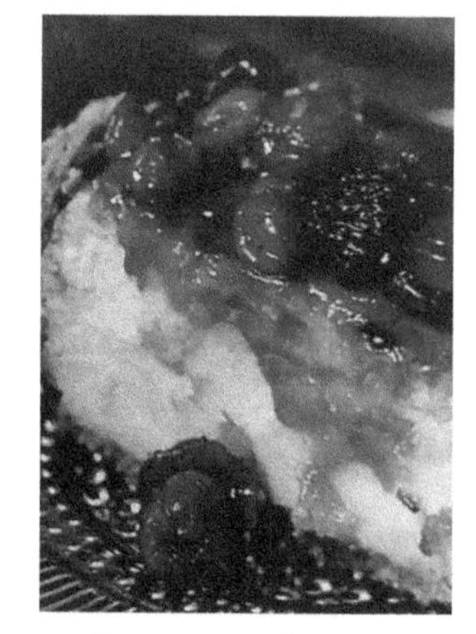

Cherry Cheesecake

Preheat oven to 350-degrees
Prepare a cheesecake crust, covering the bottom and sides of a 10-inch springform pan.

Filling
1½ lb cream cheese
1 cup xylitol sugar
½ cup granulated sugar
Cream together on a medium speed of your mixer.
6 eggs
Add and mix thoroughly.
1 tbsp juice of a lemon
1 tsp vanilla
2 cups sour cream
Add to the mixer, ix well, pour the mixture into prepared crust and bake for 1 hour.
While the cheesecake is being baked, prepare the topping.

Topping
8 oz cherry pie filling
½ cup frozen dark cherries, defrost
1 tbsp juice of a lemon
1 tsp orange zest
Mix well in a bowl
After baking the cheesecake for 1 hour, pour topping over the top, return to oven, turn the oven off and let sit for 45 minutes longer. Refrigerate 12 to 14 hours before removing from the pan.

18 servings

Throughout the years, people asked me about my favorite foods and favorite desserts. When you create recipes, you love them all; they are part of your existence, part of your family. However, if I had the choice of the last meal, I do not have to think much; Greek Peasant Salad, Goat Shrimp and the largest piece of Cinnamon Stick Cake, or maybe the entire cake.

Cinnamon Stick Cake

Preheat oven to 350-degrees

Prepare a cheesecake crust, covering the bottom and sides of a 10-inch springform pan. Use a tall springform pan. If not available, use a long piece of aluminum foil and wrap it around the pan to create a taller pan size.

This cake will rice over a shorter springform pan.

16 sheets of fillo dough

Place the 10-inch springform pan on the center of the fillo sheets and with a sharp knife cut the fillo on the outer edges of the pan. Cover the 16-inch fillo rounds with a towel and discard or save the excess fillo for another use.

Filling

2 lb cream cheese

1 cup xylitol sugar

Cream together on a medium speed of your mixer.

4 eggs

Add and mix thoroughly.

1 tbsp juice of a lemon

1 tsp vanilla

1 cup sour cream

1 cup heavy cream

1 tbsp flour

1 tsp cinnamon

1 tsp corn starch

Add to the mixer, ix well, pour the mixture into prepared crust.

Topping

⅓ cup melted butter

Lay the 8 sheets of the fillo round on top of the cake, brushing on every couple sheets with the butter.

3 cups pecan pieces

¼ cup sugar

The remaining butter – save about a tbsp to brush the remaining fillo.

1 tsp cinnamon

1 tsp ground cloves

Mix ingredients in a mixing bowl and spread evenly on top of the fillo.

8 sheets of fillo rounds

Lay on top of the pecan filling, brushing on every couple sheets with the butter.

With your sprinkle a few drops of water on top of the fillo, place the cake on top of a baking pan, add 1 cup of water in the baking pan and bake in the preheated oven and bake for 75 minutes.

Syrup

While cake is in the oven, prepare the syrup.

2 cups water

2 cinnamon sticks

1 tsp cinnamon

4 whole cloves

¼ cup sugar

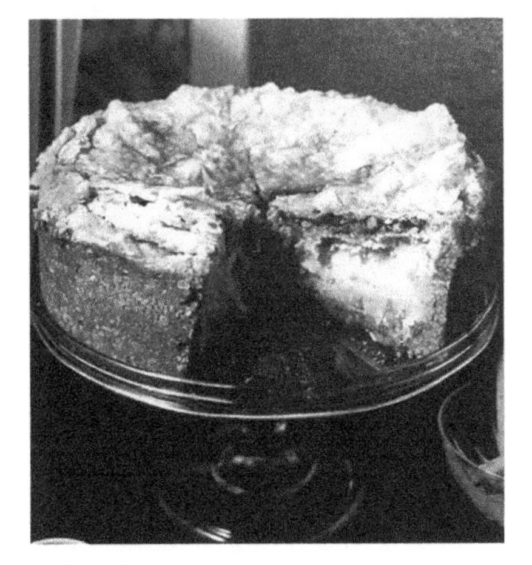

4 tbsp honey

1 tsp juice of a lemon

1 tsp juice of an orange

Bring it to a boil in a small sauté pan, reduce heat and simmer for about 10 minutes. Remove cinnamon sticks and cloves. You should have about 1 cup syrup.

Set aside.

After the cake is baked, remove from the oven and, evenly, pour syrup on top of the cake.

Turn oven off and return the cake into the oven.

Let it sit for about 30 minutes.

Remove and refrigerate for at least 12 hours before serving.

18 servings

Forget the calories here. Just close your eyes, take a bite and dream.

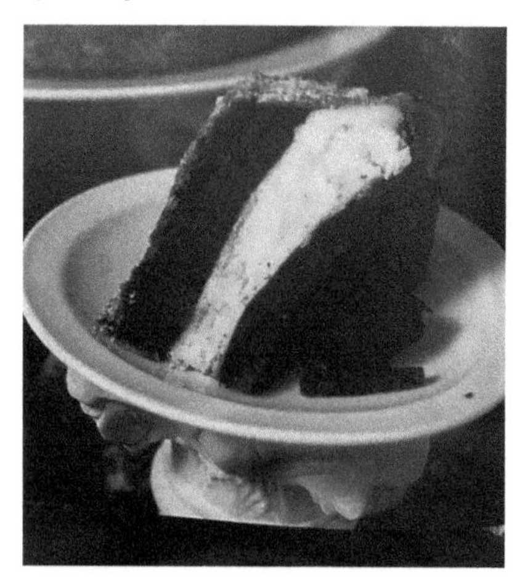

Sinful Act

Preheat oven to 325-degrees

8 oz frozen raspberries

Defrost the raspberries, place the raspberries with their liquid in the food processor and pulse 2 times.

Remove and press the mixture through a sieve, discard the pulp and save the liquid.

12 fillo sheets

Place a 10-inch high border springform pan over the fillo and cut at the outer periphery of the pan to create ten fillo rounds. Cover and set aside.

Chocolate raspberry cake

1 lbs semisweet chocolate
1 lb milk chocolate
½ lb unsweetened butter
⅛ cup raspberry juice

Place on a double boiler and melt over low heat.

Remove and place in your mixer.

8 eggs
¼ cup sugar

Beat well on slow speed.

Pour half of the chocolate mixture into the springform pan.

Lay 6 of the fillo rounds on top of the chocolate.

White chocolate cake

¾ lb cream cheese
¼ cup sugar

Cream in your mixer.

16 oz white chocolate, melted
½ cup sour cream
2 eggs

Add to the mixer and blend well.

Pour batter on top of the fillo.

Lay the rest of the fillo rounds on top of the white chocolate and pour the remaining dark chocolate batter on top.

Place the springform pan on a baking tray filled with a couple cups of water and bake in the preheated oven for 75 minutes.

Turn off oven and let the cake set in the oven for about 30 minutes longer.

Carefully, pour the remaining raspberryliquid on top of the cake and refrigerate for at least 12 to 14 hours before serving.

22 servings.

The batter of my version of the chocolate cake looks thinner than what you are used to making. No worries. It will take a bit longer to bake but in the end you will love the texture and moistness of this cake.

Chocolate Cake

Preheat oven to 350 degrees

2 cups baking flour
1 cup granulated sugar
½ cup xylitol sugar
2 tsp baking soda
1½ tsp baking powder
¾ cup cocoa powder

Place in the bowl of your mixer and blend.

½ cup vegetable oil
1½ cups milk
½ cup hot water
2 eggs
1 tsp vanilla extract

Add to the mixer and blend on medium speed until batter is smooth.

Lightly oil a 10-inch springform pan and poured the cake batter in it.

Bake in the preheated oven for about 60 to 62 minutes.

How to make chocolate shavings

Melt chocolate in a double boiler. For a double boiler, Place the chocolate in a mixing bowl. Set the bowl over a stockpot with barely simmering a small amount of water. I like to use a mixing bowl larger than the size of the stockpot, so the bottom of the mixing bowl does not touch the water.

Occasionally stir the chocolate. Do not overheat. To make the shavings place 3 or 4 tbsp of melted chocolate on a large piece of parchment paper. Cover it with another large piece of parchment paper.

With a rolling pin roll out the chocolate into paper-thin. Place it into your freezer for at least 1 hour, or when is time to use the chocolate shavings. Take out the parchment paper from the freezer, remove the top paper and break the thin chocolate into preferred pieces.

It is exactly as the name suggests

Symphony of Chocolates

Preparation

Make a 10-inch chocolate cake.
Symphony of chocolate image here

8 oz semisweet chocolate
Please, do not break up this recipe
Melt on a double boiler. Set aside

16 oz white chocolate
Melt on a double boiler. Set aside

Chocolate shavings

Use 3 tbsp of the melted chocolate.

Simple syrup

½ cup water
2 tbsp sugar
½ tsp vanilla extract
Bring to a boil in a small sauté pan reduce heat and simmer for 3 to 4 minutes. Set aside.

2 cups pastry pride, or 3 cups whipping cream
With the wire whip of your mixer beat the liquid on high speed until it forms stiff peaks. Set cream aside.

Assembling the cake

The 10-inch chocolate cake
Sliced in half lengthwise and place in a springform pan. Save the other half for another use or to make chocolate truffles. Pour the simple syrup over the cake.

White chocolate filling

½ cup unsalted butter
1 tbsp sugar
Cream in your mixer.

1 cup prepared cream
1 tsp vanilla extract
Add and mix on slow speed.

½ of the melted white chocolate
Add and blend well. Pour the filling over the cake and smooth the top with a spatula.

Semisweet chocolate filling

½ cup unsalted butter
1 tbsp sugar
Cream in your mixer

1½ cups prepared cream
Add and mix on slow speed

The melted semisweet chocolate
Add and blend well. Pour the filling over the white chocolate filling and smooth the top with a spatula.

Chestnut chocolate filling

½ cup unsalted butter
1 tbsp sugar
Cream together

the other ½ of the melted white chocolate
Add and blend well. Pour the filling over the cake and smooth the top with a spatula.

1 tsp Kahlua
½ cup chestnut puree
Add mix well and pour over the semisweet chocolate filling. Refrigerate the cake for 1 hour.

Chocolate orange icing

6 oz white chocolate
Melt in a double boiler

8 oz cream cheese
Cream in the mixer

2 cups of the prepared cream
¼ cup sour cream
1 tbsp orange zest
¼ tsp cinnamon
1 tbsp black coffee
Add to the mixer and blend well.

The melted chocolate
Add and mix on slow speed until icing is smooth.
Remove cake from the springform pan. Smooth the top and sides with a pastry spatula and spread the icing on the top and sides of the cake.

The chocolate shavings
Take out the parchment paper from the freezer, remove the top paper and break the thin chocolate into pieces. Sprinkle the chocolate shavings on the side and top of the cake.

2 tbsp chocolate vermicelli, or any other chocolate sprinkles
Sprinkle on the side and top of the cake.

20 servings

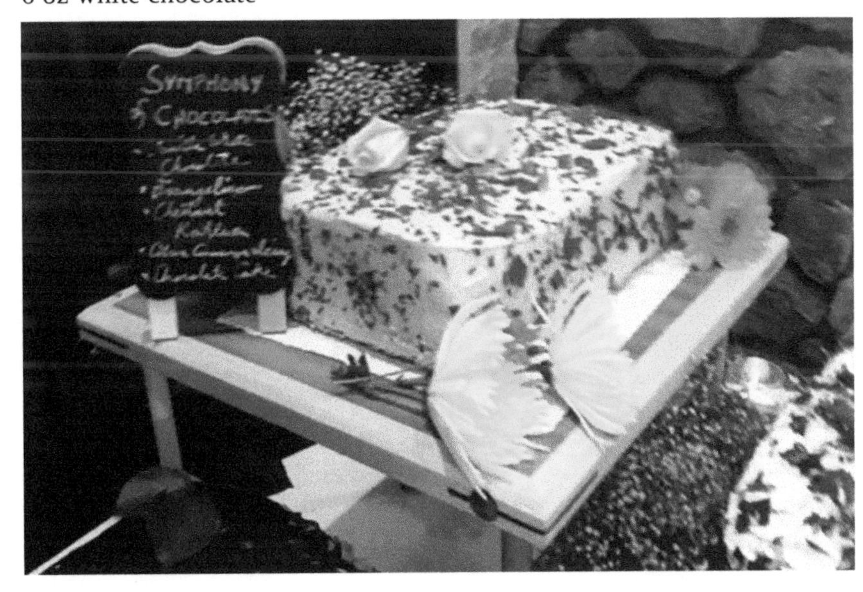

Easy to make and difficult to resist.

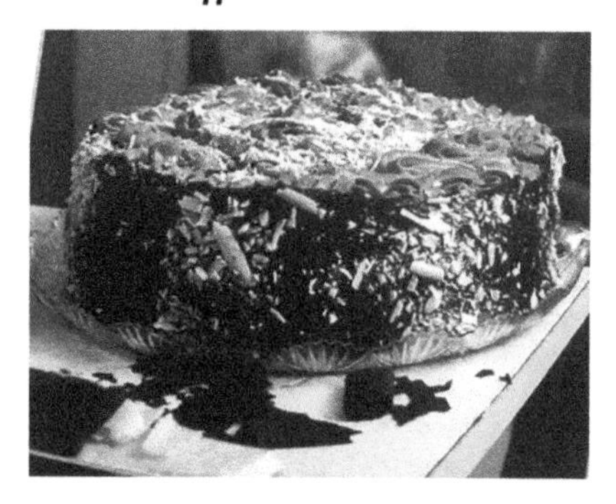

Cappuccino Mousse Cake

Make a 10-inch chocolate cake.

6 oz semisweet chocolate

Melt on a double boiler. Set aside

Simple syrup

1 cup water

3 tbsp sugar

1 tsp ground espresso or any other coffee

Bring to a boil in a small sauté pan reduce heat and simmer for 3 to 4 minutes. Set aside.

1½ cups pastry pride, or 2 cups whipping cream

With the wire whip of your mixer beat the liquid on high speed until it forms stiff peaks. Set cream aside.

Assembling the cake

The 10-inch chocolate cake

Sliced lengthwise ½ inch from the top of the cake.

Place cake on a serving plate and pour the simple syrup over the top of the cake.

Cappuccino mousse

The melted chocolate

2 cups of the prepared cream

1 tbsp ground coffee

1 tbsp orange zest, finely chopped

Place in a mixing bowl and blend well with a spatula. Place on top of the cake smooth the top and sides of the cake.

Topping

The remaining cream

2 tbsp ground cocoa

1 tsp vanilla extract

Place in a mixing bowl and blend well.

Use a large pastry bag with a star tip to decorate the top of the cake. Fill the pastry bag with the cream. Hold your pastry bag at an angle. Starting from the edge of the cake, squeeze the bag, move your hands, slightly, up and down while you move around the edge of the cake and towards the center of the cake. It is relatively simple, but it takes a bit of practice.

If you don't like your design, scrape the cream from the top of the cake, put it back in the bag and repeat.

Icing

4 oz semisweet chocolate

Melt on a double boil.

¼ cup heavy cream

Add, stir well and remove. Let cool for a few minutes. With a pastry spatula, cover the sides of the cake with the icing.

18 servings

White Cake

Preheat oven to 350-degrees

2¼ cups baking flour

2 tsp baking powder

1 tsp baking soda

½ cup granulated sugar

½ cup xylitol sugar

Place in the bowl of your mixer and blend.

¼ cup unsalted butter, soft

¼ cup vegetable oil

1 tsp vanilla extract

1 cup milk

¼ cup vegetable oil

Add to the mixer and blend on medium speed until mixture is fluffy, about 2 minutes.

6 egg whites

Add to the mixer, one at a time and blend until the batter is smooth.

Lightly oil a 10-inch springform pan and pour the cake batter in it.

Bake in the preheated oven for about 60 to 62 minutes.

This cake is the most requested special occasion cake in our family. Reading the ingredients, you may say; What? But wait until you taste it.

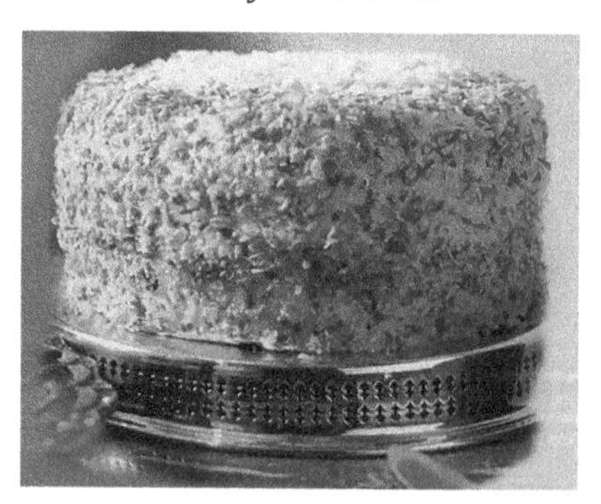

White Passion Cake

2 cups of shredded coconut

Place on a baking pan and toast in a 350-degree oven, 5 to 6 minutes until golden brown. Occasionally stir the coconut to be baked evenly. Set aside.

3 kiwis, peeled and chopped, set aside.

1 ripe mango, peeled, chopped and drain. Set aside.

Simple syrup

1 cup water

¼ cup coconut sugar

1 tsp rum vanilla extract

Bring to a boil in a small pan reduce heat and simmer for 3 to 4 minutes. Set aside.

18 oz white chocolate

Melt in a double boil over low heat. When chocolate is melted, turn off the heat.

Chocolate shavings

2 large pieces of parchment paper.

Use 3 tbsp of the melted chocolate.

Assembling the cake

2 cups pastry pride, or 3 cups whipping cream

½ tsp pure vanilla extract

With the wire whip of your mixer beat the liquid on high speed until it forms stiff peaks. Set cream aside.

White cake

Slice it in three horizontal slices. Place one slice on a serving platter. With a spoon, sprinkle some of the simple syrup to moisten the cake.

Mango mousse

3 oz cream cheese

2 tbsp xylitol sugar

Cream in your mixer.

3 tbsp sour cream

The chopped mango

Add to the mixer and blend gently. Remove bowl from the mixer.

½ cup of the prepared whipping cream

⅓ of the melted chocolate

Add to the mixer and thoroughly blend on low speed. Pour filling on the first slice of the cake and top it with the second cake slice. Pour some of the simple syrup over to soak the cake.

Kiwi white chocolate

3 oz cream cheese

2 tbsp xylitol sugar

Cream in your mixer.

3 tbsp sour cream

The chopped kiwi

Add to the mixer and blend on slow speed. Remove bowl from the mixer.

1 cup of the prepared whipping cream

⅓ of the melted chocolate

Add to the mixer and thoroughly blend on low speed. Pour filling on to the second slice of cake and top it with the third cake slice. Pour some of the simple syrup over to soak the cake.

Decorating the cake

Remaining whipped cream

Remaining melted white chocolate

½ cup sour cream

Blend with your mixer on low speed. Use it to iced the sides and top of the cake.

The toasted coconut

Cover the sides of the cake with it.

White chocolate shavings

Take out the parchment paper from the freezer, remove the top paper and break the thin chocolate into pieces. Cover the top of the cake with the chocolate shavings.

Refrigerate for at least 6 to 8 hours before serving.

Makes a 10-inch round cake or a 7.5"x6" rectangle for special occasions.

20 servings

Pastry Pride®

I used Pastry Pride® ready to whip topping for some of my cake recipes. It is versatile, creamy and easy to work with. Many pastry chefs use it for its consistency. Pastry Pride® is a non-dairy whipped topping that comes frozen. When you need it, thaw it in the refrigerator and then whip it up, just like whipping cream. Pastry Pride® is difficult to find. It is available on large wholesale/retail stores.

2 cups make 5 cups cream.

Precious Memories

In many cultures, the cuisine is as essential as religion, politics, and history. In my opinion, there is no celebration of life's special moments without food. Food offerings express love and hospitality; therefore, most familiar tastes of the past are associated with life's intriguing moments. The childhood aromas, tastes and textures of foods are ingrained into our senses, and often transport us back to a cherished place and time. Those who were fortunate to taste such special foods remember the surroundings and the people who prepared such stimulating aromas. Those precious memories recollect the charming places when parents, grandparents and friends cultivated the art of cooking and raised it to a memorable, succulent level. I am one of those fortunate people who grew up around such an environment. This is the main reason that I cherish our family's celebrations, knowing that the young ones will carry these special moments for the rest of their lives.

Every once in a while, we have to take time out of our busy days and celebrate life's special moments, to feed the soul and the body with familiar indulgences. There is no better way to celebrate these special times than with family and friends; with the house full of enticing aromas and tables laden with special foods.

Most of the recipes in the section, *Foods to Celebrate Life's Special Moments*, are foods used for our family celebrations and gatherings. Their tastes and aromas remind us of togetherness and precious moments of the past. Now there are new tastes to be introduced. Our family has grown large and engaging. Our special dinners are not dinners for two or four; now we almost fill out a small restaurant. Each one of us has their favorite dishes; flavors that intrigued good memories.

The writing of this book has been rewarding for me on so many levels; above all it is a labor of love. But now I must go. Tonight, there is another family birthday to celebrate. There will be new and familiar tastes; more memories for the young ones to cherish. I hope you do the same. Go ahead and create new flavors, add new precious memories with your family and friends.

I know that the art of fabricating seductive aromas and memorable tastes is complex in culinary art. Creativity seems more challenging in culinary art than any other because it involves the satisfaction of all the senses and the involvement of thousands of ingredients. And, it concerns the selection of foods, the manner of preparation, the savoring of the foods, and the ceremony of eating; these are the four steps that make up a healthier cuisine.

I hope my new recipes and knowledge about those four steps will help you to create new tastes and new precious memories.

Recipe index

Nikos Ligidakis

Nationally recognized chef Nikos Ligidakis demonstrates in this book his priceless culinary knowledge. There are over 250 original recipes in this unique book, each carefully crafted for those who are eating healthy diets such as elimination, gluten-free, vegetarian, vegan, recipes to celebrate life's special moments and much more. Included in this book is the nutritional information of each ingredient used, calorie-counts for the main ingredients of each recipe, information about flavors and textures of foods and various cooking techniques to intensify the flavors. Also, included are historical facts about several foods, especially the ancient grains, and tips on how to simplify your cooking process and create new tastes. There is abundant information in this book to help you enhance your cooking skills and help you to follow a healthy diet without compromising the taste.

Ligidakis gained national acclaim for combining the full tantalizing flavors of the Mediterranean region with an imaginative presentation. His success is credited to the fact that he has created a cuisine that is at once both exotic and familiar. Nikos has become a legend locally both for his selfless charitable involvement and his idiosyncratic style of cooking. He prides himself on his culinary creativity, use of quality ingredients, freshness, consistency, and the fact that he prepares everything from scratch.

Award winning author, Nikos Ligidakis, writes with clarity and passion in an ardent voice, not to just recount adventures, but with an expression of feelings, to encourage the reader to think, to find hope in the eternal struggle for the meaning of life and the awareness of harmony. Nikos is the author of several historical fiction and biography books.

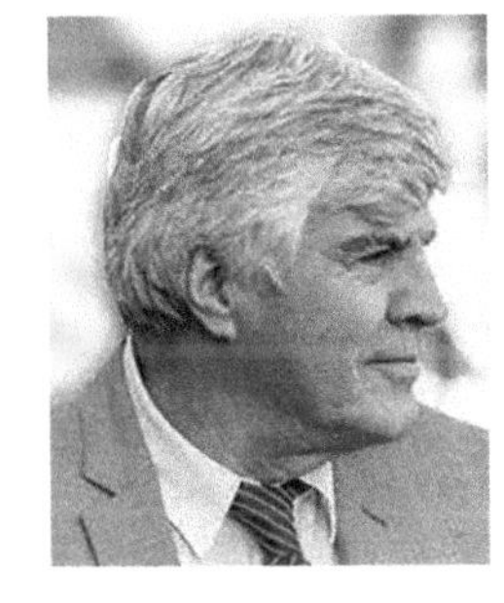

"As a writer, my aspiration has always been to share my perspective on what it means to be a human being, in all its complexities. I wanted to tell a story that reflects a comparative importance of political structures, religions and histories of the past. My books represent a lifelong dream of putting into narrative form, my many observations of the brilliance and kindness of the human spirit: people at their worst and people at their best. It is my intention to engage the reader in the process of observing history in both times past and in current day happenings for the sole purpose of gaining greater clarity in the shaping of one's own approach to life and the deepening of individual insight."

~Nikos Ligidakis

CPSIA information can be obtained
at www.ICGtesting.com
Printed in the USA
BVHW021035020120
568327BV00003B/15/P

9 780578 500331